Infectious Diseases of the Bovine

Infectious Diseases of the Bovine

Edited by George Allen

SYRAWOOD
PUBLISHING HOUSE
New York

Published by Syrawood Publishing House,
750 Third Avenue, 9th Floor,
New York, NY 10017, USA
www.syrawoodpublishinghouse.com

Infectious Diseases of the Bovine
Edited by George Allen

International Standard Book Number: 978-1-64740-373-7 (Hardback)

Cataloging-in-publication Data

Infectious diseases of the bovine / edited by George Allen.
p. cm.
Includes bibliographical references and index.
ISBN 978-1-64740-373-7
1. Cattle--Diseases. 2. Cattle--Diseases--Epidemiology.
3. Communicable diseases in animals. I. Allen, George.

SF961 .I54 2023
636.208 96--dc23

TABLE OF CONTENTS

PREFACE

The purpose of the book is to provide a glimpse into the dynamics and to present opinions and studies of some of the scientists engaged in the development of new ideas in the field from very different standpoints. This book will prove useful to students and researchers owing to its high content quality.

Bovine infections are a group of infectious diseases caused by pathogens in cattle. There are various types of bovine infections such as bluetongue, botulism, bovine tuberculosis, bovine viral diarrhea (BVD), brucellosis, foot and mouth disease, actinobacillosis, Johne's disease, psoroptic mange, Schmallenberg virus, and transmissible spongiform encephalopathies (TSE). Wooden tongue or Actinobacillosis is one of the most common types of bovine infection caused by Actinobacillosis Lignieresii bacteria. This disease affects the soft tissues present in the mouth region in adult cattle. The most common symptoms of wooden tongue include the inability to eat or drink, drooling, painful and swollen tongue, and ulcers on tongue. Iodine therapy or tetracyclines are commonly used to treat this disease. This book outlines the diagnosis, treatment, and prevention of infectious diseases of the bovine in detail. For all readers who are interested in veterinary science, the studies included herein will serve as an excellent guide to develop a comprehensive understanding.

At the end, I would like to appreciate all the efforts made by the authors in completing their chapters professionally. I express my deepest gratitude to all of them for contributing to this book by sharing their valuable works. A special thanks to my family and friends for their constant support in this journey.

Editor

1

Bovine Tuberculosis (*Mycobacterium bovis*) Outbreak Duration in Cattle Herds in Ireland

Andrew W. Byrne [1,*,†], Damien Barrett [1], Philip Breslin [2], Jamie M. Madden [3], James O'Keeffe [2] and Eoin Ryan [2,*,†]

1 One-Health Scientific Support Unit, Surveillance, Animal by-products, and TSEs (SAT) Division, Department of Agriculture, Food and the Marine, Agriculture House, Dublin 2 D02 WK12, Ireland; damien.barrett@agriculture.gov.ie
2 Ruminant Animal Health Division, Department of Agriculture, Food and the Marine, Backweston, Co. Kildare W23 VW2C, Ireland; philip.breslin@agriculture.gov.ie (P.B.); james.okeeffe@agriculture.gov.ie (J.O.)
3 Centre for Veterinary Epidemiology and Risk Analysis (CVERA), School of Veterinary Medicine, University College Dublin, Belfield, Dublin 4 D04 W6F6, Ireland; jamie.madden@ucd.ie
* Correspondence: ecologicalepidemiology@gmail.com (A.W.B.); eoin.ryan@agriculture.gov.ie (E.R.)
† Current address: Department of Health, Baggot Street, Dublin 4 D02 XW14, Ireland.

Abstract: Bovine tuberculosis (bTB) outbreaks, caused by *Mycobacterium bovis* infection, are a costly animal health challenge. Understanding factors associated with the duration of outbreaks, known as breakdowns, could lead to better disease management policy development. We undertook a retrospective observational study (2012–2018) and employed Finite Mixture Models (FMM) to model the outcome parameter, and to investigate how factors were associated with duration for differing subpopulations identified. In addition to traditional risk factors (e.g., herd size, bTB history), we also explored farm geographic area, parcels/farm fragmentation, metrics of intensity via nitrogen loading, and whether herds were designated controlled beef finishing units (CBFU) as potential risk factors for increased duration. The final model fitted log-normal distributions, with two latent classes (k) which partitioned the population into a subpopulation around the central tendency of the distribution, and a second around the tails of the distribution. The latter subpopulation included longer breakdowns of policy interest. Increasing duration was positively associated with recent (<3 years) TB history and the number of reactors disclosed, (log) herd size, beef herd-type relative to other herd types, number of land parcels, area, being designated a CBFU ("feedlot") and having high annual inward cattle movements within the "tails" subpopulation. Breakdown length was negatively associated with the year of commencement of breakdown (i.e., a decreasing trend) and non-significantly with the organic nitrogen produced on the farm (N kg/hectare), a measure of stocking density. The latter finding may be due to confounding effects with herd size and area. Most variables contributed only moderately to explaining variation in breakdown duration, that is, they had moderate size effects on duration. Herd-size and CBFU had greater effect sizes on the outcome. The findings contribute to evidence-based policy formation in Ireland.

Keywords: bovine TB; risk factors; disease control; animal health policy; veterinary epidemiology; evidence-based policy

1. Introduction

Bovine tuberculosis remains a priority pathogen of cattle in Ireland [1,2] and elsewhere [3–6] and one that expends considerable resources from farmers, the state, and, for member states, the EU

Commission. As an example, direct annual programme costs in Ireland were estimated at €92 million in 2018, €47 million from the Exchequer, €9.7 million co-financed by the EU, and €35.2 million paid by farmers [7]. A key challenge is to ensure that disease policy is evidence-based and adapts in response to changes in risk patterns so that programme effectiveness is maximised and stakeholders can be assured that decisions affecting them are underpinned by a coherent epidemiological analysis of the data [8].

The duration of breakdowns can have a significant financial impact on stakeholders [9,10], and furthermore, prolonged duration breakdowns can be a risk factor for future recrudesce [2]. Therefore, understanding risk factors associated with prolonged duration can be of benefit to tailoring policy to local conditions, with the intentions of reducing the spread of infection within and between herds.

In Ireland, a significant expansion of the dairy sector took place from 2015 onwards following the removal of EU milk quotas, with an increase of 54% in milk production from 2005 to 2018 [11]; this has been temporally correlated with an increase in TB herd incidence. The increase in dairy production has been associated with an increase in stocking density and herd size, while studies characterised the scale of cattle movements within Ireland [12], it is unclear whether the nature of how these factors relate to TB risk has also changed in that period [13]. However, data from Britain suggest such movement increases may increase inter-herd *M. bovis* spread [14].

Duration data are positive integers (natural numbers) data with often unusual distributions which can be difficult to model using conventional statistical means. Previous attempts to model breakdown duration has used categorical models where duration is split into binary outcomes [15] or ordinal outcomes [10]. Breakdown duration has also been modelled as a count of days, using a negative binomial random-effects model [10]. Time to event modelling (survival) models can be used to model the interval between failures [15,16]. Alternatively, the duration of time over a fixed period can be modelled by generalised linear models, using various distribution types (e.g., hospitalisation length of stay [17]). Breakdown duration that is the period over which herds are not able to trade due to the presence of TB infection within the herd, in Ireland is both leptokurtic and positively skewed. To explore the variation in breakdown length, a two-class Finite Mixture Model (FMM) was fitted to the data. FMMs are probabilistic models that partition populations into unobserved subpopulations, known as classes or components, without explicitly identifying the subpopulation for which observations belong. Instead, subpopulation membership is modelled as a latent class, from which the posterior class probability of membership can be estimated, and mixtures of continuous probability distributions of various types (regression models) are used to model the outcome allowing for statistical inference at the subpopulation level. Therefore, the FMM is a flexible approach to modelling heterogeneous data [18].

The study also aimed to investigate different characteristics of herds that may impact on their ability to clear the infection, and thus impact breakdown duration so that the controls may be tailored to the risk of persistence of infection. We investigated parameters that have been found to be associated with breakdown duration in other countries, including previous breakdown history, herd type, and herd size, but also explored additional potential predictors. Herd size (i.e., the number of animals on the farm) has been consistently found to be associated with TB breakdown risk, recurrence and duration [9,10,19–24]. However, herd size could be a proxy for several other farm characteristics [25], for example, the density of animals (e.g., animals per hectare) and the intensity of farming (e.g., high input-high output farms) which could be associated with TB transmission dynamics and maintenance. The geographic area of the farm and configuration (e.g., number of land parcels) could also impact on farm risk of exposure to *M. bovis* from contiguous spread from neighbours or wildlife sources [23]. Therefore, we have added additional proxies for these factors as potential risk factors in our model. This work, therefore, also helps to tease out what aspects of herd size that are associated with breakdown duration in Ireland. Controlled beef finishing units (CBFU), colloquially known as "feedlot" herds, were also identified and modelled as a factor influencing breakdown duration. Previous research elsewhere has shown how such farming systems can be associated with increase prolongation of breakdown duration, associated with increasing genotype diversity of *M. bovis* facilitated through trade movements [10,26]. Animals from such herds go straight to slaughter, and therefore, are limited in terms of onward interherd transmission but are important to identify to explain variation in our outcome of interest. Overall, this study contributes towards informing evidence-based changes to bTB policy to address the risks associated with changing herd dynamics.

2. Results

The final dataset included 17,312 breakdowns. The mean breakdown length was 177.85 days (SD: 105.25; Median: 147; IQR: 135–187; Figure 1). The distribution of breakdown durations was both leptokurtic (kurtosis: 68.24) and positively skewed (skewness: 5.90; Figure 1).

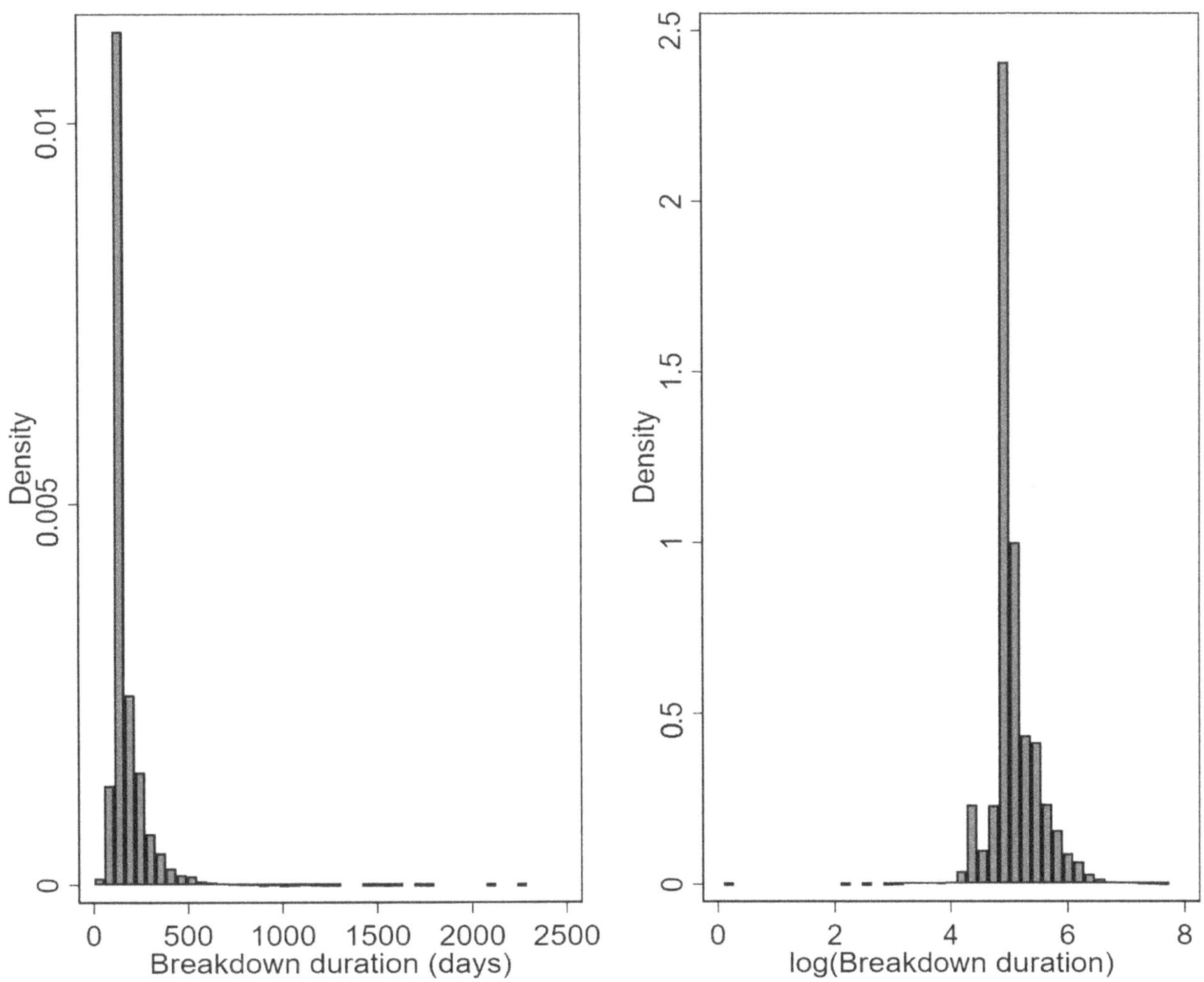

Figure 1. Breakdown duration days (**left**) and with duration log-transformed (**right**).

2.1. Model Distribution and Class Probability

Distribution fits to null models (that is, without covariates) were compared using BIC and AIC, with the following FMM models compared (Figure 2): 1. Ordinary Least Squares (OLS) log-linear; 2. GLM lognormal; 3. Gamma distribution; 4. Weibull distribution (Table 1). GLM Poisson and Negative binomial models did not converge. OLS models, where the outcome was natural logarithm transformed, were best-fitting models with the smallest AIC and BIC. There was evidence also that FMM models (with k > 1) were favoured in comparison with a model without latent subpopulation classes.

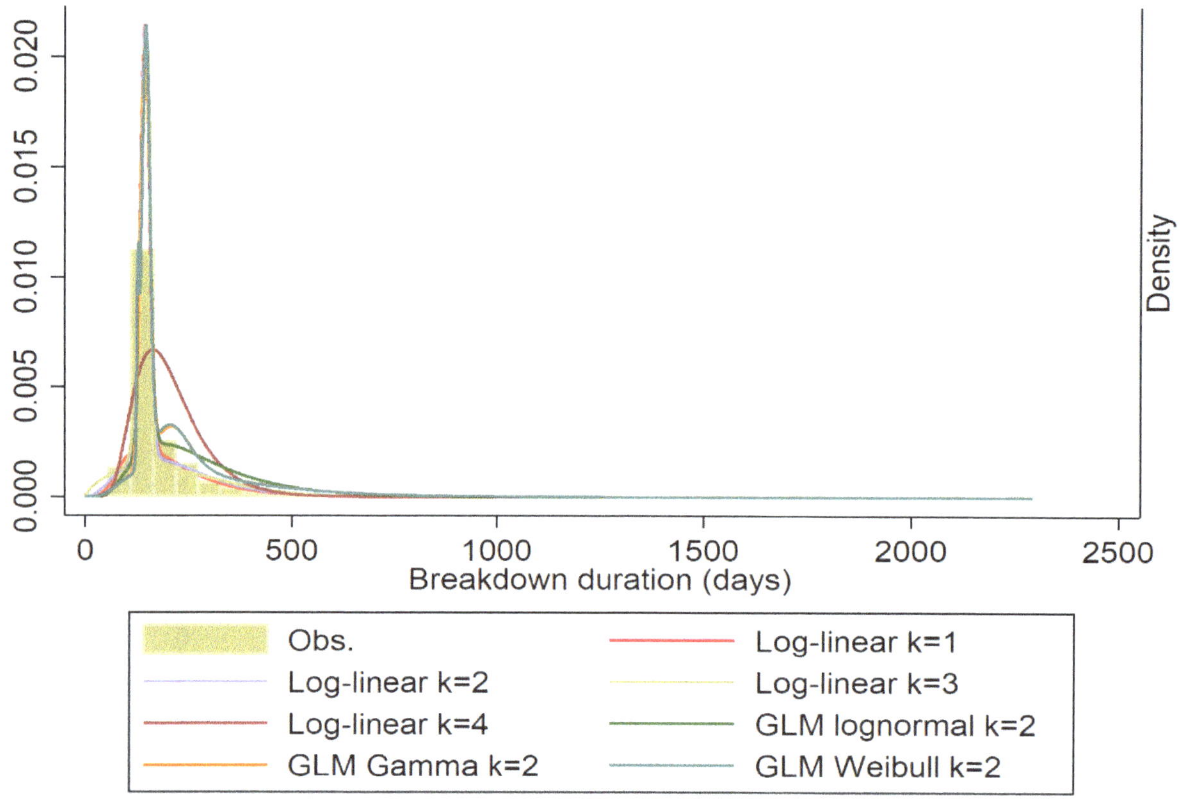

Figure 2. A comparison of Finite Fixture Models (FMMs) with differing distributions to model classes (OLS log-linear k = 1; OLS log-linear k = 2; OLS log-linear k = 3; OLS log-linear k = 4, GLM lognormal k = 2; GLM gamma distribution model k = 2; GLM Weibull distribution model k = 2).

Table 1. Comparison of Bayesian and Akaike's Information Criterion values for finite mixture models fitted to bovine TB breakdown duration data. k = number of latent classes (subpopulations).

Model	BIC	AIC
Log(duration), k = 1	17,678.83	17,663.32
Log(duration), k = 2	6532.47	6493.67
Log(duration), k = 3	6092.97	6030.90
Log(duration), k = 4	5737.85	5652.50
GLM lognormal, k = 2	182,664.06	182,625.26
GLM gamma, k = 2	183,161.31	183,122.52
GLM Weibull, k = 2	185,397.98	185,359.19

Comparing the number of classes (k) to fit the data, a three-class and four-class model fitted the data better, with a lower BIC and AIC relative to the two-class model (Table 1). However, the parsimony of the two-class models was preferred. Furthermore, research has shown the overfitting may be an issue for mixture models where k > 2, and convergence for more complicated models can be an issue for mixture models. The best-fitting model with k = 2 was the log-linear regression model [outcome variable was log-transformed before fit using the REGRESS command].

The two latent distributions fitted to different parts of data distribution (Figure 3). Figure 3 presents the predicted posterior probability of class membership for class 1 (black line) and class 2 (blue). The probability of class 1 membership (relative to class 2 membership) was very high for very large and small values. Class 2 membership was limited primarily to a narrow range around the central tendency. These data are visualised in Figure 4 by plotting the histograms of data with > 20% probability of membership for PR2 class (clear) and PR1 class (red) (Figure 4).

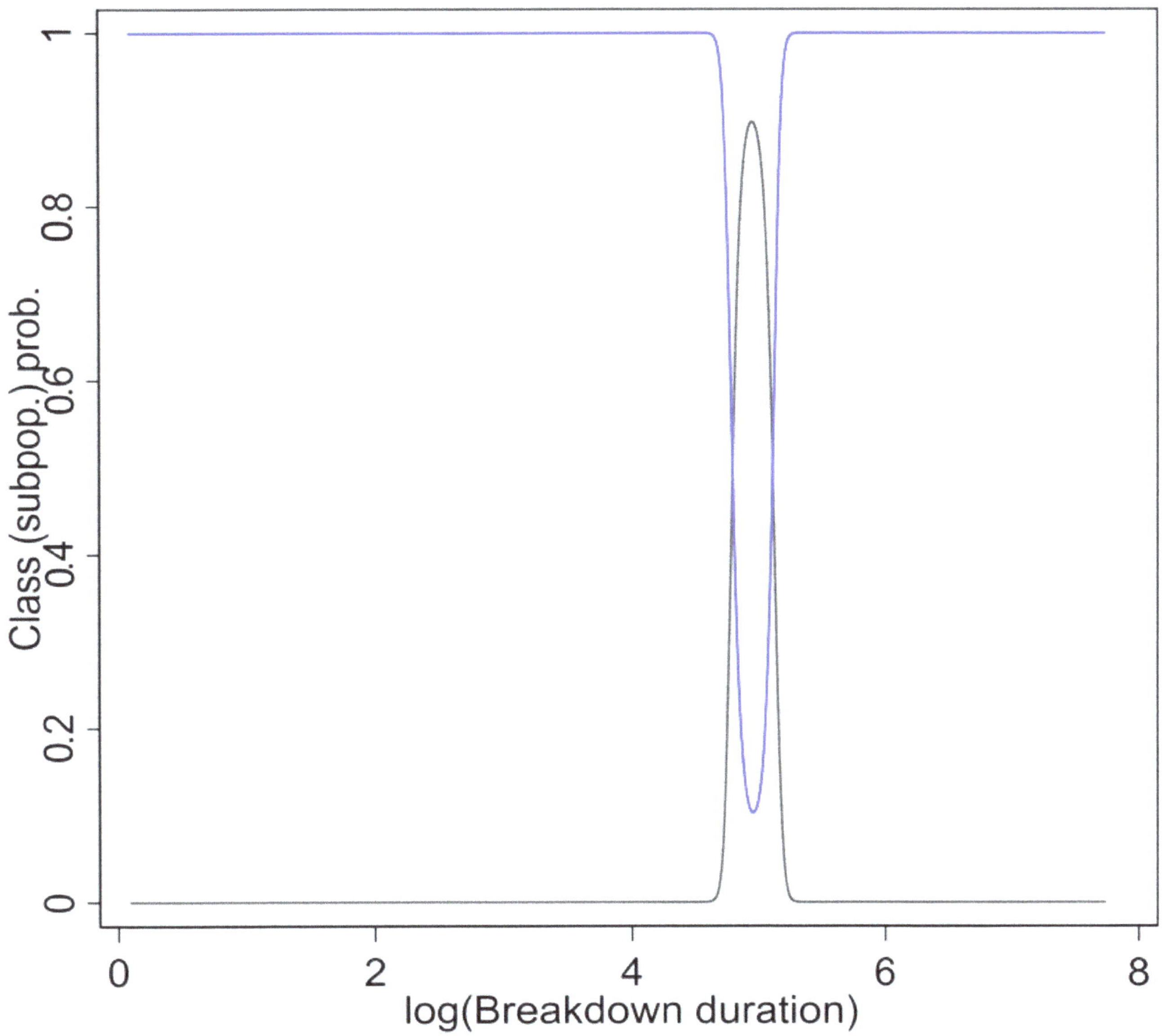

Figure 3. The predicted probability of class membership for a two-latent class FMM null model fitted to bovine tuberculosis (TB) breakdown duration data. Grey line represents class 1; blue line represents class 2.

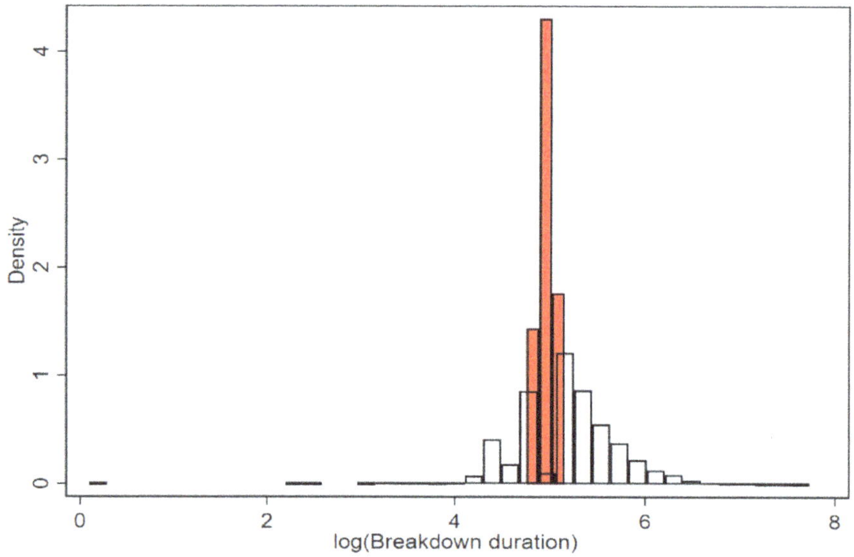

Figure 4. The predicted density from an FMM with two classes fitted to bovine TB breakdown duration data; class 1 is represented as red bars which cluster around the central tendency of the distribution; class 2 is represented as clear bars in the histogram which encapsulated more of the variance in the dataset away from the mean.

2.2. Development of a Multivariable Log-Normal FMM

A baseline model was developed with a fixed set of covariates log-herd size, herd-type, and herd history (breakdown history over the previous 3 years), as potential predictors of log-breakdown length based on previous research. The probability of being class/component 1 or 2 was modelled as a function of log-herd size, herd history and herd type, as we hypothesized that breakdown duration may be associated with these factors. Comparisons were made using BIC and AIC with baseline models with the inclusion or exclusion of these factors, separately and respectively. Baseline models had the lowest BIC values when all three factors were retained to explain variation in breakdown length, and when both log-herd size and herd type were retained as factors explaining some variation in the probability of being associated with class 1 or 2 (Baseline vs. class prob (log_hs, herd_type) ΔBIC: 43.75; Table 2). The model with the lowest AIC included herd-history as an additional predictor of class probability, but the more parsimonious (BIC) model was selected.

Table 2. Comparison of base FMM models using Bayesian and Akaike's Information Criteria.

Model	Class Probability	Regression Predictors	BIC	AIC
Log(duration), k = 2	.	log_hs herd_history herd_type	5893.03	5730.09
Log(duration), k = 2	log_hs	log_hs herd_history herd_type	5858.36	5687.66
Log(duration), k = 2	herd_type	log_hs herd_history herd_type	5853.46	5667.24
Log(duration), k = 2	herd_history	log_hs herd_history herd_type	5924.37	5730.39
Log(duration), k = 2	log_hs, herd_type	log_hs herd_history herd_type	5849.29	5655.31
Log(duration), k = 2	log_hs, herd_history	log_hs herd_history herd_type	5884.57	5682.83
Log(duration), k = 2	herd_type, herd_history	log_hs herd_history herd_type	5879.33	5662.08
Log(duration), k = 2	log_hs, herd_type, herd_history	log_hs herd_history herd_type	5872.54	5647.52

The final model outputs are presented in Tables 3 and 4. Predictions from the model (Figure S1) showed that class 1 were tightly bound around the central tendency of the distribution, "central" subpopulation; class 2 had greater representation at the tails of the distribution, "tail" subpopulation. The entropy value, which discerns how distinct subpopulation classes were, was estimated at 0.58, which is moderate but reasonable for a large population size with 2-classes. The subpopulations were reasonably balanced, with 51% of the population classified as Class 1 "central" subpopulation, and 49% being falling into the Class 2 "tail" subpopulation. The (geometric) mean breakdown duration for Class 1 subpopulation was 142 days (exp(4.96)), while for subpopulation Class 2 the mean duration was 183 days (exp(5.21)).

Table 3. Concomitant variables as predictors of class/component probabilities; coefficients represent associations with Class 2 relative to Class 1.

	Coef.	exp(Coef.)	SE	z	p	Lower 95%	Upper 95%
log_hs	0.070	1.073	0.018	3.860	<0.001	0.035	0.106
herd_type_num							
Beef	<0.001	1.000					
Dairy	0.158	1.171	0.061	2.590	0.010	0.039	0.277
Other	−0.331	0.718	0.099	−3.350	0.001	−0.525	−0.137
Suckler	−0.096	0.909	0.051	−1.870	0.061	−0.196	0.005

Table 4. Estimated associations between factors and breakdown duration (log_length) for Class 1 and Class 2 subpopulations from a finite mixture model.

Log_Length	Class 1 "Central"				Class 2 "Tail"			
	Coef.	p	Lower 95%	Upper 95%	Coef.	p	Lower 95%	Upper 95%
log_hs	<0.001	0.835	−0.003	0.002	0.090	<0.001	0.077	0.102
herd_history								
TB free	ref				ref			
Zero reactors	−0.001	0.787	−0.009	0.007	0.115	<0.001	0.068	0.162
1 reactors	0.015	<0.001	0.007	0.023	0.129	<0.001	0.076	0.182
2–4 reactors	0.017	<0.001	0.009	0.025	0.219	<0.001	0.166	0.273
≥5 reactors	0.017	0.004	0.005	0.029	0.226	<0.001	0.155	0.296
herd_type_num								
Beef	ref				ref			
Dairy	0.025	<0.001	0.018	0.031	−0.075	<0.001	−0.114	−0.036
Other	0.003	0.560	−0.006	0.012	−0.095	0.003	−0.157	−0.033
Suckler	0.006	0.015	0.001	0.011	−0.014	0.373	−0.046	0.017
Controlled finishing units								
Never	ref				ref			
Designated	−0.001	0.932	−0.030	0.027	0.710	<0.001	0.603	0.818
log_NPH	−0.003	0.040	−0.005	<0.001	−0.014	0.054	−0.028	<0.001
parcel_cut								
1	ref				ref			
2	<0.001	0.902	−0.006	0.006	0.026	0.177	−0.012	0.063
3	0.004	0.224	−0.002	0.010	0.031	0.110	−0.007	0.069
4	0.005	0.116	−0.001	0.012	0.064	0.002	0.023	0.105
≥5	0.001	0.736	−0.005	0.007	0.049	0.006	0.014	0.084
med_area	<0.001	<0.001	<0.001	<0.001	<0.001	0.299	<0.001	0.001
cut_mmoves								
<90	ref				ref			
>90	−0.039	<0.001	−0.047	−0.032	0.108	<0.001	0.062	0.155
bd_start_yr	<0.001	0.470	−0.001	0.001	−0.023	<0.001	−0.029	−0.017

The preferred model with the lowest BIC retained both log-herd size and herd type as explaining variation in the probability of herds being associated with either latent class component. Table 3 shows the output of this part of the mixture model. The model suggested that increasing log-herd size was significantly associated with having a greater probability of being in Class 2 "tail" subpopulation.

Dairy herds had a significantly greater probability of being represented in Class 2 "tail" component, relative to Class 1 "central", in comparison with beef rearing/finishing production type ($p = 0.010$). "Other" herd types had a lower probability of being in class 2 relative to beef herd types ($p < 0.001$). There was no significant difference in class probabilities between beef rearing/finishing and beef suckler ($p = 0.061$) herd type.

The associations between factors hypothesized to impact breakdown duration for Class 1 and Class 2 are presented in Table 4. All predictors were retained in the log-normal regression parts of the model explaining breakdown duration for both components/class 1 and 2. Comparing coefficients between Class 1 and Class 2 suggests that risk factors may have a different associated effect on breakdown duration.

Class 1 breakdowns duration tend to decrease with increasing nitrogen load per hectare (log; log_NPH) and for breakdowns commencing later in the time series (bd_start_yr). The duration was positively associated with herd history (herd_history), with herds with breakdowns during the previous three years having a longer duration than those without breakdowns. There was not, however, a clear dose-dependency in terms of breakdown size (i.e., number of reactors disclosed). Herds with 1, 2–4, or > 4 reactors were a significantly higher risk for longer breakdowns within this "central" subpopulation, relative to herds without reactors. There was no difference in breakdown duration between herds without a previous breakdown and "zero-reactor" breakdowns (i.e., historic breakdowns that were disclosed due to a TB lesion detected at routine slaughter and in which no additional reactors were disclosed at follow-up herd tests). There was no significant association between duration and herd size, CBFU (feedlot) status or farm fragmentation (parcel_cut). Inward movements were dichotomised into herds which had high mean yearly inward movements (>90 moves) or lower mean inward movements (<90). In Class 1 subpopulation, there was a negative association between high inward movements and breakdown length (−0.039; 95% CI: −0.04–−0.032; 3.8% reduction in duration).

Herds associated with class 2 "tail" subpopulation exhibited significantly increased breakdown duration with increasing herd-size (log_hs), and if designated with a "feedlot" status (CBFU). Duration of breakdowns increased by 9.4% (β: 0.090; 95% CI: 0.077–0.102) for every log-unit increase in herd size. Feedlot herds within class 2 subpopulation were 203.4% (β: 0.710; 95% CI: 0.603–0.818) longer duration relative to non-feedlot herds. The median predicted duration for feedlot herds was 451 days, whereas as the median duration was 182 days for non-feedlot designated herds. The predicted relationship for this subpopulation for herd size and feedlot designation is presented in Figure 5.

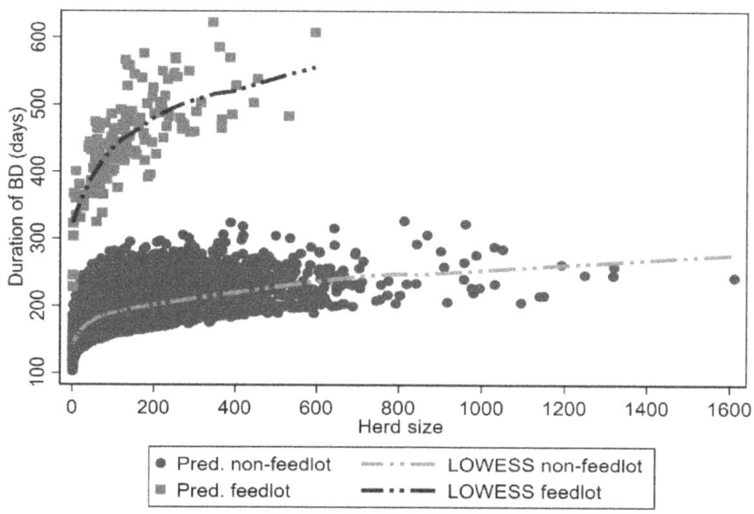

Figure 5. Relationship between herd size and breakdown duration as predicted for Class 2 subpopulation of a finite mixture model. Squares are predictions for herds with a controlled beef finishing unit "feedlot" designation; Points are predictions for herds without "feedlot" designation. Lines are Local Weighted Scatterplot Smoothing (LOWESS) curves fitted to the data.

Duration increased if a herd had previously experienced a breakdown during the previous 3-years. There was a trend towards dose-dependency, with increasing duration associated with a greater number of reactors disclosed during the previous breakdown (Figure 6), however, the size effect was reasonably small. For example, there was a 25% (β: 0.226; $p < 0.001$; 95% CI: 0.155–0.296) increase in mean duration for the herd with five or more reactors relative to herds which did not experience a breakdown during the previous 3 years.

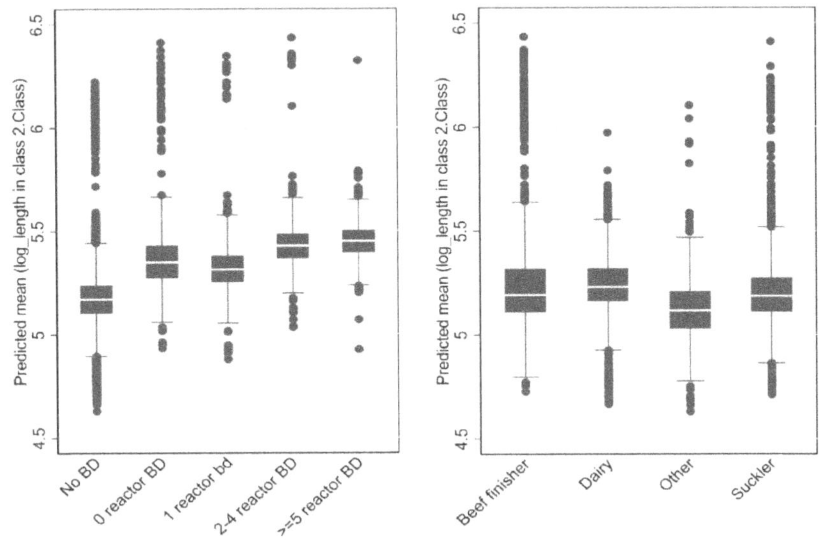

Figure 6. Relationship between breakdown history during the previous 3 years and predicted mean breakdown duration (top). Relationship between herd type and predicted mean breakdown duration (bottom). Note, log scale.

Parcel number (parcel_cut), a measure of farm fragmentation, was positively associated with increased breakdown length, though only for herds with 4 or more parcels relative to herds with 1. Again, the effect size was moderate, for example, a 6.6% (β: 0.064; $p < 0.001$; 95% CI: 0.023–0.105) increasing duration for herds with 4 parcels relative to herds with only 1 parcel.

Beef rearing/finishing herds had significantly longer breakdown duration relative to dairy, suckler or "other" herd types (herd_type) (Table 4; Figure 6). For example, dairy herds experienced mean breakdown log-lengths the were 7.2% shorter (exp(β: −0.138)-1) relative to beef herds.

The linear predictor for start year of breakdown (bd_start_yr) suggested that breakdown lengths decreased slightly per year of the study for Class 2 subpopulation (0.5% reduction per year; β: −0.023; $p < 0.001$; 95% CI: −0.017––0.029).

Controlling for herd size, intensity metric based on nitrogen loading (NPH) was negatively associated with breakdown length, though this effect was not significant (β: −0.014; $p = 0.054$; 95% CI: −0.028 < 0.001). It was likely that the effect was impacted by confounding with herd size and area.

In Class 2 subpopulation, there was a positive association between breakdown length and high inward movement (0.108; 0.062–0.155; 11.4% increase in duration). The size effects for both subpopulations are reasonably small, for example, herds in subpopulation 2 increase their mean duration by approximately 20.8 days if they make > 90 inward moves per annum (i.e., mean [183 days] × 0.114).

3. Discussion

This study was the first to explore variation in breakdown duration explicitly in Ireland, and more generally the first to use finite mixture models (FMM) to explore the variation in breakdown duration for bTB. It is also the first study to investigate cattle production of nitrogen per hectare (a common measure of the intensity of livestock production within the EU) as a potential factor associated with bovine TB breakdown duration. The significance of this approach lies in enabling the adaption of disease policies to change risks based on an evidence base which is inclusive of larger trends such as livestock intensification.

Previous research has dichotomised breakdown duration and modelled using logit distributions (e.g., [9,15,26,27]), have broken down duration into ordered categories of increasing duration and modelled using ordinal regression models [10] or have modelled duration as a count of days using a negative binomial discrete distribution [10] or using simulation approaches [28]. The durations recorded in the present study exhibited an unusual distribution, with both positive skewness and kurtosis. The mixture model allowed for two different distributions to be fit to the data, with class associations being modelled via a latent class model.

The latent classification of the data into two classes suggested that observations were clustering tightly around the central tendency and a second which captured more of the variation in the outcome, especially at the tails of the distribution. The latent component of the model suggested that larger herds and dairy, relative to beef, herds had a higher probability to be represented by the tail subpopulation, relative to the central subpopulation. This may indicate that such herd characteristics are associated with more unusual breakdowns away from the central tendency. Previous research has found that chronic breakdowns, which would be represented by our tails subpopulation, can be associated with both increasing numbers of animals within the herd (e.g., [9]) and dairy enterprises ([27,29]) relative to other herd types.

In terms of interpretation, the latent classification and the "tail" subpopulation log-normal regression model are informative. The log-normal regression for the 'central' subpopulation is less informative, from a policy perspective, as 1. It seeks to explain variation over a narrow range; that is, the variance in the outcome was low, 2. Larger breakdowns are of greater significance from a disease policy development perspective, assuming that at least partially the speed at which average breakdowns clear may be more related to breakdown management/compliance and response times (e.g., actions by the farmer and operational delivery by veterinarians) as well as epidemiologically relevant factors. However, it is interesting to note the differences in the relationship between the outcome and predictors between subpopulations. In the central subpopulation, there was no significant association with duration and herd-size, number of land parcels, controlled finishing units (feedlots) or breakdown starting year. Dairy herds varied in their association with breakdown duration across subpopulations, with longer durations relative to beef herds in subpopulation 1, and shorter durations relative to beef herds in subpopulation 2. However, it should be borne in mind that dairy herds have a higher class-probability for subpopulation two. Furthermore, dairy herds tend to be larger and have older age profile animals, both of which are associated with bTB risk [22,28].

The class 2 log-normal part of the FMM suggested that breakdown lengths were significantly increased with increasing numbers of reactors disclosed at the breakdown during the previous 3 years. Herd history has been associated with breakdown length in previous studies outside of Ireland, though metrics of TB history were not always analogous to what was done in the present study [10,15]. A history of TB in a herd was associated with large (>13 reactors) bTB breakdowns, relative to small (2–4 reactors) in a case-control study in Ireland [30]. Interestingly, recent work suggested that that previous breakdown size was not associated with recurrence risk in Ireland [2].

The factors that appeared to have the largest effects on breakdown duration were herd-size and whether the herd was ever designated a controlled beef finishing unit "feedlot" herd. Controlled finishing unit herds are non-breeding beef finishing units which are only permitted to move cattle directly to slaughter and fulfil certain criteria to receive the designation, for example, biosecurity protocols are in place, and boundaries are double fenced or equivalent to prevent any direct contact with cattle on neighbouring lands/premises/holdings. Such herds may apply for controlled finishing unit herd designation upon breakdown, subject to there being no evidence of within-herd spread; breakdowns are typically due to lesions detected at routine slaughter from cattle bought-in and fattened over a relatively short period of time for finishing. This status enables them to continue to buy in beef cattle for finishing during breakdowns. These herds are deemed of lower risk for onward infection transmission due to high turnover of animals within the herds before going direct to slaughter. The effectiveness of controls to prevent such herd enterprises posing a risk to neighbouring herds via wildlife spillover or contiguous spread is subject to another ongoing study (J. Madden pers. comm.). Beef fattening herds in Northern Ireland, which can buy-in animals during breakdowns, have increased strain diversity of *M. bovis* and increased breakdown duration time, linked to inward animal movements from a wide geographical area [10,31]. The association between such herds and increased breakdown length identified in this study and in Northern Ireland may be explained by the ability of the business model to continue while under restriction; the length of breakdown does not reflect a chronic disease problem on these farms per se but rather the reality that a farm practice which involves purchasing in large numbers of beef cattle for fattening and slaughter makes it likely that the detection of bTB lesions at routine slaughter would be a regular occurrence, given the background level of bTB in Ireland. Each such detection extends the breakdown again, lengthening breakdown duration but not necessarily reflecting the continuing spread of infection within the herd.

Herd size has been found to be a significant factor for TB breakdown risk in general for many studies (e.g., see [3,23]). Brooks-Pollock and Keeling [22] showed how herd size was associated with breakdown persistence, which the authors interpreted as indicating a lack of clearance of infection within herds after a breakdown. We have attempted to explore what correlates and related variables of herd size that might be important for breakdown duration with the inclusion of nitrogen load (a measure of agricultural intensity, based on organic nitrogen per hectare), land area, and parcel number. For Class 2, "tail" subpopulation, there were significant increases in log-length of breakdown with increasing land area and the number of parcels (primarily 4 or more parcels, relative to single parcel units), while controlling for herd size. However, for both factors, the effect size was small. Despite this, previous work elsewhere has found significant positive associations between farm fragmentation [32–34] and land area [33,35] and TB breakdown risk, though there are little comparative data on these factors relationship with breakdown duration.

Surprisingly, controlling for herd size there was a negative relationship with increasing nitrogen load. This outcome is most likely affected by the significant confounding relationship between herd size, area and nitrogen load (see Figure S2). Indeed, nitrogen per hectare (NPH) was positively and significantly associated with breakdown duration at the univariable level but not significantly in a multivariable model without area or herd size (Figure S3; Table S1). The final multivariable model suggested that herd size, that is the number of animals/potential hosts, appears to be the key herd-level factor for predicting breakdown length.

It was encouraging that for both subpopulations that the temporal trend was for a reduction in mean duration over time. This suggests that interventions aimed at clearing infection once reactors are identified are being more effective over time. However, it should be noted that the estimated reduction is very small, being less than a day reduction in mean duration for the class 2 subpopulation. Previous work in Ireland has found a decreasing trend also in breakdown recurrence from 1998–2015 [36], though recent trends suggest the incidence is increasing.

In conclusion, our work has suggested breakdown duration in Ireland is related to several herd and farm characteristics, including the herd size, type, area (acreage), fragmentation, and trading frequency. Given that herd size and acreage contributed additively to increasing breakdown duration, trends in farming including farm expansion and consolidation may signal future increases in breakdown duration, causing a greater challenge to the bTB control program.

4. Materials and Methods

4.1. Data

The dataset used is a breakdown herd dataset where each line in the dataset represents a discrete breakdown [37]. Throughout, the start date and end date within that file was used to define breakdown durations (see [37] for additional detail). All breakdowns were initiated by the disclosure of (i) bTB reactors from Single Intradermal Comparative Cervical Tuberculin test (SICCTT) or (ii) the disclosure of a bTB lesion found at slaughter (factory lesion). End dates were when herds were derestricted, in compliance with the EU regulations on bovine TB. The dataset included breakdowns that were ongoing between January 2012 and December 2018 and were initiated from January 2012–December 2018. Follow-up period ended in August 2019.

Two inclusion criteria were employed to the data. Only the most recent breakdowns per herd were selected; this was to avoid repeated measures per herd and therefore simplify the analysis. All breakdowns that were censored by the follow-up (i.e., they were still experiencing a breakdown when follow-up finished in August 2019) were removed from the dataset.

All data are available upon reasonable request from corresponding authors.

4.2. Model

Finite Mixture Models (FMM) are a flexible modelling framework that have been applied to several biological problems, including clustering, estimation of diagnostics performance, and for modelling heterogeneous data [18]. In addition, FMM is an approach that can be applied to duration models [17,18,38]. Applications of an FMM model to duration include modelling length of stay in hospitals [17] and age-at-onset for various conditions in human medicine including migraine or bipolar disorder (e.g., [39–41]). FMMs give flexibility to fit the data by allowing admixture of distributions, called classes (k) to explain the variation in the data. Furthermore, different continuous probability distribution types can be fitted, including normal, log-normal, Poisson, negative binomial, Gamma and Weibull. For example, log-normal distributions have been applied to "survival" type data, as an alternative to Cox proportional hazard models [42]. Here we developed a model of breakdown duration without repeated measures using an FMM approach.

Models were compared using Bayesian information criteria (BIC) and Akaike's Information Criteria (AIC) values, which favour models which explain variation in our outcome while penalising models with many vaguely informative parameters. Where BIC and AIC did not support the same model configuration, the model with the least parameters were preferred, which was generally the BIC preferred model. Simulation studies have shown that BIC is generally preferred to AIC for FMM, as AIC can tend to select for too many classes [43].

Entropy value, which discerns how distinct subpopulation [latent] classes were, was estimated [44]. The higher the number the greater the separations between classes, "rule of thumb" threshold of 0.8 has been proposed. However, recent simulation analysis has shown that entropy values are sensitive to sample size. Entropy values < 0.2 might be expected in large sample studies (e.g., >3000 observations, 1500 per subpopulation) with balanced spilt between 2-classes and where true sample separation has been simulated [44].

Our process was to plot out the distribution of breakdown durations and fit differing FMM types, including log-normal, normal, and count distributions. We explored $k > 2$ class models, but only retained a two-class model for multivariable models to ensure a more parsimonious model that was more meaningful from an epidemiological perspective. Furthermore, a higher number of components in FMMs are associated with overfitting [45].

The steps involved in the construction of the model is depicted in Figure S4. Once we developed a well-fitting null model without covariates, we built multivariable FMMs. Initially, baseline models were fit with the parameters: herd size, herd history, and herd types. Then additional parameters were added sequentially. Comparisons between model configurations were made using AIC/BIC values; lower values indicated better performing models. Outcome and covariate parameter summary statistics are presented in Table 5.

Table 5. Summary statistics of outcome and covariate parameters for the FMM model of bTB breakdown duration.

Variable	n	Mean	Std. Dev.	exp(Mean)	Min	Max
log_length	17,312	5.087	0.403	161.869	0.095	7.736
log_hs	17,312	4.058	1.162	57.887	<0.001	7.385
log_NPH	17,312	4.397	0.986	81.210	−4.605	6.733
med_area	17,312	49.360	39.962		<1.000	754.900
herd_history						
TB free	13,833	80%			0	1
Zero reactors	1156	7%			0	1
1 reactor	896	5%			0	1
2–4 reactors	935	5%			0	1
≥5 reactors	492	3%			0	1
herd_type						
Beef	3576	21%			0	1
Dairy	4743	27%			0	1
Other	830	5%				
Suckler	8163	47%			0	1
Feedlot						
0	17,173	99%				
1	139	1%			0	1
parcel_cut						
1	3030	18%				
2	3299	19%			0	1
3	3069	18%			0	1
4	2425	14%			0	1
≥5	5489	32%			0	1
cut_mmoves						
0	15,660	90%				
1	1652	10%			0	1
bd_start_yr						
2012	1231	7%				
2013	2473	14%			0	1
2014	2466	14%			0	1
2015	2486	14%			0	1
2016	2571	15%			0	1
2017	2935	17%			0	1
2018	3150	18%			0	1

Additional predictors of breakdown duration were added to this model. The model fitted a controlled beef finishing unit proxy "feedlot" status (binary; 1 if herd ever had designation as a controlled beef finishing unit; 0 otherwise), an intensity metric based on nitrogen loading per hectare (logarithm of median bovine nitrogen per hectare over 2015–2018), the number of parcels (recorded per herd in 2018 using LPIS at a resolution of 7 m), land area (median hectares over 2015–2018), and breakdown start year, and inward animal movement metric. The mean number of inward animal moves (2013–2018) into a farm was dichotomised into "large" (mean ≥90 per annum) and other (<90 mean moves).

Herd size was log-transformed. Herd history was a categorical variable indicating whether the herd had previously had a breakdown within 3-years, and if so, the size of the breakdown in terms of reactors disclosed (0, 1, 2–4, ≥5). Breakdowns with 0 reactors would have been initiated by lesions found during slaughter at abattoir during post-mortem surveillance [37]. Herd types were taken from the AHCS dataset, as beef, dairy, "other" or sucker herds. Herd type was based on standard definitions used by DAFM: dairy herds are self-explanatory; beef herds are non-breeding herds; suckler herds are beef breeding herds; the designation "other" reflects herds which engage in a combination of such activities.

Other variables offered to the models included: controlled finishing unit (colloquially referred to in Ireland as "feedlots") status, nitrogen loading, number of farm fragments/parcels, number of moves into the herd, and year of breakdown initiation.

"Feedlot" status was assigned if a herd was ever designated a controlled beef finishing unit (CBFU) by DAFM at the breakdown from 2006–2018 (see Discussion).

Nitrogen, measured as the organic nitrogen loading per hectare (NPH) from bovines, was measured as the median NPH per herd over 2015–2018 assigned to each herd. Because of the skew of this variable (a small number of herds with very large NPH values) the parameter was log-transformed. These data were estimated by DAFM in accordance with Nitrogen Regulations in Ireland.

The number of farm parcels was measured from the Land Parcel Identification System (LPIS) 2018, with discrete land-parcels being classified if parcels were >7 m from each other. This buffer was chosen to ensure that parcels that effectively were single units were not counted as separate parcels. Land parcels were categorised into 1, 2, 3, 4 or ≥5 parcels.

Land area was measured as the mean hectares land area declared during 2015–2018 for Basic Payment Scheme (BPS) purposes. The median of these values per herd was assigned as a metric of geographic footprint for each herd in the dataset. There was a 99% correlation between individual yearly and median land area.

Movement of animals into herds were measured by a single metric in this instance, as the mean of total inward moves per annum from 2013–2018, inclusive. Univariable models suggested that most variation in the relationship between breakdown length and inward moves was whether herds brought in large numbers of cattle or not. Therefore, the data were categorised into herds with an average of >90 inward moves per year and those with <90 inward moves per year.

Year of breakdown initiation was entered into models initially as categorical variables but added many parameters (n = 7 parameters; 2012–2018). The exploratory analysis suggested that trends could be modelled as a single linear predictor.

All analysis was undertaken in Stata 15.1 MP–Parallel Edition (Stata Corp., 2017) using the FMM suite of commands.

Author Contributions: Conceptualization, A.W.B., P.B. and E.R.; methodology, A.W.B.; formal analysis, A.W.B., J.M.M.; investigation, A.W.B. and J.M.M.; data curation, J.M.M.; writing—original draft preparation, A.W.B.; writing—review and editing, A.W.B., D.B., J.O., J.M.M., P.B. and E.R.; supervision, D.B. All authors have read and agreed to the published version of the manuscript.

Acknowledgments: The authors would like to acknowledge the support of the One-health Scientific Support Unit and the provision of nitrogen data by colleagues in the Nitrates, Biodiversity and Engineering Division, DAFM.

References

1. Clarke, A.; Maher, J.; Byrne, A.W.; More, S.J.; Horan, M.; Barrett, D. Development and application of a prioritisation tool for animal health surveillance activities in Ireland. *Front. Vet. Sci.* **2020**, *5*. in review.
2. Byrne, A.W.; Barrett, D.; Breslin, P.; Madden, J.M.; O'Keeffe, J.; Ryan, E. Future risk of bovine tuberculosis breakdown: A dominance analysis approach. *BioRxiv* **2020**.
3. Allen, A.R.; Skuce, R.A.; Byrne, A.W. Bovine tuberculosis in Britain and Ireland–A perfect storm? The confluence of potential ecological and epidemiological impediments to controlling a chronic infectious disease. *Front. Vet. Sci.* **2018**, *5*, 109. [CrossRef] [PubMed]
4. De Garine-Wichatitsky, M.; Caron, A.; Kock, R.; Tschopp, R.; Munyeme, M.; Hofmeyr, M.; Michel, A. A review of bovine tuberculosis at the wildlife–livestock–human interface in sub-Saharan Africa. *Epidemiol. Infect.* **2013**, *141*, 1342–1356. [CrossRef] [PubMed]
5. De Kantor, I.N.; Ritacco, V. An update on bovine tuberculosis programs in Latin American and Caribbean countries. *Vet. Microbiol.* **2006**, *112*, 111–118. [CrossRef] [PubMed]
6. Cawley, A.; Cronin, A. Spending Review Animal Health: TB Eradication. Irish Government Economic and Evaluation Service (IGEES), Government of Ireland. Available online: http://budget.gov.ie/Budgets/2020/Documents/Budget/Animal%20Health%20-%20TB%20Eradication.pdf (accessed on 15 July 2020).
7. More, S.J. Perspectives from the science-policy interface in animal health and welfare. *Front. Vet. Sci.* **2019**, *6*, 382. [CrossRef]
8. Karolemeas, K.; McKinley, T.J.; Clifton-Hadley, R.S.; Goodchild, A.V.; Mitchell, A.; Johnston, W.T.; Conlan, A.J.K.; Donnelly, C.A.; Wood, J.L.N. Predicting prolonged bovine tuberculosis breakdowns in Great Britain as an aid to control. *Prev. Vet. Med.* **2010**, *97*, 183–190. [CrossRef]
9. Milne, G.; Allen, A.; Graham, J.; Lahuerta-Marin, A.; McCormick, C.; Presho, E.; Reid, N.; Skuce, R.; Byrne, A.W. Bovine tuberculosis breakdown duration in cattle herds: An investigation of herd, host, pathogen and wildlife risk factors. *PeerJ* **2020**, *8*, e8319. [CrossRef]
10. Kelly, P.; Shalloo, L.; Wallace, M.; Dillon, P. The Irish dairy industry–Recent history and strategy, current state and future challenges. *Int. J. Dairy Technol.* **2020**, *73*, 309–323. [CrossRef]
11. Ashe, S.; More, S.J.; O'Keeffe, J.; White, P.; McGrath, G.; Aznar, I. Survival and dispersal of a defined cohort of Irish cattle. *Ir. Vet. J.* **2009**, *62*, 1–6. [CrossRef]
12. Brown, E.; Marshall, A.H.; Mitchell, H.J.; Byrne, A.W. Cattle movements in Northern Ireland form a robust network: Implications for disease management. *Prev. Vet. Med.* **2019**, *170*, 104740. [CrossRef] [PubMed]
13. Gilbert, M.; Mitchell, A.; Bourn, D.; Mawdsley, J.; Clifton-Hadley, R.; Wint, W. Cattle movements and bovine tuberculosis in Great Britain. *Nature* **2005**, *435*, 491–496. [CrossRef] [PubMed]
14. Doyle, L.P.; Courcier, E.A.; Gordon, A.W.; O'Hagan, M.J.H.; Menzies, F.D. Bovine tuberculosis in Northern Ireland: Risk factors associated with duration and recurrence of chronic herd breakdowns. *Prev. Vet. Med.* **2016**, *131*, 1–7. [CrossRef]
15. Wolfe, D.M.; Berke, O.; Kelton, D.F.; White, P.W.; More, S.J.; O'Keeffe, J.; Martin, S.W. From explanation to prediction: A model for recurrent bovine tuberculosis in Irish cattle herds. *Prev. Vet. Med.* **2010**, *94*, 170–177. [CrossRef]
16. Moran, J.L.; Solomon, P.J. ANZICS Centre for Outcome and Resource Evaluation (CORE) of the Australian and New Zealand Intensive Care Society (ANZICS). A review of statistical estimators for risk-adjusted length of stay: Analysis of the Australian and New Zealand intensive care adult patient data-base, 2008–2009. *BMC Med. Res. Methodol.* **2012**, *12*, 68. [CrossRef]
17. McLachlan, G.J.; Peel, D. *Finite Mixture Models*; John Wiley & Sons: Hoboken, NJ, USA, 2004.
18. Griffin, J.M.; Martin, S.W.; Thorburn, M.A.; Eves, J.A.; Hammond, R.F. A case-control study on the association of selected risk factors with the occurrence of bovine tuberculosis in the Republic of Ireland. *Prev. Vet. Med.* **1996**, *27*, 75–87. [CrossRef]
19. Olea-Popelka, F.J.; White, P.W.; Collins, J.D.; O'Keeffe, J.; Kelton, D.F.; Martin, S.W. Breakdown severity during a bovine tuberculosis episode as a predictor of future herd breakdowns in Ireland. *Prev. Vet. Med.* **2004**, *63*, 163–172. [CrossRef]
20. Green, L.E.; Cornell, S.J. Investigations of cattle herd breakdowns with bovine tuberculosis in four counties of England and Wales using VETNET data. *Prev. Vet. Med.* **2005**, *70*, 293–311. [CrossRef]

21. Brooks-Pollock, E.; Keeling, M. Herd size and bovine tuberculosis persistence in cattle farms in Great Britain. *Prev. Vet. Med.* **2009**, *92*, 360–365. [CrossRef]
22. Skuce, R.A.; Allen, A.R.; McDowell, S.W. Herd-level risk factors for bovine tuberculosis: A literature review. *Vet. Med. Int.* **2012**, *2012*. [CrossRef]
23. Bessell, P.R.; Orton, R.; White, P.C.; Hutchings, M.R.; Kao, R.R. Risk factors for bovine tuberculosis at the national level in Great Britain. *BMC Vet. Res.* **2012**, *8*, 51. [CrossRef] [PubMed]
24. Griffin, J.M.; Hahesy, T.; Lynch, K.; Salman, M.D.; McCarthy, J.; Hurley, T. The association of cattle husbandry practices, environmental factors and farmer characteristics with the occurrence of chronic bovine tuberculosis in dairy herds in the Republic of Ireland. *Prev. Vet. Med.* **1993**, *17*, 145–160. [CrossRef]
25. Milne, G.M.; Graham, J.; Allen, A.; Lahuerta-Marin, A.; McCormick, C.; Presho, E.; Skuce, R.; Byrne, A.W. Spatiotemporal analysis of prolonged and recurrent bovine tuberculosis breakdowns in Northern Irish cattle herds reveals a new infection hotspot. *Spat. Spatio Temporal Epidemiol.* **2019**, *28*, 33–42. [CrossRef] [PubMed]
26. Reilly, L.A.; Courtenay, O. Husbandry practices, badger sett density and habitat composition as risk factors for transient and persistent bovine tuberculosis on UK cattle farms. *Prev. Vet. Med.* **2007**, *80*, 129–142. [CrossRef]
27. Brooks-Pollock, E.; Conlan, A.J.; Mitchell, A.P.; Blackwell, R.; McKinley, T.J.; Wood, J.L. Age-dependent patterns of bovine tuberculosis in cattle. *Vet. Res.* **2013**, *44*, 97. [CrossRef]
28. Milne, M.G.; Graham, J.; Allen, A.R.; Lahuerta-Marin, A.; McCormick, C.; Presho, E.; Skuce, R.A.; Byrne, A.W. Herd Characteristics, Wildlife Risk and Bacterial Strain Genotypes in Persistent Breakdowns of Bovine Tuberculosis in Northern Irish Cattle Herds. In Proceedings of the SVEPM 2018 Conference Society of Veterinary Epidemiology and Preventive Medicine, Tallinn, Estonia, 21–23 March 2018.
29. Clegg, T.A.; Good, M.; Hayes, M.; Duignan, A.; McGrath, G.; More, S.J. Trends and predictors of large tuberculosis episodes in cattle herds in Ireland. *Front. Vet. Sci.* **2018**, *5*, 86. [CrossRef]
30. Milne, M.G.; Graham, J.; Allen, A.; McCormick, C.; Presho, E.; Skuce, R.; Byrne, A.W. Variation in Mycobacterium bovis genetic richness suggests that inwards cattle movements are a more important source of infection in beef herds than in dairy herds. *BMC Microbiol.* **2019**, *19*, 154. [CrossRef]
31. Johnston, W.T.; Gettinby, G.; Cox, D.R.; Donnelly, C.A.; Bourne, J.; Clifton-Hadley, R.; Le Fevre, A.M.; McInerney, J.P.; Mitchell, A.; Morrison, W.I.; et al. Herd-level risk factors associated with tuberculosis breakdowns among cattle herds in England before the 2001 foot-and-mouth disease epidemic. *Biol. Lett.* **2005**, *1*, 53–56. [CrossRef]
32. Mill, A.C.; Rushton, S.P.; Shirley, M.D.F.; Murray, A.W.A.; Smith, G.C.; Delahay, R.J.; McDonald, R.A. Farm-scale risk factors for bovine tuberculosis incidence in cattle herds during the Randomized Badger Culling Trial. *Epidemiol. Infect.* **2012**, *140*, 219–230. [CrossRef]
33. Broughan, J.M.; Maye, D.; Carmody, P.; Brunton, L.A.; Ashton, A.; Wint, W.; Alexander, N.; Naylor, R.; Ward, K.; Goodchild, A.V.; et al. Farm characteristics and farmer perceptions associated with bovine tuberculosis incidents in areas of emerging endemic spread. *Prev. Vet. Med.* **2016**, *129*, 88–98. [CrossRef]
34. Vial, F.; Johnston, W.T.; Donnelly, C.A. Local cattle and badger populations affect the risk of confirmed tuberculosis in British cattle herds. *PLoS ONE* **2011**, *6*, e18058. [CrossRef] [PubMed]
35. Houtsma, E.; Clegg, T.A.; Good, M.; More, S.J. Further improvement in the control of bovine tuberculosis recurrence in Ireland. *Vet. Rec.* **2018**, *183*, 622. [CrossRef] [PubMed]
36. Byrne, A.W.; Barrett, D.; Breslin, P.; Madden, J.M.; O'Keeffe, J.; Ryan, E. Post-mortem surveillance of bovine tuberculosis in Ireland: Herd-level variation in the probability of herds disclosed with lesions at routine slaughter to have skin test reactors at follow-up test. *Vet. Res. Commun.* **2020**, 1–6. [CrossRef]
37. McLachlan, G.J.; McGiffin, D.C. On the role of finite mixture models in survival analysis. *Stat. Methods Med. Res.* **1994**, *3*, 211–226. [CrossRef] [PubMed]
38. Asuni, C.; Manchia, M.; Deidda, A.; Stochino, M.E.; Cherchi, A.; Del Zompo, M. Mixture analysis of age at onset in migraine without aura: Evidence for three subgroups. *Headache* **2010**, *50*, 1313–1319. [CrossRef]
39. Gortazar, C.; Vicente, J.; Boadella, M.; Ballesteros, C.; Galindo, R.C.; Garrido, J.; Aranaz, A.; de La Fuente, J. Progress in the control of bovine tuberculosis in Spanish wildlife. *Vet. Microbiol.* **2011**, *151*, 170–178. [CrossRef]
40. Manchia, M.; Zai, C.C.; Squassina, A.; Vincent, J.B.; De Luca, V.; Kennedy, J.L. Mixture regression analysis on age at onset in bipolar disorder patients: Investigation of the role of serotonergic genes.

Eur. Neuropsychopharmacol. **2010**, *20*, 663–670. [CrossRef]
41. Nowrouzi, B.; Kamhi, R.; Hu, J.; Kennedy, J.L.; Matmari, M.; de Luca, V. Age at onset mixture analysis and systematic comparison in schizophrenia spectrum disorders: Is the onset heterogeneity dependent on heterogeneous diagnosis? *Schizophr. Res.* **2015**, *164*, 83–91. [CrossRef]
42. Royston, P. The lognormal distribution as a model for survival time in cancer, with an emphasis on prognostic factors. *Stat. Neerl.* **2001**, *55*, 89–104. [CrossRef]
43. Van Horn, M.L.; Smith, J.; Fagan, A.A.; Jaki, T.; Feaster, D.J.; Masyn, K.; Hawkins, J.D.; Howe, G. Not quite normal: Consequences of violating the assumption of normality in regression mixture models. *Struct. Equ. Model.* **2012**, *19*, 227–249. [CrossRef]
44. Jaki, T.; Kim, M.; Lamont, A.; George, M.; Chang, C.; Feaster, D.; Van Horn, M.L. The effects of sample size on the estimation of regression mixture models. *Educ. Psychol. Meas.* **2019**, *79*, 358–384. [CrossRef] [PubMed]
45. Magnussen, S.; Næsset, E.; Gobakken, T. An application niche for finite mixture models in forest resource surveys. *Can. J. For. Res.* **2019**, *49*, 1453–1462. [CrossRef]

2

PRMT5 is Required for Bovine Leukemia Virus Infection In Vivo and Regulates BLV Gene Expression, Syncytium Formation and Glycosylation In Vitro

Wlaa Assi [1,2,3], Tomoya Hirose [1,2], Satoshi Wada [3], Ryosuke Matsuura [1,2], Shin-nosuke Takeshima [1,2,3,4] and Yoko Aida [1,2,5,*]

1 Laboratory of Viral Infectious Diseases, Department of Computational Biology and Medical Sciences, Graduate School of Frontier Sciences, The University of Tokyo, 2-1 Hirosawa, Wako, Saitama 351-0198, Japan; wlaa.pharma92@yahoo.com (W.A.); kamaboko517tmp@gmail.com (T.H.); oinari.atsuage@gmail.com (R.M.); takesima@jumonji-u.ac.jp (S.-n.T.)

2 Viral Infectious Diseases Unit, RIKEN, 2-1 Hirosawa, Wako, Saitama 351-0198, Japan

3 Photonics Control Technology Team, RIKEN Center for Advanced Photonics, 2-1 Hirosawa, Wako, Saitama 351-0198, Japan; swada@riken.jp

4 Department of Food and Nutrition, Jumonji University, Niiza, Saitama 352-8510, Japan

5 Nakamura Laboratory, Baton Zone program, Riken Cluster for Science, Technology and Innovation Hub, 2-1 Hirosawa, Wako, Saitama 351-0198, Japan

* Correspondence: aida@riken.jp

Abstract: Bovine leukemia virus (BLV) is the causative agent of enzootic bovine leukosis, which is the most common neoplastic disease of cattle and is closely related to human T-cell leukemia viruses. We investigated the role of a new host protein, PRMT5, in BLV infection. We found that PRMT5 is overexpressed only in BLV-infected cattle with a high proviral load, but not in those with a low proviral load. Furthermore, this upregulation continued to the lymphoma stage. PRMT5 expression was upregulated in response to experimental BLV infection; moreover, PRMT5 upregulation began in an early stage of BLV infection rather than after a long period of proviral latency. Second, siRNA-mediated PRMT5 knockdown enhanced BLV gene expression at the transcript and protein levels. Additionally, a selective small-molecule inhibitor of PRMT5 (CMP5) enhanced BLV gene expression. Interestingly, CMP5 treatment, but not siRNA knockdown, altered the gp51 glycosylation pattern and increased the molecular weight of gp51, thereby decreasing BLV-induced syncytium formation. This was supported by the observation that CMP5 treatment enhanced the formation of the complex type of *N*-glycan more than the high mannose type. In conclusion, PRMT5 overexpression is related to the development of BLV infection with a high proviral load and lymphoma stage and PRMT5 inhibition enhances BLV gene expression. This is the first study to investigate the role of PRMT5 in BLV infection in vivo and in vitro and to reveal a novel function for a small-molecule compound in BLV-gp51 glycosylation processing.

Keywords: bovine leukemia virus; PRMT5; proviral load; BLV gene expression; PRMT5 inhibitor; gp51; glycosylation; syncytia formation

---

1. Introduction

Bovine leukemia virus (BLV) is the causative agent of enzootic bovine leukosis, a B-cell leukemia and lymphoma [1,2], which occurs worldwide and causes serious losses in the cattle industry [3]. Approximately 70% of infected cattle, the natural host of BLV, remain asymptomatic, whereas the major portion of the remaining infected cattle develops persistent lymphocytosis (PL) and only 1–5% develop leukemia/lymphoma after a relatively long period of latency [1]. Therefore, BLV infection results not only in enzootic bovine leukosis development, but also in reductions in lifetime milk production, reproductive efficiency, and lifespan [3–5].

BLV belongs to the *Deltaretrovirus* genus of the Retroviridae family and is closely related to human T-cell leukemia viruses types 1 and 2 (HTLV-1 and -2) [1,2]. The HTLV-1 proviral load (PVL), which represents the retroviral genome integrated into the host genome, is an important risk factor of viruses-associated disease prediction [6]. Similarly, BLV PVL correlates strongly not only with the BLV infection capacity as assessed by syncytium formation [7,8], but also with BLV disease progression [7,9,10]. For example, BLV-infected cattle at the PL stage are known to carry a significantly increased number of PVL compared to the number of the PVL in aleukemic cattle. A further increase was observed at the lymphoma stage [7,9]. Additionally, BLV PVL is a useful index for estimating transmission risk [11]. A previous report demonstrated that cows with a PVL of greater than 14,000 copies/10^5 cells and 18,000 copies/10^5 cells in blood samples secreted BLV into the nasal mucus [12]. Furthermore, we recently determined that BLV provirus in infected cows was detected in milk samples only when the PVL in the blood samples exceeded 10,000 copies/10^5 cells [13]. These findings suggest that a PVL of approximately 10,000 copies/10^5 peripheral blood cells is a relatively high number and indicates BLV spreading within the whole body. Thus, a PVL of 10,000 copies/10^5 cells was used in our study as a threshold to classify BLV-infected cattle into high-PVL (HPVL) or low-PVL (LPVL). In contrast, a low PVL (LPVL) is known to prevent natural BLV infection in cattle [14]. One of the host factors affecting BLV PVL is the genetic variation of bovine leukocyte antigen (*BoLA*). Several studies have identified *BoLA-DRB3* alleles and single-nucleotide polymorphisms in the *BoLA* region that are associated with BLV PVL and disease progression [9,15–20]. However, other factors contributing to the susceptibility to BLV-induced lymphoma and PVL, in addition to *BoLA-DRB3* polymorphism, remain to be identified.

In addition to the structural genes *gag*, *pro*, *pol*, and *env*, the BLV genome contains the regulatory genes *tax* and *rex* and genes R3 and G4 [1,2]. *gag* of BLV is translated as the precursor Pr70 Gag and is processed into three mature proteins: p15 is the matrix protein, p24 is the most abundant capsid protein, and p12 is the nucleocapsid protein [21,22]. *env* of BLV encodes a Pr72 envelope (Env) precursor that is glycosylated in the rough endoplasmic reticulum and Golgi apparatus [21,23]. This precursor is cleaved by cellular proteases into two mature proteins—the surface subunit gp51 and transmembrane subunit gp30—which are associated by disulfide bonds [21,24]. BLV infection is mediated by the interaction of gp51 with the recently identified cellular receptor cationic amino acid transporter 1 [25]. This gp51 is highly glycosylated because the molecular weight of its peptide backbone without glycans is 30.5 kDa and it contains eight asparagine (N) residues that are putative *N*-glycosylation sites [23]. BLV surface subunit gp51-linked *N*-glycosylation appeared to regulate viral replication, antigenic conformation, and syncytium forming capacity in vitro [26,27] and infectivity in vivo [26]. In general, retroviral Env glycosylation mediates virion attachment to cell membranes, transport of Env proteins to the cell membrane, and cell-to-cell fusion [28–30]. In contrast, Env-associated glycans act as a shield that confers resistance to neutralizing antibodies [30,31].

Arginine methylation is an important posttranslational modification with crucial roles in chromatin regulation, transcription control, RNA processing, nuclear/cytoplasmic shuttling, DNA repair, and other biological processes [32,33]. Arginine methylation is catalyzed by members of the protein arginine-*N*-methyltransferase (PRMT) family. PRMTs are divided into four types of enzymes. Type I, which is the most common, induces asymmetric dimethylation; Type II catalyzes symmetric dimethylation; Type III produces monomethyl arginine as its final product; and Type IV is found only in fungi [34]. In the virology field, protein arginine methylation has been determined to play critical roles in the biology of several viruses, including hepatitis delta virus [35], hepatitis B virus [36–38], human immunodeficiency virus type-1 (HIV-1) [39–43], HTLV-1 [44], Epstein-Barr virus (EBV) [45,46], and Kaposi's sarcoma associated herpesvirus [47].

PRMT5 is a type II arginine methyltransferase that was recently shown to be crucial in EBV-driven B-cell transformation [46] and HTLV-1-mediated T-cell transformation [44]. Additionally, PRMT5 regulates various steps in virus lifecycles. For example, PRMT5 restricts hepatitis B virus replication via two mechanisms: epigenetic suppression of covalently closed circular DNA and interference with pregenomic RNA encapsidation [38]. Further studies showed that PRMT5 regulates nuclear import of hepatitis B virus core (HBc) in which PRMT5 overexpression increases the nuclear accumulation of HBc and in which PRMT5 inhibition reduces HBc levels in the nuclei [36]. Moreover, the early lytic protein of Kaposi's sarcoma-associated herpesvirus, ORF59, associates with PRMT5 and disrupts its binding with the chromatin, which in turn disrupts its repressive effect to move to the lytic reactivation phase [47]. A recent study also demonstrated that PRMT5 supports HIV-1 replication by maintaining Vpr protein stability [48]. However, it remains unclear whether PRMT5 acts as a host cell factor that is important in BLV gene expression and infection.

In this study, we investigated the role of PRMT5 in various aspects of BLV infection in vivo and in vitro. First, we focused on the correlation between the PRMT5 expression level and BLV PVL, an index of virus infectivity, in peripheral blood from infected animals in various stages, such as the lymphoma and asymptomatic stages. Second, we revealed the impact of PRMT5 inhibition on BLV gene expression, gp51 glycosylation, and syncytium formation. This is the first study to investigate the role of PRMT5 in BLV infection.

2. Materials and Methods

2.1. Cell Culture and Transfection

FLK-BLV cells, which are permanently infected with BLV (kindly provided by Prof. Onuma, M.), were cultured in Dulbecco's modified Eagle's Medium (Thermo Fisher Scientific, Waltham, MA, USA) containing 10% heat-inactivated fetal bovine serum (Sigma-Aldrich, St. Louis, MO, USA). PK15-BLV cells, which were produced by stably transfecting the pig kidney-15 (PK15) cells (National Institutes of Biomedical Innovation, Health and Nutrition: JCRB9040) with CMVΔU3-pBLV-IF2, were cultured in Minimum Essential Medium Eagle (Thermo Fisher Scientific) containing 10% fetal bovine serum and 1% non-essential amino acids (Gibco, Grand Island, NY, USA). CMVΔU3-pBLV-IF2 is the modified version of the BLV-infectious molecular clone pBLV-IF2, which was used previously [25,49]. CMVΔU3-pBLV-IF2 was modified by replacing the U3 region that contains the BLV promoter with the strong CMV promoter to enhance BLV expression. FLK-BLV and PK15-BLV were selected because they stably express BLV-viral proteins and produce BLV-virus particles, enabling analysis of several aspects of the virus life cycle related to the expression of viral proteins.

For transfection of small interfering RNA (siRNA), we used Lipofectamine RNAiMax Reagent (Thermo Fisher Scientific) according to the manufacturers' instructions and RNA was extracted from these cells using TRIzol reagent (Thermo Fisher Scientific) according to the manufacturer's protocol.

2.2. Animal Samples and Isolation of Genomic DNA and RNA

Blood samples were collected from 62 Holstein cattle including BLV-negative cattle and BLV-infected cattle, which were maintained in Japan. These cows were classified into three groups according to their PVL as follows: (i) BLV-negative cattle (PVL = 0; $N = 20$), (ii) BLV-infected cattle with LPVL (PVL $\leq$10,000 copies/10^5 cells; $N = 15$), and (iii) BLV-infected cattle with HPVL (PVL >10,000 copies/10^5 cells; $N = 27$). Blood samples were also collected from BLV-infected Holstein cows with lymphoma ($N = 20$). Lymphoma was diagnosed by both gross and histological observation and by detecting atypical mononuclear cells in the slaughterhouse. All animal experiments were conducted in accordance with the guidelines for Laboratory Animal Welfare and Animal Experiment Control established by the RIKEN Animal Experiments Committee (H29–2-104, 14 February 2017). For experimental infection, five BLV-negative one-year-old Japanese black calves carrying susceptible alleles *BoLA-DRB3*1601/*1601* were experimentally challenged intravenously with blood containing a PVL of 4×10^7 copies/10^5 cells. This study was approved by the Animal Ethical Committee and Animal Care and Use Committee of the Kyoto Biken Institute.

Blood samples were collected and diluted in a 1:1 ratio with Ambion® nuclease-free water before adding TRIzol LS in a 3:1 ratio of TRIzol LS to the diluted whole blood. The mixtures of whole blood with TRIzol LS were transported to the lab and stored at −80°C. An equal volume of the mixture was used to extract RNA from the samples using TRIzol LS protocol (Thermo Fisher Scientific) according to the manufacturer's instructions. Genomic DNA for PCR amplification was isolated from EDTA-treated whole blood samples using the Wizard Genomic DNA Purification Kit (Promega Corporation, Madison, WI, USA).

2.3. Measurement of the BLV PVL

The BLV PVL was measured by BLV-CoCoMo-qPCR-2 (RIKEN Genesis, Kanagawa, Japan) using genomic DNA as described previously [50]. Briefly, the BLV long terminal repeat (LTR) region was amplified in a reaction mixture containing THUNDERBIRD Probe qPCR Mix (Toyobo, Osaka, Japan) and the degenerate primer pair: CoCoMo FRW primer and CoCoMo REV primer. FAM-LTR was used as a probe. *BoLA-DRA* (internal control) was amplified using the primer pair DRA-F and DRA-R. FAM-DRA was used as a probe. The PVL was calculated using the following equation: (number of BLV-LTR copies/number of *BoLA-DRA* copies) $\times 10^5$ cells.

2.4. Quantitative Reverse Transcription–Polymerase Chain Reaction (qRT-PCR)

RNA was reverse-transcribed for cDNA synthesis using a High Capacity RNA-to-cDNA kit (Thermo Fisher Scientific) according to the manufacturer's instructions. Primers for PRMT5, GAPDH, *gag*, and *tax* were designed using the primer-designing tool provided by the National Center for Biotechnology Information. The primer list is shown in Table S1. RT-PCR was performed with the KAPA SYBR® FAST qPCR Kit (KAPA BIOSYSTEMS, Wilmington, MA, USA) using an Applied Biosystems 7500 Fast Real-Time PCR system (Foster City, CA, USA). The following thermal cycling program was used: 95 °C for 3 min, followed by 40 cycles of 95 °C for 10 s and 60 °C for 30 s. Samples were evaluated in duplicate and data analysis was performed using the comparative CT method (ΔΔCT) with normalization to GAPDH mRNA expression.

2.5. siRNA Transfection

siRNA designed to target PRMT5 (si-PRMT5) of FLK-BLV or PK15-BLV was constructed by Silencer Select siRNAs (Ambion, Austin, TX, USA). To knock down PRMT5 in FLK-BLV cells, Silencer® select Product # s20376 was used. For PK15-BLV knockdown, Silencer® select Product # s20377 was used. siRNA negative control (si-NC) was constructed by Ambion (catalog# 4390843). On the day of transfection, 3×10^5 cells of FLK-BLV or PK15-BLV were seeded into a 6-well plate and transfected with si-PRMT5 or si-NC using Lipofectamine RNAiMAX reagent (Thermo Fisher Scientific) according to the manufacturer's instructions. After 48 or 72 h of incubation, cell lysates were prepared and knockdown efficiency was evaluated by RT-PCR or Western blotting analysis.

2.6. PRMT5 Inhibitor Treatment

CMP5, a selective PRMT5 inhibitor [46], was purchased from Merck KGaA (Darmstadt, Germany). Cells were grown for 24 h at 37 °C, after which the medium was collected and replaced with fresh medium with or without 5, 10, or 20 μM of CMP5 and the cells were grown for an additional 24 h. After a total of 48 h, cell lysates were prepared to determine intracellular expression of PRMT5 by Western blotting analysis.

2.7. Western Blotting Analysis

Cells were lysed for 30 min on ice in 20 mM Tris-HCl (pH 7.4), 300 mM NaCl, 2 mM EDTA, and 2% NP40 supplemented with a protease inhibitor cocktail (Roche Diagnostics, Mannheim, Germany). Lysates were mixed with SDS buffer and boiled for 5 min. Protein concentrations were determined with Pierce™ BCA Protein Assay Kit (Thermo Fisher Scientific). Equal amounts of protein were electrophoresed via SDS-polyacrylamide gel electrophoresis (PAGE). The proteins were then transferred onto a polyvinylidene difluoride membrane (Millipore, Billerica, MA, USA) using a Trans-Blot Turbo apparatus (Bio-Rad, Hercules, CA, USA) and incubated with anti-BLV gp51 monoclonal antibody (Mab) (BLV 2) (1:200; VMRD, Pullman, WA, USA), anti-BLV Gag Mab (BLV 3) (1:200; VMRD), polyclonal anti-PRMT5 (1:1000; Abcam, Cambridge, UK), or anti-α-tubulin clone B-5-1-2 Mab (1:2000; Sigma). After washing, the membranes were incubated with horseradish peroxidase-conjugated AffiniPure goat anti-mouse IgG (1:2000; Jackson ImmunoResearch, West Grove, PA, USA) or horseradish peroxidase-conjugated goat anti-rabbit IgG (1:1000; Amersham Biosciences, Amersham, UK). Signals were visualized after treating the membrane with SuperSignal™ West Pico PLUS Chemiluminescent Substrate (Thermo Fisher Scientific). Images were acquired using a MultiImage TM light Cabinet (Alpha Innotech Corporation, San Leandro, CA, USA). Band intensity was quantitated using the analysis tool provided with the AlphaEaseFC™ software (Alpha Innotech Corporation).

2.8. *Deglycosylation by PNGase F or Endo H*

FLK-BLV or PK15-BLV were cultured in the absence or presence of 20 μM CMP5 for 48 h. Thereafter, the cell lysates were treated in the absence or presence of PNGase F (Promega, Madison, WI 53711-5399, USA) for 3 h or Endo H (Promega) overnight according to the manufacturer's protocol (catalog# V483A and catalog #V4871), respectively.

2.9. *Cell Viability Assay*

A Premix WST-1 Cell Proliferation Assay Kit (Takara, Shiga, Japan) was used to assess the effect of CMP5 on cell viability. For each cell line, 3×10^4 cells were seeded into a 96-well plate at a final volume of 100 μL in the absence or presence of different concentrations of CMP5. The assay was conducted according to the manufacturer's instructions.

2.10. *Immunofluorescence Confocal Microscopy*

FLK-BLV cells were grown on coverslips with or without CMP5 treatment. After 48 h, the cells were fixed with 4% paraformaldehyde for 15 min at room temperature; next, they were permeabilized with 0.5% Triton X for 5 min and then blocked with 5% skim milk for 30 min. The gp51 staining in the cell membrane was performed without the permeabilization step. The cells were incubated with anti-BLV gp51 Mab (BLV 2) (1:100; VMRD) or anti-BLV Gag Mab (BLV 3) (1:100; VMRD) for 1 h at room temperature followed by 30 min incubation with Alexa Fluor 488 rabbit anti-mouse for Gag or Alexa Fluor 594 rabbit anti-mouse for Env (1:300; Invitrogen, Carlsbad, CA, USA). Nuclei were stained with Hoechst 33342 (1:2000; ImmunoChemistry Technologies LLC. Bloomington, MN, USA) for 5 min in the dark. After each staining step, the samples were washed three times with PBS. The coverslips were mounted on glass slides and fluorescence images were obtained using an FV1000 confocal laser-scanning microscope (Olympus, Tokyo, Japan).

2.11. *gp51 Cell Membrane Staining by Flow Cytometry*

FLK-BLV cells were collected using 2 mM ethylenediaminetetraacetic acid (EDTA)/PBS for 5 min at 37 °C and washed twice with PBS and 5×10^5 cells were stained with anti-BLV gp51 Mab (BLV 2) (1:50; VMRD) for 1 h on ice. The cells were then stained with APC rat anti-mouse (1:100; APC-anti mouse, BD Pharmingen, Franklin Lakes, NJ, USA) for 30 min on ice. Propidium Iodide (PI) was used for live/dead staining. Stained cells were analyzed using a BD AccuriTM C6 Plus with a sampler flow cytometer (BD Biosciences, Franklin Lakes, NJ, USA). The data were analyzed using FlowJo v10 (FlowJo, LLC, Ashland, OR, USA).

2.12. *Luminescence Syncytium Induction Assay (LuSIA)*

The luminescence syncytium induction assay (LuSIA) using CC81-GREMG cells was performed as described previously [51]. CC81 GREMG (1×10^5 cells) were co-cultured with 5×10^4 FLK-BLV cells in a 12-well plate in LuSIA medium, after which the indicated concentrations of CMP5 were added. After 48 h incubation, the cells were washed with PBS and fixed with 4% formaldehyde/PBS containing 10 μg/mL Hoechst 33342 (Thermo Fisher Scientific). The fluorescent syncytia were visualized by EVOS2 fluorescence microscopy (Thermo Fisher Scientific) and 9 fields of view in each well were automatically scanned with a 4× objective. Syncytia were detected by enhanced green fluorescent protein (EGFP) expression and counted using HCS Studio Cell Analysis software (Thermo Fisher Scientific).

2.13. *Statistical Analysis*

All data were expressed as the mean ± standard deviation based on at least 3 independent experiments. Statistical significance was evaluated using Student's *t*-test. Differences were estimated to be significant at $p \leq 0.05$ (*) and strongly significant at $p \leq 0.01$ (**) and $p \leq 0.001$(***). The *p* value in the animal experiments was calculated by the Kruskal-Wallis test and Dunn's multiple comparisons test.

3. Results

3.1. *PRMT5 Is Overexpressed in BLV-Infected Cattle with High* PVL *In Vivo*

BLV PVL is an important index of the risk of BLV transmission and infectivity as well as disease progression [7,8,10,12,13]. To investigate the correlation between PRMT5 expression and BLV PVL, we collected blood samples from 62 cows which were asymptomatic and had not developed symptoms of lymphoma at the time of blood collection. First, we performed CoCoMo-qPCR-2 to calculate the BLV PVL, which was used to classify the cows into three groups: BLV-negative cattle (control group), BLV-infected cattle with a low-PVL (LPVL group), and BLV-infected cattle with a high-PVL (HPVL group). As described previously [9,15], a BLV-PVL of 10,000 copies/10^5 was used as a threshold to distinguish between the HPVL and LPVL groups. Next, we evaluated PRMT5 expression at the RNA levels by qRT-PCR. The mean fold-change in PRMT5 was 1.12 ± 0.62 in the control group, 1.18 ± 0.64 in the LPVL group, and 1.64 ± 0.62 in the HPVL group (Figure 1A). PRMT5 expression was significantly higher in the HPVL group than in the uninfected group ($p = 0.0014$) and LPVL group ($p = 0.012$) (Figure 1). Our results showed that PRMT5 was significantly overexpressed only in BLV-infected cattle with a high PVL, but not in those with a low PVL. Furthermore, a positive correlation was obtained between the BLV PVL and PRMT5 expression fold-change ($r = 0.52$) (Figure 1B).

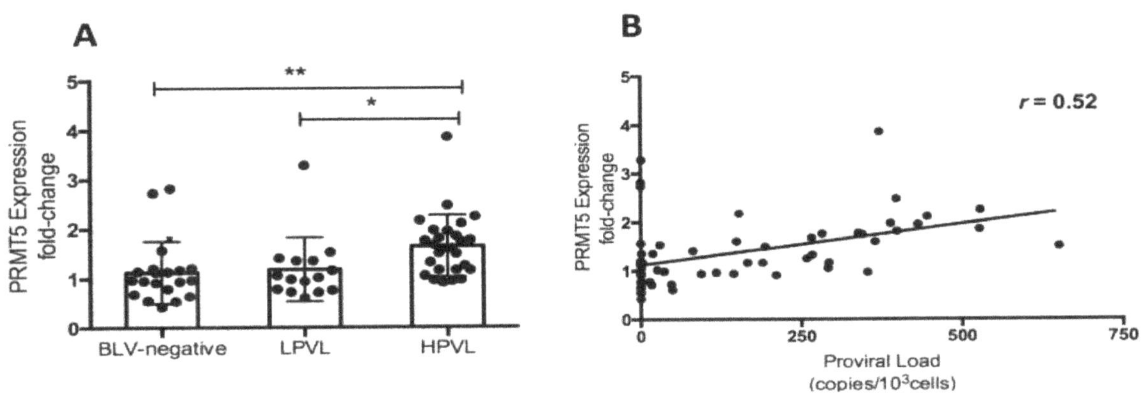

Figure 1. Change in PRMT5 expression at the RNA level in bovine leukemia virus (BLV) infection. (**A**) PRMT5 expression at the RNA level of 20 BLV-negative cattle (PVL, proviral load = 0), 15 BLV-infected but clinically normal cows with a low PVL (LPVL; PVL ≤ 10,000 copies/10^5 cells), and 27 BLV-infected but clinically normal cows with a high PVL (HPVL; PVL > 10,000 copies/10^5 cells) was measured by qRT-PCR and the fold-change was calculated using the ΔΔCT method with normalization to GAPDH

expression as an internal control. Samples were run in duplicate. A scatter plot with bar showing the mean of PRMT5 expression fold-change in the three groups. BLV PVL was measured by CoCoMo-qPCR. Error bars represent the standard deviation of the biological replicates (20 BLV-negative, 15 LPVL, 27 HPLV). The p value was calculated using the Kruskal-Wallis test (<0.0006). Dunn's multiple comparisons test was used to evaluate the significance between groups. The asterisk indicates a significant difference (* $p \leq 0.05$, ** $p \leq 0.01$). (**B**) Correlation between BLV PVL of each cattle and the corresponding PRMT5 expression fold-change (62 in total), Spearman r was used to evaluate the strength of the correlation.

3.2. PRMT5 Overexpression Starts from an Early Stage of BLV Infection In Vivo

As shown in Figure 1, PRMT5 was upregulated only in BLV-infected cattle with a high PVL. To further investigate the role of PRMT5 in BLV infection in vivo, we examined whether PRMT5 is overexpressed in the early stage of BLV infection. Therefore, we performed experimental infection of five BLV-negative Japanese black calves carrying the susceptible alleles *BoLA-DRB3*1601/1601*, which are related to a high PVL in BLV infection [52] and we collected blood samples at different time points during the first month of infection (0, 0.5, 1, 2, 3, and 4 weeks). Next, we monitored BLV PVL and PRMT5 expression at each time point. The mean of BLV PVL was 0 copies/10^5 cells before infection (0 week), 34 copies/10^5 cells after 3 days, 1158 copies/10^5 cells after 1 week, 26,760 copies/10^5 cells after 2 weeks, 90,150 copies/10^5 cells after 3 weeks, and 62,440 copies/10^5 cells after 4 weeks (Figure 2a, line graph). The mean fold-change in PRMT5 was 1 before infection, 1.44 after 3 days, 1.48 after 1 week, 2.6 after 2 weeks, 3.7 after 3 weeks, and 2.3 after 4 weeks. The highest expression of PRMT5 was observed during the third week (fold-change = 3.74, p = 0.0008) and then the expression slightly decreased after 4 weeks (fold-change = 2.3, p = 0.01) (Figure 2A, bar graph). Interestingly, and consistently with the data shown in Figure 1A, a strong positive correlation was found between the fold-upregulation of PRMT5 and BLV PVL (r = 0.79) (Figure 2B). Thus, PRMT5 expression was upregulated in response to BLV infection and the level of upregulation was positively correlated with the BLV PVL. Moreover, PRMT5 upregulation began in an early stage of BLV infection rather than being established after a long period of proviral latency.

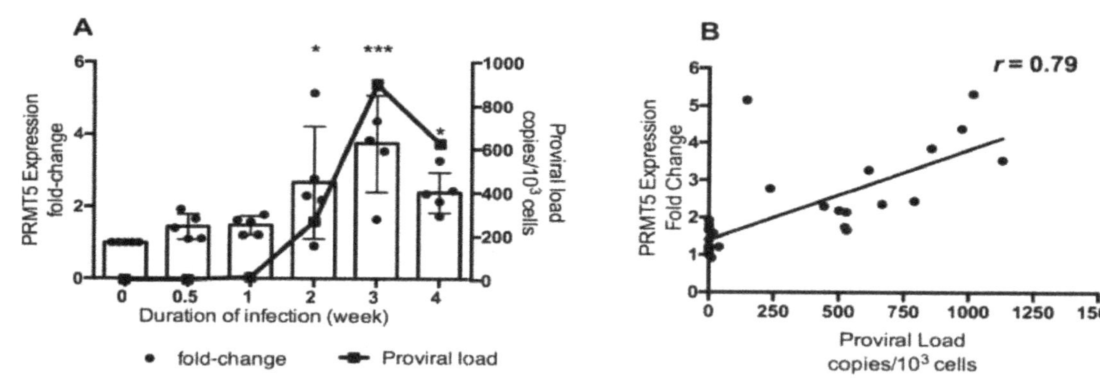

Figure 2. Change in PRMT5 expression at the RNA level in response to experimental BLV infection during the early stage of infection. (**A**) Five BLV-negative Japanese black calves carrying susceptible alleles *BoLA-DRB3*1601/*1601* were experimentally challenged intravenously with BLV, and RNA and DNA were extracted from these animals at six time points during the first month of infection. The BLV PVL was measured by CoCoMo-qPCR using genomic DNA. PRMT5 expression was measured by qRT-PCR using RNA and the fold-change was calculated using the ΔΔCT method with normalization to GAPDH expression as an internal control. Samples were run in duplicate. A combined bar and line graph show the mean of PRMT5 expression fold-change at each point (bar graph and left axis) with the corresponding mean of proviral load (line graph and right axis). Error bars represent the standard deviation of the PRMT5 fold-change of five cattle, p value was calculated using the Kruskal-Wallis test

(0.002), and Dunn's multiple comparisons test was used to compare the mean of the PRMT5 fold-change at each time point of infection with the mean before infection. The asterisk indicates a significant difference (* $p \leq 0.05$ and *** $p \leq 0.001$). (**B**) Correlation between BLV PVL of each cattle at each time point and the corresponding PRMT5 expression fold-change, Spearman r was used to evaluate the strength of the correlation.

3.3. *PRMT5 Overexpression Continues to Lymphoma Stage of BLV Infection In Vivo*

Finally, we investigated whether the change in PRMT5 expression in BLV-infected cattle occurred in the lymphoma stage of disease. We compared PRMT5 expression at the RNA level among three groups of cattle: 20 BLV-negative cattle, 42 BLV-infected but clinically normal cattle, and 20 BLV-infected cattle with lymphoma. The fold-change in PRMT5 expression was 1.12 ± 0.62 in BLV-negative cattle, 1.48 ± 0.66 in the asymptomatic group, and 2.45 ± 1.1 in the lymphoma group (Figure 3). This strongly indicates that PRMT5 upregulation continues until the lymphoma stage of BLV. Additionally, we confirmed the positive correlation between BLV PVL and PRMT5 expression fold-change ($r = 0.524$).

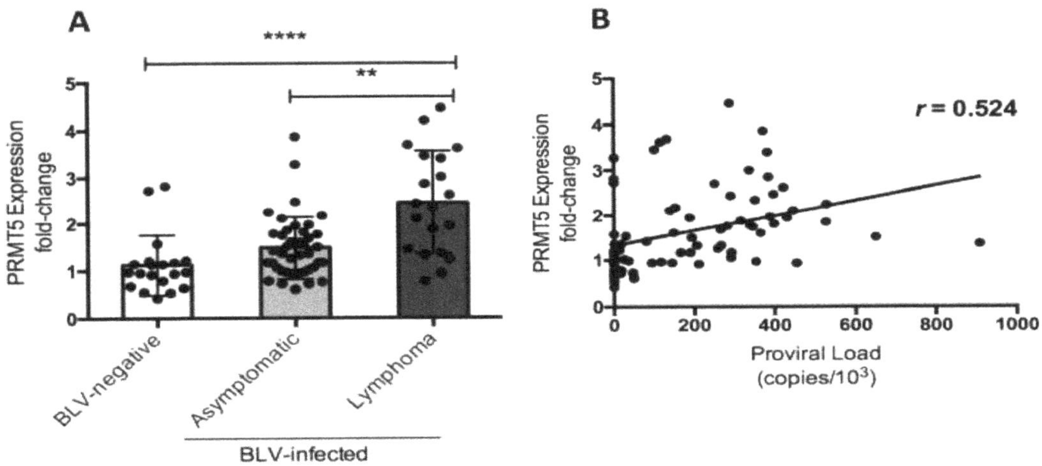

Figure 3. PRMT5 gene expression at the RNA level in BLV-infected cattle with lymphoma. (**A**) PRMT5 expression at the RNA level of 20 BLV-negative cattle, 42 BLV-infected but clinically normal cows, and 20 BLV-infected cattle with lymphoma were measured by qRT-PCR and the fold-change was calculated using the ΔΔCT method with normalization to GAPDH expression as an internal control. Samples were run in duplicate. A scatter plot with a bar showing the mean of the fold-change in PRMT5 expression of the three groups of cattle. BLV PVL was measured by CoCoMo-qPCR. The p value was calculated using the Kruskal-Wallis test (<0.0001) and Dunn's multiple comparisons test was used to evaluate the significance among groups. The asterisk indicates a significant difference (** $p \leq 0.001$ and **** $p \leq 0.0001$). (**B**) Correlation between BLV PVL of each cow and corresponding PRMT5 expression fold-change (81 in total), Spearman r was used to evaluate the strength of the correlation.

3.4. *PRMT5 Knockdown Enhances BLV Gene Transcription In Vitro*

The data shown in Figures 1–3 indicate that PRMT5 overexpression contributes to developing BLV infection with a high proviral load and may influence which infected cows progress from the asymptomatic stage to the lymphoma stage. Next, we examined the impact of PRMT5 inhibition on BLV infection in vitro. PRMT5 is a well-known regulator of gene transcription either by catalyzing symmetric dimethylarginine of histone proteins to generate repressive histone markers, including

H2AR3me2s, H3R8me2s, and H4R3me2s, or by methylation of nonhistone proteins, such as transcription factors [33,53]. To investigate the effect of PRMT5 inhibition on BLV gene expression, we knocked down PRMT5 in two cell lines, FLK-BLV, a permanently BLV-infected cell line, and PK15-BLV, a stably transfected cell line with CMVΔU3-pBLV-IF2, by siRNA. Next, we measured the mRNA of two viral transcripts, *gag*, which is produced by the un-spliced mRNA, and *tax*, which is produced by the double splicing event (Figure 4). We found that PRMT5 knockdown significantly enhanced the *gag* and *tax* transcription levels. In the FLK-BLV cell line, the fold-change of *gag* was 1.3 ($p = 0.03$) and of *tax* was 1.33 ($p = 0.04$). In the PK15-BLV cell line, the fold-change of *gag* was 1.72 ($p = 0.01$) and of *tax* was 1.6 ($p = 0.0014$).

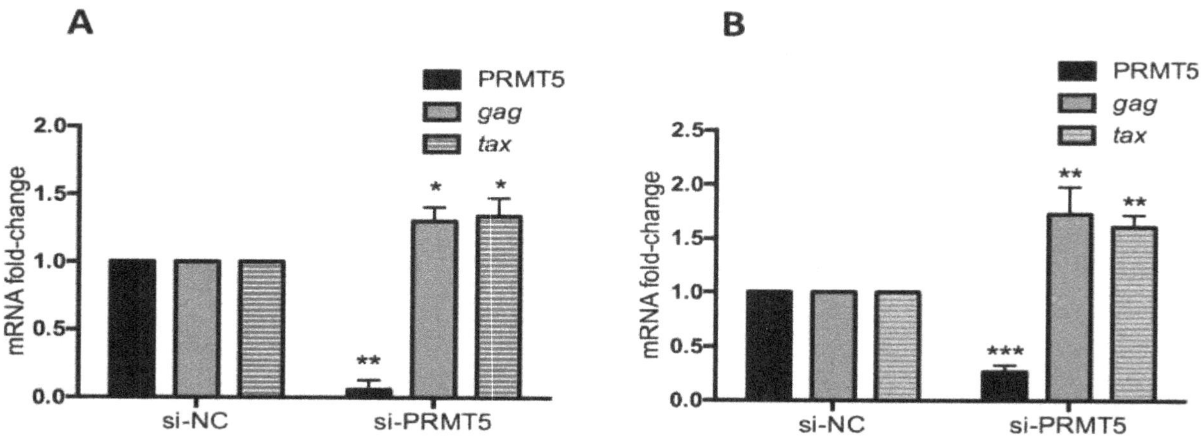

Figure 4. Effect of PRMT5 knockdown on BLV gene transcription. FLK-BLV (**A**) or PK15-BLV (**B**) cells were transfected with scramble siRNA (si-NC) or siRNA targeting PRMT5 (si-PRMT5) for 48 h for FLK-BLV or 72 h for PK15-BLV. BLV gene transcription (mRNA-*gag* and mRNA-*tax*) in addition to PRMT5 gene expression at the RNA level was evaluated by qRT-PCR. The ΔΔCT method was used to calculate the fold-change and GAPDH expression was used as an internal control. Error bars represent the standard deviation of three experiments. The p value was calculated using the Student's t-test. The asterisk indicates a significant difference (* $p \leq 0.05$, ** $p \leq 0.01$, and *** $p \leq 0.001$).

3.5. *PRMT5 Knockdown Enhances BLV Protein Expression In Vitro*

To confirm the finding shown in Figure 4 at the protein level, FLK-BLV or PK15-BLV were transfected with siRNA targeting PRMT5 or mock siRNA for 48 or 72 h and then cell lysates were prepared and the expression levels of two viral proteins (Env gp51and Gag p24) were evaluated by Western blotting with anti-BLV gp51 Mab or anti-BLV p24 Mab. We confirmed that siRNA-mediated inhibition of PRMT5 in FLK-BLV significantly enhanced intracellular Env expression ($p = 0.02$) (Figure 5A). Moreover, the expression of both of Env and Gag in PK15-BLV were significantly enhanced as a result of PRMT5 knockdown ($p = 0.05$ and 0.02 for Env and Gag, respectively) (Figure 5B). The bands corresponding to unprocessed Gag are shown in Figure S2A,B for FLK-BLV and PK15-BLV, respectively. These results show that there was no defect in Gag processing after PRMT5 knockdown.

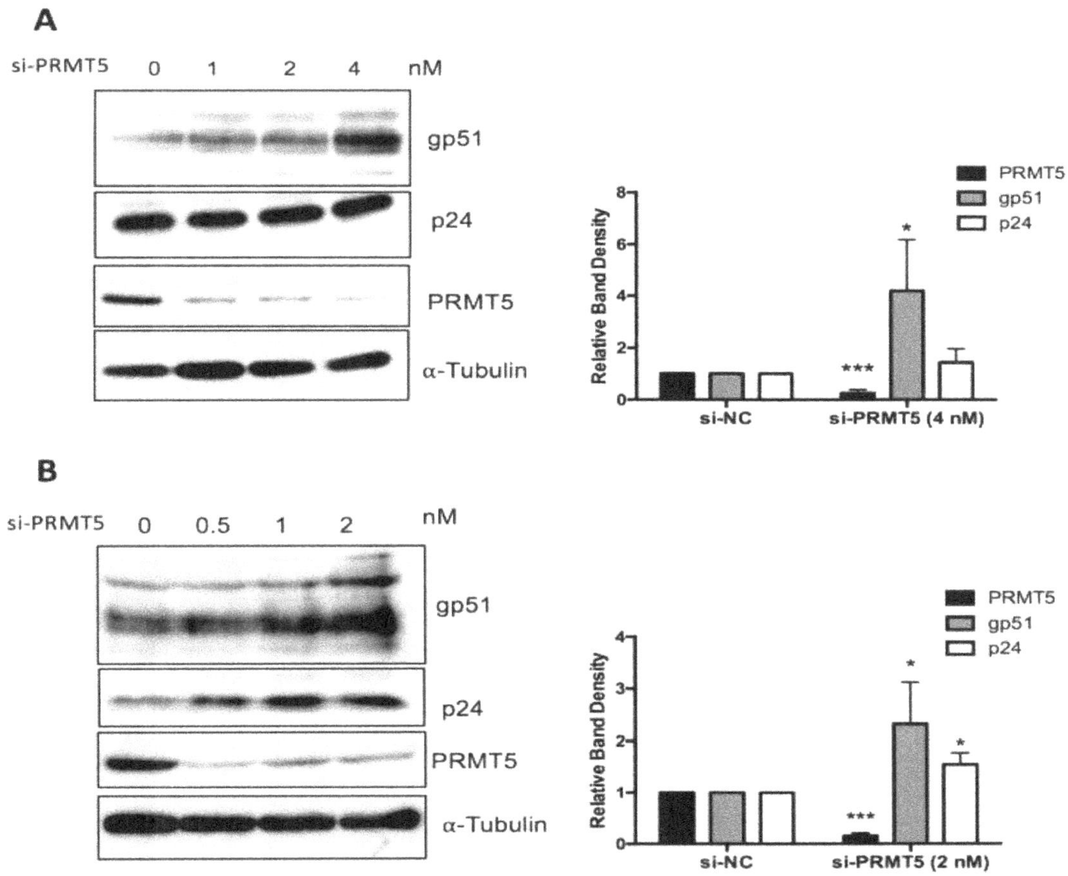

Figure 5. Effect of PRMT5 knockdown on BLV protein expression. FLK-BLV (**A**) or PK15-BLV (**B**) cells were transfected with scramble siRNA (si-NC) or siRNA targeting PRMT5 (si-PRMT5) at the indicated concentrations for 48 h for FLK-BLV or 72 h for PK15-BLV. Cell lysates were prepared and the expression of two viral proteins (Env gp51 and Gag p24) were assessed by Western blotting. Knockdown efficiency was evaluated by evaluating PRMT5 protein expression by Western blotting. The relative band density of each protein normalized to α-tubulin expression is shown for each cell line. Error bars represent the standard deviation of three experiments. The p value was calculated by Student's t-test. The asterisk indicates a significant difference (* $p \leq 0.05$, and *** $p \leq 0.001$). Positions of BLV gp51 and p24, PRMT5, and α-tubulin proteins are indicated.

3.6. Selective PRMT5 Inhibitor Enhances BLV Protein Expression and Alters gp51 Mobility over SDS-PAGE In Vitro

Next, we examined the effect of a pharmacological PRMT5 inhibitor on BLV protein expression. We used a small-molecule PRMT5 inhibitor (CMP5), which was described previously by Alinari et al. [46]. We examined the effect of CMP5 on FLK-BLV and PK15-BLV. FLK-BLV or PK15-BLV was cultured in fresh medium with or without 5, 10, or 20 μM of CMP5 for 48 h. Cell lysates were prepared and the viral protein expression levels of Env and Gag were evaluated by Western blotting analysis with anti-BLV gp51 Mab or anti-BLV p24 Mab. Consistently, CMP5 treatment enhanced the protein expression of both gp51 and p24 in a dose-dependent manner in FLK-BLV, showing significance at a concentration of 20 μM (Figure 6A). In contrast, in PK15-BLV, BLV expression was not significantly affected (Figure 6B). The bands corresponding to unprocessed Gag are shown in Figure S2C,D for FLK-BLV and PK15-BLV, respectively. These results also revealed that there was no defect in Gag processing after CMP5 treatment.

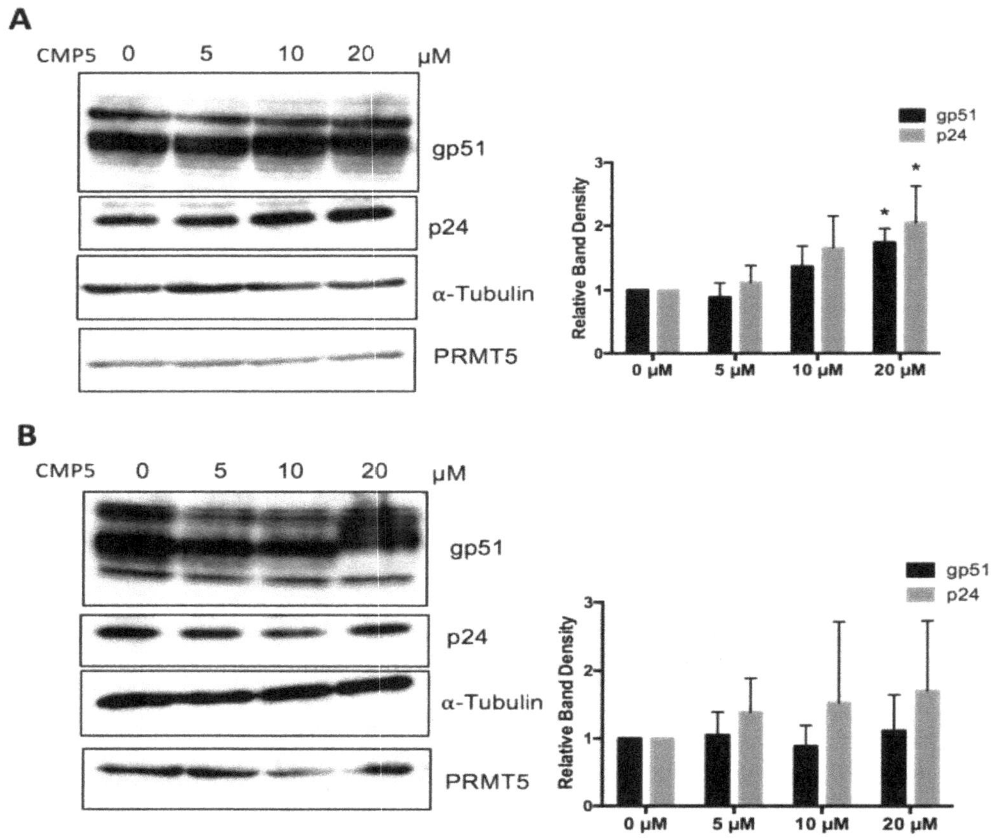

Figure 6. Effect of a small molecular PRMT5 inhibitor (CMP5) on BLV protein expression. FLK-BLV (**A**) or PK15-BLV (**B**) were cultured in the absence or the presence of the indicated concentrations of CMP5 for 48 h. Cell lysates were prepared and viral proteins (Env gp51 and Gag p24) in addition to PRMT5 were evaluated by Western blotting. The relative band density of each protein normalized to α-tubulin expression is shown for each cell line. The PRMT5 expression level was not changed as a result of CMP5 treatment and was excluded from analysis. All band layers of gp51 were calculated. Error bars represent the standard deviation of three independent experiments. The p value was calculated using the Student's t-test. The asterisk indicates a significant difference (* $p \leq 0.05$). Positions of BLV gp51 and p24, PRMT5, and α-tubulin proteins are indicated.

Unexpectedly, we found that CMP5 treatment altered gp51 electrophoretic mobility in SDS-PAGE and formed gp51 with a higher apparent molecular weight than gp51 in untreated cells (Figure 6A,B). The change in the apparent molecular weight was more evident at 20 µM. Thus, we further investigated the possible impact of this inhibitor on BLV envelope protein glycosylation.

3.7. Selective PRMT5 Inhibitor Alters gp51 Glycosylation Processing In Vitro

N-Glycan structures are classified into three types: high mannose, hybrid, and complex types. All types share a common tri-mannosyl core (Man3GlcNAc2). However, they differ in the structure of the remaining branches [54,55]. The complex type of *N*-glycan typically runs slower in SDS-PAGE than the high mannose type. To further illustrate the effect of CMP5 treatment on gp51 electrophoretic mobility in SDS-PAGE, we examined whether the slow migration of gp51 in the presence of CMP5 resulted from an increase in the complex type of *N*-glycan. We cultured FLK-BLV or PK15-BLV in the absence (CMP5–) or presence of 20 µM of CMP5 (CMP5+) for 48 h. Cell lysates of each cell line were collected and divided into three parts: one part was not treated (PNGase F−/Endo H−), the second part was treated with PNGase F (PNGase F+), and the third part was treated with Endo H (Endo H+). As illustrated in Figure 7A, PNGase F removed all types of *N*-linked glycosylation from the glycoprotein: high mannose, hybrid, and complex.

Additionally, PNGase F severs the bond between *N*-acetylglucosamine (GlcNAc) and asparagine (Asn), liberating the entire sugar chain and converting asparagine (Asn) to aspartic acid (Asp). In contrast, Endo H cleaves only the high mannose and hybrid types of *N*-glycans and the complex type remains resistant to Endo H deglycosylation. Endo H cleaves the bond between the two GlcNAc residues in the core region, leaving one GlcNAc bound to the protein [56].

Consistent with the observation shown in Figure 6, we found that CMP5 treatment (CMP5+) altered the electrophoretic mobility of gp51, forming a higher apparent molecular weight smear of gp51 in both FLK-BLV and PK15-BLV (Figure 7B,C, PNGase F−/Endo H−). PNGase F treatment led to the accumulation of an approximately 30 KDa product in both FLK-BLV and PK15-BLV (Figure 7B,C, PNGase F+). This corresponds to the calculated molecular weight of the envelope peptidic core in the absence of any glycosylation of BLV gp51. Thus, after PNGase F treatment, the change in the migration pattern of gp51 disappeared, indicating that CMP5 affects the gp51 glycosylation pattern. Additionally, endo H treatment in PK15-BLV showed that the complex type of *N*-glycan of gp51 may increase after CMP5 treatment (Figure 7C, Endo H+), whereas in FLK-BLV, the complex type did not appear to be affected (Figure 7B, Endo H+). Our results show that CMP5 treatment altered gp51 glycosylation processing.

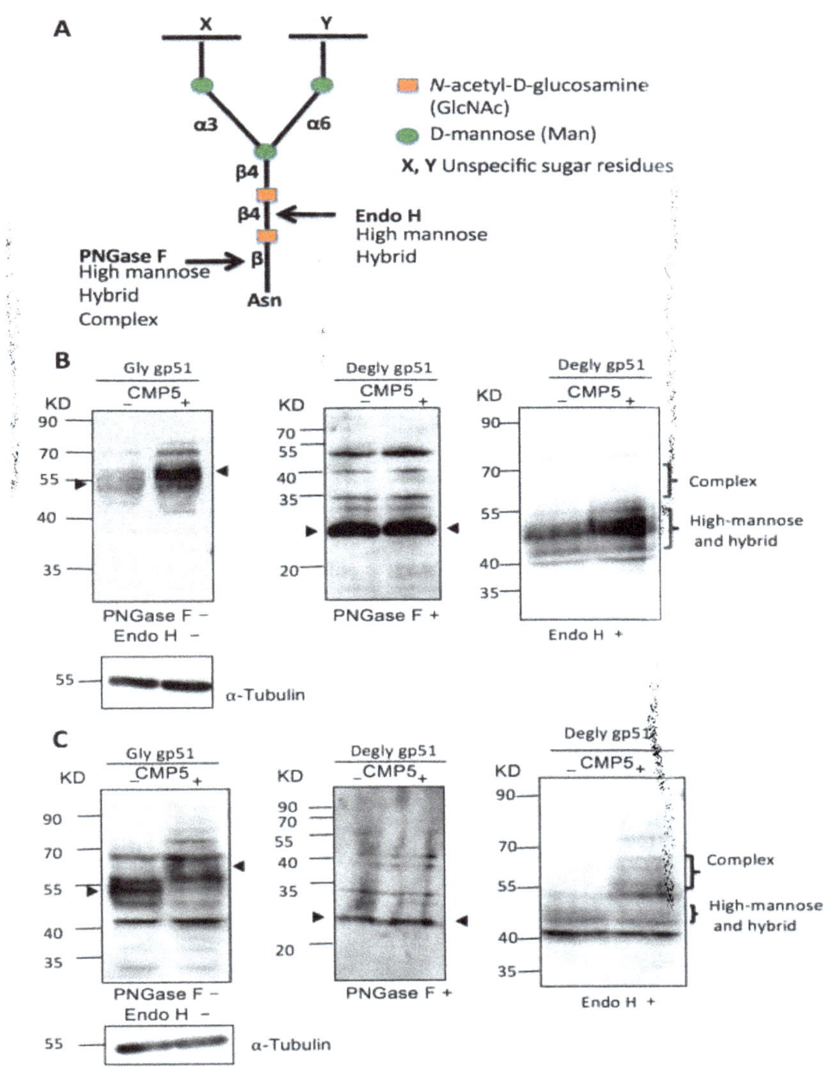

Figure 7. Deglycosylation assay of BLV gp51 using PNGase F and endo H. (**A**) Schematic representation of PNGase F and Endo H sensitive bonds in the core of *N*-glycans. (**B**) FLK-BLV or (**C**) PK15-BLV were

treated with Milli-Q water (CMP5−) or 20 μM CMP5 (CMP5+) for 48 h. Cell lysates were divided into three parts: one part was untreated (PNGase F−/Endo H−), the second part was deglycosylated by PNGase F (PNGase F+), and the third part was deglycosylated by Endo H (Endo H+). The cell lysates from the three conditions were subjected to Western blotting analysis with anti BLV gp51 (BLV2). α-Tubulin was used as a loading control. The data are a representation of at least three experiments. The positions of BLV gp51 protein with or without glycosylation, gp51 glycosylation pattern such as complex, and high-mannose and hybrid pattern, in addition to α-tubulin protein, are indicated.

3.8. CMP5 Treatment Does Not Change Env Localization at the Plasma Membrane

Next, we examined whether CMP5 treatment affects Gag or Env localization or Env trafficking to the cell membrane. FLK-BLV cells were grown on coverslips in the absence (CMP5–) or presence of 20 μM of CMP5 (CMP5+) for 48 h; Gag was stained with a green fluorescent marker, Env was stained with a red fluorescent marker, and DAPI was used to stain the nucleus. Gag and Env localization were evaluated by fluorescence confocal microscopy. The cellular membrane staining of gp51was performed without the permeabilization step and the intracellular staining was conducted after the permeabilization with 0.5% Triton X-100 for 5 min. We observed a large accumulation of Gag after CMP5 treatment (Figure 8A). Additionally, the intracellular Env protein accumulated near to the nucleus after the treatment (Figure 8B). In contrast, the cell membrane expression of gp51 was not severely affected, as demonstrated by the fluorescence confocal microscopy (Figure 8C) and by flow cytometry (Figure 8D).

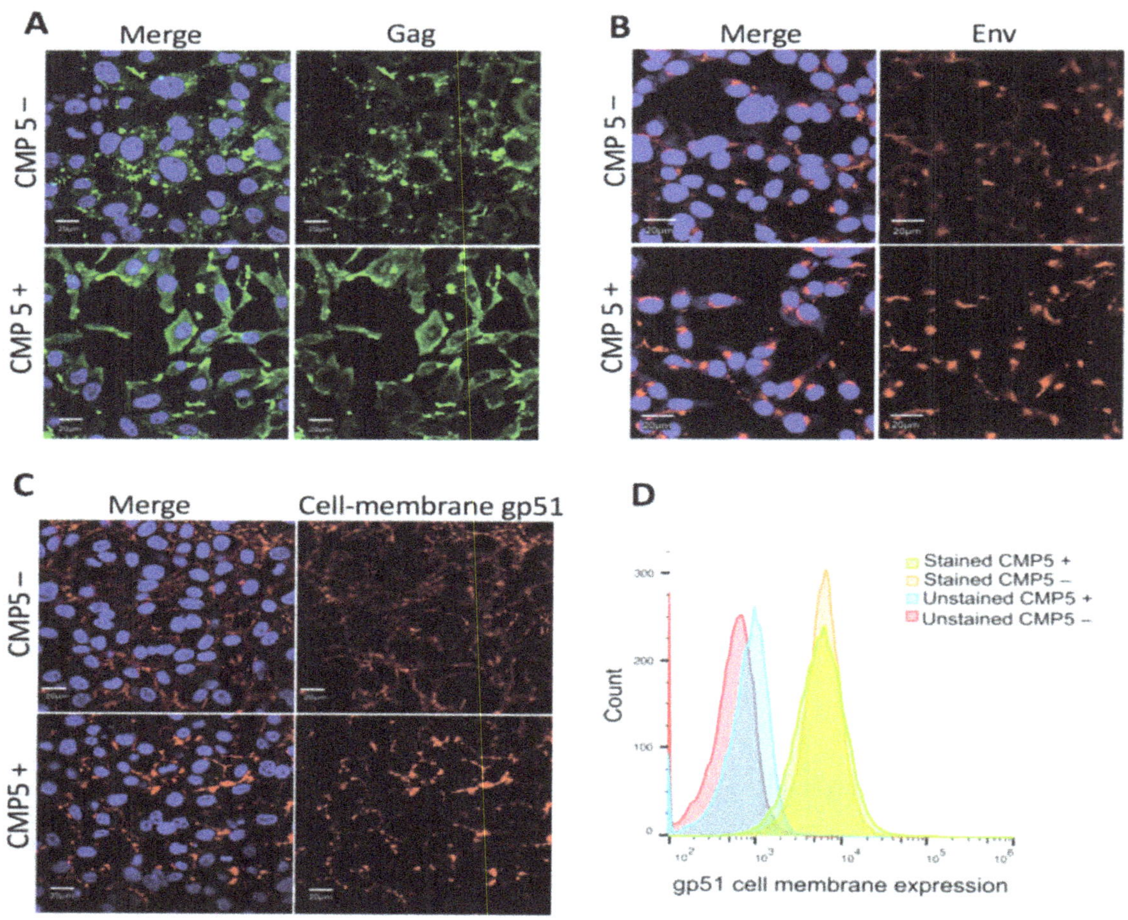

Figure 8. Effect of CMP5 on Gag and Env localization. (**A**,**B**) FLK-BLV were grown on coverslips and treated with Milli-Q water (CMP5–) or CMP5 20 μM (CMP5+), Gag was stained with green fluorescence (**A**), Env was stained with red fluorescence (**B**), The cellular membrane staining of gp51 was performed without the permeabilization step (**C**). DAPI (blue fluorescence) was used to stain the nucleus and the merge picture represents Gag or Env with DAPI. The data are a representation of three experiments.

Images were acquired with a 60X objective and the scale bar is equal to 20 µm. (**D**) FLK-BLV were treated with Milli-Q water (CMP5−) or CMP5 20 µM (CMP5+), the cells were collected, and gp51 cell membrane expression was assessed by flow cytometry. The data are a representation of two experiments. Scale bar—20 µm.

3.9. Selective PRMT5 Inhibitor Impedes BLV ENV-Mediated Syncytia formation In Vitro

Previous studies showed that perturbation of the *N*-linked glycan structure of the HIV and HTLV-1 envelope proteins affects syncytia formation [57,58]. Therefore, we examined the impact of the PRMT5 inhibitor CMP5 on the syncytium formation ability. We used LuSIA to quantify the syncytia [8,51]. Because examining the syncytia formation ability of PK15-BLV cells was not possible because of the relatively longer time required for forming the syncytia, we only assessed the effect of CMP5 on syncytia formation using the FLK-BLV cell line. The LuSIA depends on a new reporter cell line (CC81-GREMG) stably transfected with a reporter plasmid in which the EGFP reporter gene is expressed under control of the glucocorticoid response element (GRE)-mutated long terminal repeat (LTR)-U3 promoter and enables direct visualization of syncytia. CC81-GREMG expresses EGFP in response to BLV trans-activator p38tax expression and forms fluorescent syncytia when cultured with BLV-producing cells.

FLK-BLV cells were co-cultured with CC81-GREMG cell in the absence or presence of different concentrations of CMP5. Interestingly, CMP5 treatment negatively affected syncytia formation; this was detected by fluorescence microscopy (Figure 9A) and automated quantification showing that the syncytia counts were decreased in a dose-dependent manner, showing significance at concentrations of 10 µM ($p = 0.017$) and 20 µM ($p = 0.0002$) (Figure 9B). In contrast, the total cell count during the assay remained unaffected (Figure 9C). In addition, the maximum used concentration of CMP5 (20 µM) did not severely affect the viability of FLK-BLV or CC81-GREMG (Figure 9D). These observations exclude the toxic effect of CMP5 on FLK-BLV or CC81-GREMG. Our results obtained by LuSIA using CC81-GREMG cells strongly suggest that PRMT5 regulates the induction of the syncytia by BLV Env.

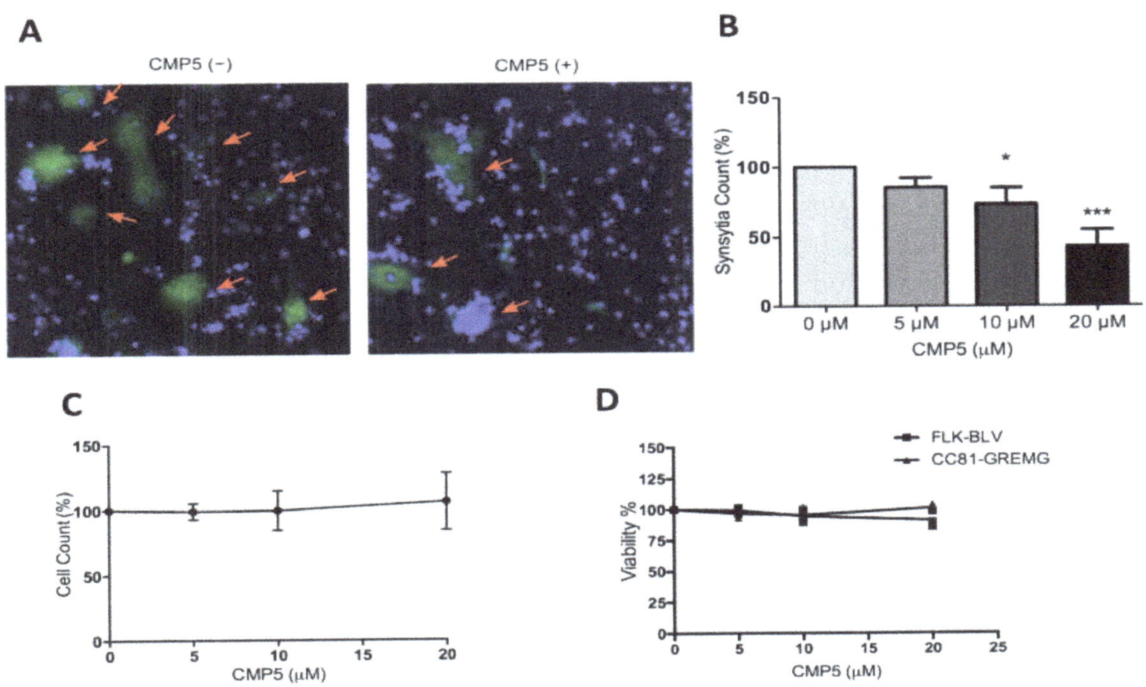

Figure 9. CMP5 effect on BLV ENV-mediated syncytia formation. A BLV-producing cell line FLK-BLV was co-cultured with a reporter cell line CC81-GREMG and treated with Milli-Q water (CMP5−) or

CMP5 at the indicated concentrations (CMP5+) for 48 h. (**A**,**B**). Fluorescent syncytia in nine fields of view in each well were automatically scanned by EVOS2 fluorescence microscopy with a 4× objective. Fluorescent syncytia were recognized by enhanced green fluorescent protein (EGFP) expression and gated by their area and intensity. Red arrows indicate positions of fluorescent syncytia. Hoechst 33342 was used to stain the nucleus. Each picture is a representation of nine pictures acquired for each well. (**B**) Data analysis of (**A**) shows syncytia count using HCS Studio Cell Analysis software. Error bars represent the standard deviation of three independent experiments, the p value was calculated by ANOVA (0.00031), and Dunnett's multiple comparisons test showed a significant decrease in the syncytia count at 10 μM (* $p = 0.017$) and 20 μM (*** $p = 0.0002$). (**C**) Effects of CMP5 on the total cell count taken from gating and counting of Hoechst 33342 staining using HCS Studio Cell Analysis software (Thermo Fisher Scientific). (**D**) CMP5 effect on cell viability according to WST-1 assay.

4. Discussion

BLV-mediated pathogenicity depends on a delicate balance between viral gene expression and certain host-related genetic and epigenetic events [2]. The mutation rate of BLV is relatively low [59] and spontaneous variations in the BLV genome have a limited impact on the biological properties of the virus [60]. Thus, host factors are thought to play crucial roles in determining the BLV infection profile. Herein, we investigated the role of the host protein PRMT5 in BLV infection in vivo and in vitro. Our study revealed three major conclusions as follows. First, our data suggested that PRMT5 overexpression is involved in the development of BLV infection with a high proviral load, thus affecting which infected cows progress from the asymptomatic stage to the lymphoma stage, and that PRMT5 overexpression may serve as an index of disease progression in vivo. Second, we demonstrated that PRMT5 acts as a novel negative regulator of BLV protein expression in vitro. Knockdown PRMT5 or its inhibition with an inhibitor enhanced BLV gene expression at the RNA and protein levels in BLV-infected cell lines. Finally, CMP5 inhibition demonstrated that the gp51 glycosylation pattern was altered under CMP5 treatment among different BLV-producing cell lines, thereby decreasing BLV-induced syncytium formation mediated by Env glycosylation. Our findings provide insight into the role of PRMT5 in the BLV viral life cycle and for the development of new anti-BLV drugs.

In this study, we found that PRMT5 was significantly upregulated in BLV-infected cattle with HPVL (PVL >10,000 copies/10^5), but not in those with LPVL (PVL ≤10,000 copies/10^5) (Figure 1). This finding indicates that PRMT5 upregulation is related to transmission. Furthermore, this upregulation continued to the lymphoma stage (Figure 3). We also performed experimental infection of five cattle carrying the susceptible alleles *BoLA-DRB3*1601/*1601*, which are associated with an increased risk of developing BLV infection with HPVL, and we confirmed that PRMT5 is upregulated in response to BLV infection (Figure 2A) and its level of upregulation was strongly correlated with BLV PVL (Figure 2B). Finally, we found that PRMT5 upregulation starts as early as two weeks post-infection (Figure 2A). This finding supports previous observations that PRMT5 expression increases at 4–8 days post-EBV infection [46]. Taken together, our data suggest that overexpression of PRMT5 contributes to the development and maintenance of BLV infection. Notably, PRMT5 was not the only PRMT member to be upregulated in BLV infection. PRMT1, which is Type I PRMT, was also upregulated. Additionally, our preliminary data showed that the PRMT1 expression fold-change was correlated with BLV PVL (data not shown). This indicates that PRMT5 is not specifically upregulated, but rather overexpression of other PRMTs is involved in regulating the BLV proviral load.

Our present study clearly demonstrates that PRMT5 negatively regulates BLV expression as PRMT5 inhibition including siRNA-mediated PRMT5 knockdown and treatment with CMP5 enhanced BLV gene expression at the transcriptional and protein levels in BLV-expressing cell lines, indicating that PRMT5 had an additive inhibitory effect on BLV gene expression (Figures 4–6). This result is supported by previous data showing that shRNA-mediated reduction in PRMT5 protein levels or its inhibition by a small molecule inhibitor (PRMT5i) in HTLV-1-infected lymphocytes resulted in increased viral gene expression [44]. PRMT5 catalyzes symmetric dimethylation of arginine residues in several histone and non-histone proteins [33,61]. Therefore, PRMT5 may regulate BLV gene expression either via an epigenetic mechanism and by producing repressive histone marks or methylation of non-histone proteins such as transcription factors. Additionally, our findings suggest why BLV maintains a silent state within infected cells in vivo. Indeed, PRMT5 is overexpressed in BLV-infected animals in vivo (Figures 1–3). This proviral latency represents a strategy for avoiding the host immune system and consequently allows for tumor development. Thus, numerous studies have focused on identifying compounds capable of reversing BLV latency to enhance immune clearance of the virus; previous studies also revealed histone deacetylation and DNA hypermethylation as epigenetic modifications involved in BLV transcriptional repression [62–64]. Therefore, understanding the mechanism of how PRMT5 regulates BLV expression requires further analysis.

Alinari and co-workers [46] investigated the role of PRMT5 in EBV-induced B-cell transformation and developed a small-molecule PRMT5 inhibitor (CMP5) capable of blocking EBV-driven B-cell transformation without affecting normal B cells. Interestingly, we found that CMP5 treatment of FLK-BLV and PK15-BLV affects the glycosylation pattern of BLV gp51. This was further supported by the finding that CMP5 treatment enhanced the formation of complex or hybrid types of *N*-glycan over the high-mannose type. Therefore, following CMP5 treatment, gp51 traveled more slowly than untreated gp51 in SDS-PAGE. The effects of CMP5 on gp51 glycosylation processing involve a sophisticated process requiring a large number of enzymes and organelles, named as the glycosylation machinery. The glycosylation machinery is a group of enzymes, chaperones, transporters, sugar donors, and accessory molecules necessary to form a specific glycan structure [65]. Therefore, glycosylation is a highly regulated and dynamic process that is extremely sensitive to changes in components of the glycosylation machinery. The diversity of glycans depends on not only the expression levels of the molecules involved in glycan biosynthesis, including glycosyltransferases, but also on the interplay of all regulatory molecules involved in the process. This may affect both the number of glycans (macroheterogeneity) and nature of these glycan chains (microheterogeneity) [65]. Thus, CMP5 treatment may alter the expression levels of some components of the glycosylation machinery, thereby altering the gp51 glycosylation pattern.

Notably, the effect of CMP5 treatment on the gp51 glycosylation pattern differs between the two cell lines (FLK-BLV and PK15-BLV), which belong to different host species. In the PK15-BLV cell line, CMP5 treatment enhanced the formation of the complex type of *N*-glycan over the high mannose type. In FLK-BLV, however, the results did not reveal that the irregular type of *N*-glycan resulted from CMP5 treatment. Similarly, a previous report clearly showed distinct differences in the glycosylation profiles of HIV-1 ENV gp120 expressed in CHO, which originated from hamsters, and 293T cells, which originated from humans [66]. Therefore, this variation in different cell lines is expected as the nature of *N*-linked glycans attached to a glycoprotein is determined not only by the peptide backbone of a protein, but also by the cell in which it is expressed.

Although CMP5 affects the gp51 apparent molecular weight, siRNA knockdown of PRMT5 did not appear to induce the same effect (Figure S1). The reason why this difference arose between siRNA-mediated PRMT5 knockdown and CMP5 treatment was unclear, but there are two possibilities. First, the impact of CMP5 treatment on gp51 glycosylation may be non-specific, resulting from inhibition of other PRMTs protein rather than PRMT5. Second, gp51 glycosylation is a highly dynamic process that is highly influenced by the time and efficiency of PRMT5 inhibition and differs between pharmacological inhibition and knockdown inhibition. Considering that Alinari and co-workers [46] showed that CMP5 selectively blocks S2Me-H4R3 in JeKo cells, whereas it is inactive against PRMT1, PRMT4, and PRMT7 in cellular screening assays, CMP5 appears to be selective for PRMT5 over type1 PRMTs. Additionally, the initial predicted binding interactions of CMP5 with their hPRMT5 model suggested that the pyridine ring of CMP5 forms a p-stacking interaction with the Phe327 residue, which is critical for directing PRMT5 to catalyze symmetric dimethylation of arginine, explaining the selectivity of CMP5 for type II PRMT5, not type I PRMTs. They also performed RNA-seq of PRMT5-shRNA or CMP5 treatment in transformed LCLs (60A) cells and observed significant overlap between genes de-repressed by CMP5 and genes de-repressed by PRMT5-shRNA, confirming the specificity of this compound. In contrast, we observed that CMP5 treatment increases the apparent molecular weight of gp51 at 20 μM, but not at 5 or 10 μM (Figure 6b). Therefore, the extent and duration of PRMT5 inhibition in siRNA knockdown may be insufficient to affect the glycosylation processing of gp51. Further transcriptomic or proteomic studies are required to identify the differentially expressed genes and determine the biological processes altered by CMP5 treatment or PRMT5 knockdown.

Our study showed that CMP5 treatment impeded BLV-induced syncytium formation, which was measured by LuSIA [8,51]. However, CMP5 treatment did not impair the gp51 expression at the cell membrane (Figure 8C,D). Seemingly, the intracellular expression of Env accumulated near to the nucleus after CMP5 treatment (Figure 8B). The reason of this phenomena and whether or not it is related to the observed reduction of the syncytia formation remain unclear. On the other hand, previous studies reported that the electrophoretic mobility of the surface subunit of the HIV envelope (gp120) was decreased when gp120 was synthesized in the presence of castanospermine or 1-deoxynojirimycin (inhibitors of glucosidase I). Consequently, these inhibitors blocked HIV-1-induced syncytium formation and cytopathicity [58,67,68]. Therefore, incorrect glycosylation processing of gp120 may negatively affect HIV-1 induced syncytium formation. In addition, BLV SU-linked *N*-glycosylation appeared to regulate the syncytium-forming capacity in vitro [26,27]. Taken together, CMP5 treatment likely impedes BLV-induced syncytium formation by affecting gp51 glycosylation processing.

In conclusion, we determined various roles for PRMT5 in BLV infection in vivo and in vitro; CMP5 and other PRMT5 inhibitors should be further investigated and evaluated in clinical studies as a novel antiretroviral therapy.

Author Contributions: Y.A. and W.A. conceived and designed the study. W.A., T.H., S.W., R.M., S.-n.T. and Y.A. acquired, analyzed, and interpreted the data. Y.A. contributed the reagents, materials, and analysis tools. W.A. and Y.A. drafted and revised the manuscript. All authors have read and agreed to the published version of the manuscript.

Acknowledgments: The authors thank the veterinary officers of the prefectural Livestock Hygiene Service Centers and veterinary of Kyoto Biken Institute for their help with blood sampling and the collection of epidemiological data. We thank all members of the Virus Infectious Disease Field of RIKEN and we thank Dr. Tadashi Suzuki for the useful suggestions. We are grateful to the Support Unit, Bio-material Analysis, RIKEN BSI Research Resources Center for helping with the sequence analysis. We would like to thank Editage (www.editage.com) for English language editing.

References

1. Gillet, N.; Florins, A.; Boxus, M.; Burteau, C.; Nigro, A.; Vandermeers, F.; Balon, H.; Bouzar, A.B.; Defoiche, J.; Burny, A.; et al. Mechanisms of leukemogenesis induced by bovine leukemia virus: Prospects for novel anti-retroviral therapies in human. *Retrovirology* **2007**, *4*, 18. [CrossRef] [PubMed]
2. Aida, Y.; Murakami, H.; Takahashi, M.; Takeshima, S.N. Mechanisms of pathogenesis induced by bovine leukemia virus as a model for human T-cell leukemia virus. *Front. Microbiol.* **2013**, *4*, 1–11. [CrossRef] [PubMed]
3. Polat, M.; Takeshima, S.N.; Aida, Y. Epidemiology and genetic diversity of bovine leukemia virus. *Virol. J.* **2017**, *14*, 209. [CrossRef] [PubMed]
4. Nekouei, O.; VanLeeuwen, J.; Stryhn, H.; Kelton, D.; Keefe, G. Lifetime effects of infection with bovine leukemia virus on longevity and milk production of dairy cows. *Prev. Vet. Med.* **2016**, *133*, 1–9. [CrossRef]
5. Otta, S.L.; Johnson, R.; Wells, S.J. Association between bovine-leukosis virus seroprevalence and herd-level productivity on US dairy farms. *Prev. Vet. Med.* **2003**, *61*, 249–262. [CrossRef]

6. Furtado, M.D.S.B.S.; Andrade, R.G.; Romanelli, L.C.F.; Ribeiro, M.A.; Ribas, J.G.; Torres, E.B.; Barbosa-Stancioli, E.F.; Proietti, A.B.; Martins, M.L. Monitoring the HTLV-1 proviral load in the peripheral blood of asymptomatic carriers and patients with HTLV-associated myelopathy/tropical spastic paraparesis from a Brazilian cohort: ROC curve analysis to establish the threshold for risk disease. *J. Med. Virol.* **2012**, *84*, 664–671. [CrossRef]
7. Jimba, M.; Takeshima, S.N.; Matoba, K.; Endoh, D.; Aida, Y. BLV-CoCoMo-qPCR: Quantitation of bovine leukemia virus proviral load using the CoCoMo algorithm. *Retrovirology* **2010**, *7*, 1–19. [CrossRef]
8. Sato, H.; Watanuki, S.; Murakami, H.; Sato, R.; Ishizaki, H.; Aida, Y. Development of a luminescence syncytium induction assay (LuSIA) for easily detecting and quantitatively measuring bovine leukemia virus infection. *Arch. Virol.* **2018**, *163*, 1519–1530. [CrossRef]
9. Lo, C.-W.; Borjigin, L.; Saito, S.; Fukunaga, K.; Saitou, E.; Okazaki, K.; Mizutani, T.; Wada, S.; Takeshima, S.; Aida, Y. BoLA-DRB3 Polymorphism is Associated with Differential Susceptibility to Bovine Leukemia Virus-Induced Lymphoma and Proviral Load. *Viruses* **2020**, *12*, 352. [CrossRef]
10. Ohno, A.; Takeshima, S.N.; Matsumoto, Y.; Aida, Y. Risk factors associated with increased bovine leukemia virus proviral load in infected cattle in Japan from 2012 to 2014. *Virus Res.* **2015**, *210*, 283–290. [CrossRef]
11. Juliarena, M.A.; Gutierrez, S.E.; Ceriani, C. Determination of proviral load in bovine leukemia virus-infected cattle with and without lymphocytosis. *Am. J. Vet. Res.* **2007**, *68*, 1220–1225. [CrossRef] [PubMed]
12. Yuan, Y.; Kitamura-Muramatsu, Y.; Saito, S.; Ishizaki, H.; Nakano, M.; Haga, S.; Matoba, K.; Ohno, A.; Murakami, H.; Takeshima, S.N.; et al. Detection of the BLV provirus from nasal secretion and saliva samples using BLV-CoCoMo-qPCR-2: Comparison with blood samples from the same cattle. *Virus Res.* **2015**, *210*, 248–254. [CrossRef] [PubMed]
13. Watanuki, S.; Takeshima, S.N.; Borjigin, L.; Sato, H.; Bai, L.; Murakami, H.; Sato, R.; Ishizaki, H.; Matsumoto, Y.; Aida, Y. Visualizing bovine leukemia virus (BLV)-infected cells and measuring BLV proviral loads in the milk of BLV seropositive dams. *Vet. Res.* **2019**, *50*, 102. [CrossRef] [PubMed]
14. Juliarena, M.A.; Barrios, C.N.; Ceriani, M.C.; Esteban, E.N. Hot topic: Bovine leukemia virus (BLV)-infected cows with low proviral load are not a source of infection for BLV-free cattle. *J. Dairy Sci.* **2016**, *99*, 4586–4589. [CrossRef]
15. Takeshima, S.N.; Ohno, A.; Aida, Y. Bovine leukemia virus proviral load is more strongly associated with bovine major histocompatibility complex class II DRB3 polymorphism than with DQA1 polymorphism in Holstein cow in Japan. *Retrovirology* **2019**, *16*, 10–15. [CrossRef] [PubMed]
16. Nikbakht Brujeni, G.; Ghorbanpour, R.; Esmailnejad, A. Association of BoLA-DRB3.2 Alleles with BLV Infection Profiles (Persistent Lymphocytosis/Lymphosarcoma) and Lymphocyte Subsets in Iranian Holstein Cattle. *Biochem. Genet.* **2016**, *54*, 194–207. [CrossRef] [PubMed]
17. Brym, P.; Bojarojć-Nosowicz, B.; Oleński, K.; Hering, D.M.; Ruść, A.; Kaczmarczyk, E.; Kamiński, S. Genome-wide association study for host response to bovine leukemia virus in Holstein cows. *Vet. Immunol. Immunopathol.* **2016**, *175*, 24–35. [CrossRef]
18. Takeshima, S.N.; Sasaki, S.; Meripet, P.; Sugimoto, Y.; Aida, Y. Single nucleotide polymorphisms in the bovine MHC region of Japanese Black cattle are associated with bovine leukemia virus proviral load. *Retrovirology* **2017**, *14*, 24. [CrossRef]
19. Carignano, H.A.; Roldan, D.L.; Beribe, M.J.; Raschia, M.A.; Amadio, A.; Nani, J.P.; Gutierrez, G.; Alvarez, I.; Trono, K.; Poli, M.A.; et al. Genome-wide scan for commons SNPs affecting bovine leukemia virus infection level in dairy cattle. *BMC Genomics* **2018**, *19*, 142. [CrossRef]
20. Hayashi, T.; Mekata, H.; Sekiguchi, S.; Kirino, Y.; Mitoma, S.; Honkawa, K.; Horii, Y.; Norimine, J. Cattle with the BoLA class II DRB3*0902 allele have significantly lower bovine leukemia proviral loads. *J. Vet. Med. Sci.* **2017**, *79*, 1552–1555. [CrossRef]
21. Sagata, N.; Yasunaga, T.; Ohishi, K.; Tsuzuku-Kawamura, J.; Onuma, M.; Ikawa, Y. Comparison of the entire genomes of bovine leukemia virus and human T-cell leukemia virus and characterization of their unidentified open reading frames. *EMBO J.* **1984**, *3*, 3231–3237. [CrossRef] [PubMed]
22. Hamard-Peron, E.; Muriaux, D. Retroviral matrix and lipids, the intimate interaction. *Retrovirology* **2011**, *8*, 15. [CrossRef] [PubMed]
23. De Brogniez, A.; Mast, J.; Willems, L. Determinants of the bovine leukemia virus envelope glycoproteins involved in infectivity, replication and pathogenesis. *Viruses* **2016**, *8*, 88. [CrossRef] [PubMed]

24. Johnston, E.R.; Radke, K. The SU and TM envelope protein subunits of bovine leukemia virus are linked by disulfide bonds, both in cells and in virions. *J. Virol.* **2000**, *74*, 2930–2935. [CrossRef] [PubMed]
25. Bai, L.; Sato, H.; Kubo, Y.; Wada, S.; Aida, Y. CAT1/SLC7A1 acts as a cellular receptor for bovine leukemia virus infection. *FASEB J.* **2019**, *33*, 14516–14527. [CrossRef] [PubMed]
26. De Brogniez, A.; Bouzar, A.B.; Jacques, J.-R.; Cosse, J.-P.; Gillet, N.; Callebaut, I.; Reichert, M.; Willems, L. Mutation of a Single Envelope N-Linked Glycosylation Site Enhances the Pathogenicity of Bovine Leukemia Virus. *J. Virol.* **2015**, *89*, 8945–8956. [CrossRef]
27. Rizzo, G.; Forti, K.; Serroni, A.; Cagiola, M.; Baglivo, S.; Scoccia, E.; De Giuseppe, A. Single N-glycosylation site of bovine leukemia virus SU is involved in conformation and viral escape. *Vet. Microbiol.* **2016**, *197*, 21–26. [CrossRef]
28. Mamoun, R.Z.; Morisson, M.; Rebeyrotte, N.; Busetta, B.; Couez, D.; Kettmann, R.; Hospital, M.; Guillemain, B. Sequence variability of bovine leukemia virus env gene and its relevance to the structure and antigenicity of the glycoproteins. *J. Virol.* **1990**, *64*, 4180–4188. [CrossRef]
29. Pikora, C. Glycosylation of the ENV Spike of Primate Immunodeficiency Viruses and Antibody Neutralization. *Curr. HIV Res.* **2004**, *2*, 243–254. [CrossRef]
30. Aguilar, H.C.; Matreyek, K.A.; Filone, C.M.; Hashimi, S.T.; Levroney, E.L.; Negrete, O.A.; Bertolotti-Ciarlet, A.; Choi, D.Y.; McHardy, I.; Fulcher, J.A.; et al. N-Glycans on Nipah Virus Fusion Protein Protect against Neutralization but Reduce Membrane Fusion and Viral Entry. *J. Virol.* **2006**, *80*, 4878–4889. [CrossRef]
31. Wei, X.; Decker, J.M.; Wang, S.; Hui, H.; Kappes, J.C.; Wu, X.; Salazar-Gonzalez, J.F.; Salazar, M.G.; Kilby, J.M.; Saag, M.S.; et al. Antibody neutralization and escape by HIV-1. *Nature* **2003**, *422*, 307–312. [CrossRef] [PubMed]
32. Bedford, M.T.; Richard, S. Arginine Methylation: An Emerging Regulator of Protein Function. *Mol. Cell* **2005**, *18*, 263–272. [CrossRef] [PubMed]
33. Bedford, M.T.; Clarke, S.G. Protein arginine methylation in mammals: Who, what, and why. *Mol. Cell* **2009**, *33*, 1–13. [CrossRef] [PubMed]
34. Peng, C.; Wong, C.C.L. The story of protein arginine methylation: Characterization, regulation, and function. *Expert Rev. Proteomics* **2017**, *14*, 157–170. [CrossRef]
35. Li, Y.-J.; Stallcup, M.R.; Lai, M.M.C. Hepatitis Delta Virus Antigen Is Methylated at Arginine Residues, and Methylation Regulates Subcellular Localization and RNA Replication. *J. Virol.* **2004**, *78*, 13325–13334. [CrossRef]
36. Lubyova, B.; Hodek, J.; Zabransky, A.; Prouzova, H.; Hubalek, M.; Hirsch, I.; Weber, J. PRMT5: A novel regulator of Hepatitis B virus replication and an arginine methylase of HBV core. *PLoS ONE* **2017**, *12*, e0186982. [CrossRef]
37. Benhenda, S.; Ducroux, A.; Riviere, L.; Sobhian, B.; Ward, M.D.; Dion, S.; Hantz, O.; Protzer, U.; Michel, M.-L.; Benkirane, M.; et al. Methyltransferase PRMT1 Is a Binding Partner of HBx and a Negative Regulator of Hepatitis B Virus Transcription. *J. Virol.* **2013**, *87*, 4360–4371. [CrossRef]
38. Zhang, W.; Chen, J.; Wu, M.; Zhang, X.; Zhang, M.; Yue, L.; Li, Y.; Liu, J.; Li, B.; Shen, F.; et al. PRMT5 restricts hepatitis B virus replication through epigenetic repression of covalently closed circular DNA transcription and interference with pregenomic RNA encapsidation. *Hepatology* **2017**, *66*, 398–415. [CrossRef]
39. Fulcher, A.J.; Sivakumaran, H.; Jin, H.; Rawle, D.J.; Harrich, D.; Jans, D.A. The protein arginine methyltransferase PRMT6 inhibits HIV-1 Tat nucleolar retention. *Biochim. Biophys. Acta Mol. Cell Res.* **2016**, *1863*, 254–262. [CrossRef]
40. Xie, B.; Invernizzi, C.F.; Richard, S.; Wainberg, M.A. Arginine Methylation of the Human Immunodeficiency Virus Type 1 Tat Protein by PRMT6 Negatively Affects Tat Interactions with both Cyclin T1 and the Tat Transactivation Region. *J. Virol.* **2007**, *81*, 4226–4234. [CrossRef]
41. Singhroy, D.N.; Mesplède, T.; Sabbah, A.; Quashie, P.K.; Falgueyret, J.P.; Wainberg, M.A. Automethylation of protein arginine methyltransferase 6 (PRMT6) regulates its stability and its anti-HIV-1 activity. *Retrovirology* **2013**, *10*, 73. [CrossRef] [PubMed]
42. Boulanger, M.-C.; Liang, C.; Russell, R.S.; Lin, R.; Bedford, M.T.; Wainberg, M.A.; Richard, S. Methylation of Tat by PRMT6 Regulates Human Immunodeficiency Virus Type 1 Gene Expression. *J. Virol.* **2005**, *79*, 124–131. [CrossRef] [PubMed]

43. Invernizzi, C.F.; Xie, B.; Richard, S.; Wainberg, M.A. PRMT6 diminishes HIV-1 Rev binding to and export of viral RNA. *Retrovirology* **2006**, *3*, 93. [CrossRef] [PubMed]
44. Panfil, A.R.; Al-Saleem, J.; Howard, C.M.; Mates, J.M.; Kwiek, J.J.; Baiocchi, R.A.; Green, P.L. PRMT5 is upregulated in HTLV-1-mediated T-Cell transformation and selective inhibition alters viral gene expression and infected cell survival. *Viruses* **2015**, *8*, 7. [CrossRef]
45. Leonard, S.; Gordon, N.; Smith, N.; Rowe, M.; Murray, P.G.; Woodman, C.B. Arginine methyltransferases are regulated by Epstein-Barr virus in B cells and are differentially expressed in Hodgkin's lymphoma. *Pathogens* **2012**, *1*, 52–64. [CrossRef]
46. Alinari, L.; Mahasenan, K.V.; Yan, F.; Karkhanis, V.; Chung, J.; Smith, E.M.; Quinion, C.; Smith, P.L.; Kim, L.; Patton, J.T.; et al. Selective inhibition of protein arginine methyltransferase 5 blocks initiation and maintenance of B-cell transformation. *Blood* **2015**, *125*, 2530–2543. [CrossRef]
47. Strahan, R.C.; McDowell-Sargent, M.; Uppal, T.; Purushothaman, P.; Verma, S.C. KSHV Encoded ORF59 Modulates Histone Arginine Methylation of the Viral Genome to Promote Viral Reactivation. *PLoS Pathog.* **2017**, *13*, e1006482. [CrossRef]
48. Murakami, H.; Suzuki, T.; Tsuchiya, K.; Gatanaga, H.; Taura, M.; Kudo, E.; Okada, S.; Takei, M.; Kuroda, K.; Yamamoto, T.; et al. Protein Arginine N-methyltransferases 5 and 7 Promote HIV-1 Production. *Viruses* **2020**, *12*, 355. [CrossRef]
49. Matsuura, R.; Inabe, K.; Otsuki, H.; Kurokawa, K.; Dohmae, N.; Aida, Y. Three YXXL sequences of a bovine leukemia virus transmembrane protein are independently required for fusion activity by controlling expression on the cell membrane. *Viruses* **2019**, *11*, 1140. [CrossRef]
50. Takeshima, S.N.; Kitamura-Muramatsu, Y.; Yuan, Y.; Polat, M.; Saito, S.; Aida, Y. BLV-CoCoMo-qPCR-2: Improvements to the BLV-CoCoMo-qPCR assay for bovine leukemia virus by reducing primer degeneracy and constructing an optimal standard curve. *Arch. Virol.* **2015**, *160*, 1325–1332. [CrossRef]
51. Sato, H.; Watanuki, S.; Bai, L.; Borjigin, L.; Ishizaki, H.; Matsumoto, Y.; Hachiya, Y.; Sentsui, H.; Aida, Y. A sensitive luminescence syncytium induction assay (LuSIA) based on a reporter plasmid containing a mutation in the glucocorticoid response element in the long terminal repeat U3 region of bovine leukemia virus. *Virol. J.* **2019**, *16*, 66. [CrossRef] [PubMed]
52. Miyasaka, T.; Takeshima, S.N.; Jimba, M.; Matsumoto, Y.; Kobayashi, N.; Matsuhashi, T.; Sentsui, H.; Aida, Y. Identification of bovine leukocyte antigen class II haplotypes associated with variations in bovine leukemia virus proviral load in Japanese Black cattle. *Tissue Antigens* **2013**, *81*, 72–82. [CrossRef] [PubMed]
53. Fabbrizio, E.; El Messaoudi, S.; Polanowska, J.; Paul, C.; Cook, J.R.; Lee, J.-H.; Negre, V.; Rousset, M.; Pestka, S.; Le Cam, A.; et al. Negative regulation of transcription by the type II arginine methyltransferase PRMT5. *EMBO Rep.* **2002**, *3*, 641–645. [CrossRef] [PubMed]
54. Bieberich, E. Synthesis, Processing, and Function of N-glycans in N-glycoproteins. *Adv. Neurobiol.* **2014**, *9*, 47–70. [CrossRef]
55. N-Glycans-Essentials of Glycobiology—NCBI Bookshelf. Available online: https://www.ncbi.nlm.nih.gov/books/NBK20720/ (accessed on 18 April 2020).
56. Freeze, H.H.; Kranz, C. Endoglycosidase and glycoamidase release of N-linked glycans. *Curr. Protoc. Mol. Biol.* **2010**, *2010*. [CrossRef]
57. Pique, C.; Pham, D.; Tursz, T.; Dokhélar, M.C. Human T-cell leukemia virus type I envelope protein maturation process: Requirements for syncytium formation. *J. Virol.* **1992**, *66*, 906–913. [CrossRef]
58. Gruters, R.A.; Neefjes, J.J.; Tersmette, M.; De Goede, R.E.Y.; Tulp, A.; Huisman, H.G.; Miedema, F.; Ploegh, H.L. Interference with HIV-induced syncytium formation and viral infectivity by inhibitors of trimming glucosidase. *Nature* **1987**, *330*, 74–77. [CrossRef]
59. Mansky, L.M.; Temin, H.M. Lower mutation rate of bovine leukemia virus relative to that of spleen necrosis virus. *J. Virol.* **1994**, *68*, 494–499. [CrossRef]
60. Murakami, H.; Uchiyama, J.; Suzuki, C.; Nikaido, S.; Shibuya, K.; Sato, R.; Maeda, Y.; Tomioka, M.; Takeshima, S.-N.; Kato, H.; et al. Variations in the viral genome and biological properties of bovine leukemia virus wild-type strains. *Virus Res.* **2018**, *253*, 103–111. [CrossRef]
61. Guccione, E.; Richard, S. The regulation, functions and clinical relevance of arginine methylation. *Nat. Rev. Mol. Cell Biol.* **2019**, *20*, 642–657. [CrossRef]

62. Pierard, V.; Guiguen, A.; Colin, L.; Wijmeersch, G.; Vanhulle, C.; Van Driessche, B.; Dekoninck, A.; Blazkova, J.; Cardona, C.; Merimi, M.; et al. DNA cytosine methylation in the bovine leukemia virus promoter is associated with latency in a lymphoma-derived B-cell line: Potential involvement of direct inhibition of camp-responsive element (CRE)-binding protein/cre modulator/activation transcription factor binding. *J. Biol. Chem.* **2010**, *285*, 19434–19449. [PubMed]
63. Merezak, C.; Reichert, M.; Van Lint, C.; Kerkhofs, P.; Portetelle, D.; Willems, L.; Kettmann, R. Inhibition of Histone Deacetylases Induces Bovine Leukemia Virus Expression In Vitro and In Vivo. *J. Virol.* **2002**, *76*, 5034–5042. [CrossRef] [PubMed]
64. Achachi, A.; Florins, A.; Gillet, N.; Debacq, C.; Urbain, P.; Foutsop, G.M.; Vandermeers, F.; Jasik, A.; Reichert, M.; Kerkhofs, P.; et al. Valproate activates bovine leukemia virus gene expression, triggers apoptosis, and induces leukemia/lymphoma regression in vivo. *Proc. Natl. Acad. Sci. USA* **2005**, *102*, 10309–10314. [CrossRef] [PubMed]
65. Van Kooyk, Y.; Kalay, H.; Garcia-Vallejo, J.J. Analytical tools for the study of cellular glycosylation in the immune system. *Front. Immunol.* **2013**, *4*, 1–6. [CrossRef]
66. Go, E.P.; Liao, H.X.; Alam, S.M.; Hua, D.; Haynes, B.F.; Desaire, H. Characterization of host-cell line specific glycosylation profiles of early transmitted/founder HIV-1 gp120 envelope proteins. *J. Proteome Res.* **2013**, *12*, 1223–1234. [CrossRef]
67. Montefiori, D.C.; Robinson, W.E.; Mitchell, W.M. Role of protein N-glycosylation in pathogenesis of human immunodeficieny virus type 1. *Proc. Natl. Acad. Sci. USA* **1988**, *85*, 9248–9252. [CrossRef]
68. Zhang, M.; Gaschen, B.; Blay, W.; Foley, B.; Haigwood, N.; Kuiken, C.; Korber, B. Tracking global patterns of N-linked glycosylation site variation in highly variable viral glycoproteins: HIV, SIV, and HCV envelopes and influenza hemagglutinin. *Glycobiology* **2004**, *14*, 1229–1246. [CrossRef]

3

Fatal Interstitial Pneumonia Associated with Bovine Coronavirus in Cows from Southern Italy

Maria Grazia Amoroso [1,*,†], Giuseppe Lucifora [2,†], Barbara Degli Uberti [1], Francesco Serra [1], Giovanna De Luca [1], Giorgia Borriello [3], Alessandro De Domenico [4], Sergio Brandi [1], Maria Concetta Cuomo [3], Francesca Bove [3], Marita Georgia Riccardi [3], Giorgio Galiero [3] and Giovanna Fusco [1]

1 Unit of Virology, Department of Animal Health, Experimental Zooprophylactic Institute of Southern Italy, Via Salute 2, 80055 Portici, Italy; barbara.degliuberti@cert.izsmportici.it (B.D.U.); francesco.serra@izsmportici.it (F.S.); giovanna.deluca@izsmportici.it (G.D.L.); sergio.brandi@cert.izsmportici.it (S.B.); giovanna.fusco@cert.izsmportici.it (G.F.)

2 Section of Vibo Valentia, Experimental Zooprophylactic Institute of Southern Italy, Contrada Piano di Bruno, 89852 Mileto, Italy; giuseppe.lucifora@cert.izsmportici.it

3 Department of Animal Health, Experimental Zooprophylactic Institute of Southern Italy, Via Salute 2, 80055 Portici, Italy; giorgia.borriello@izsmportici.it (G.B.); marycc@live.it (M.C.C.); francesca.bove@izsmportici.it (F.B.); maritageorgia.riccardi@izsmportici.it (M.G.R.); giorgio.galiero@cert.izsmportici.it (G.G.)

4 Freelance Veterinary, Ordine dei Veterinari di Vibo Valentia, 89900 Vibo Valentia, Italy; alessandro.dedomenico@yahoo.com

* Correspondence: mamoroso@izsmportici.it

† The two authors equally contributed to the paper.

Abstract: An outbreak of winter dysentery, complicated by severe respiratory syndrome, occurred in January 2020 in a high production dairy cow herd located in a hilly area of the Calabria region. Of the 52 animals belonging to the farm, 5 (9.6%) died with severe respiratory distress, death occurring 3–4 days after the appearance of the respiratory signs (caught and gasping breath). Microbiological analysis revealed absence of pathogenic bacteria whilst Real-time PCR identified the presence of RNA from Bovine Coronavirus (BCoV) in several organs: lungs, small intestine (jejunum), mediastinal lymph nodes, liver and placenta. BCoV was therefore hypothesized to play a role in the lethal pulmonary infection. Like the other CoVs, BCoV is able to cause different syndromes. Its role in calf diarrhea and in mild respiratory disease is well known: we report instead the involvement of this virus in a severe and fatal respiratory disorder, with symptoms and disease evolution resembling those of Severe Acute Respiratory Syndromes (SARS).

Keywords: bovine coronavirus; interstitial pneumonia; phylogenetic analysis; real time PCR

---

1. Introduction

Coronaviruses (CoVs) are enveloped viruses, with a RNA single-stranded large genome of 27.6–31 kb [1]. This big group of viruses, belonging to the order *Nidovirales*, suborder *Coronavirinae*, family *Coronaviridae*, subfamily *Orthocornavirinae*, is divided, (on the basis of the antigenic and genetic properties of these viruses [1,2] into 4 genera: alpha, beta, gamma and delta coronavirus. Coronaviruses are responsible for enteric, respiratory and neurological diseases in both birds and mammals, including humans [3]. Bats and birds are major reservoir of CoVs and some CoVs are endemic in domestic animals in different countries [4]. Several coronaviruses are well known for their ability to change tissue tropism, to pass species barriers and to adapt to new ecological niches.

These abilities are related to two factors commonly occurring during RNA replication: accumulation of point mutations (one mutation for each round of replication) caused by the low fidelity of their RNA dependent RNA polymerase (RdRp), as well as homologous and heterologous recombination events [1,2]. These features promote the emergence of novel strains with novel biological properties such as host range, tissue tropism and virulence [1,5]. The high mutation and recombination rates are indeed implicated in the emergence of new human coronaviruses, of animal origin, as occurred for the appearance of the strains HCoV-229E and HCoV-OC43 (the only two human coronaviruses known before SARS emergence), as well as for the arising of SARS-CoV Middle East Respiratory Syndrome Coronavirus Infection, (MERS-CoV) and the recent global pandemic SARS-CoV-2 [1,3,6–8]. CoVs infections in veterinary medicine are well known from a long time [1]. The most common animal CoVs are: infectious bronchitis virus (chickens), porcine transmissible gastroenteritis, porcine hemagglutinating encephalomyelitis and porcine epidemic diarrhea CoVs (swine), bovine coronavirus (BCoV, cattle), canine enteric and canine respiratory CoVs (dogs), and feline coronavirus (cats) [3]. BCoV belongs, together with human coronavirus (OC43), human enteric coronavirus (4408) and canine respiratory coronavirus (CRCoV), to subgroup A of the betacoronavirus genus [9–11]. This virus is pneumoenteric and has a dual tissue tropism, infecting both intestine and respiratory apparatus (upper and lower tracts), a feature in common with human SARS and SARS-CoV-2 [5]. It is endemic worldwide and is considered one of the major causes of neonatal calf diarrhea, with mortality related to virus ability to destroy the intestinal villi and to cause severe bloody diarrhea [2]. In adult dairy cattle, BCoV is instead associated with the well-known winter dysentery (WD), which causes severe drop in milk production and consequent significant economic losses for the herds [2]. In cattle of various ages, the virus is also responsible for respiratory infections (bovine respiratory disease complex, shipping fever) of feedlot cattle [5]. In our study we report the unusual course of a clinically diagnosed WD in a dairy cattle herd of Southern Italy, in which the disease has never been described before. The majority of affected animals showed gastrointestinal disease with bloody diarrhea and mild respiratory symptoms (cough, slight temperature increase, nasal discharge). Among them, 5 displayed a severe respiratory illness, which evolved into death within few days after the occurrence of the first respiratory difficulties. To ascertain the cause of death, animals underwent necroscopy and organs were analyzed to investigate the presence of possible bacterial and viral pathogens respectively by cultural and molecular methods.

2. Materials and Methods

2.1. Outbreak Description

The herd consisted of a total population of 52 Italian Friesian cows, 29 of which in lactation. Cattle were housed under a single canopy and separated into production groups with feeders on the central corridor and drinking bowls inside each paddock. The production system was characterized by internal recovery. No movements or purchases occurred in the three years before the occurrence of the WD outbreak. At the beginning of January 2020 most of the lactating cows, all vaccinated against bovine alpha-herpesvirus 1 (BoHV-1) and bovine viral diarrhea virus (BVD), began to experience symptoms of disease clinically diagnosed as WD. In details, 25 lactating cows (86%) showed bloody diarrhea and a decrease in milk production up to two thirds. Dry cows and juveniles showed no symptoms. After about 2days, the majority of cows with diarrhea exhibited respiratory symptoms, with cough and catarrhal secretion, dyspnea and moderate febrile rise (rectal temperature, 39.2–40.5 °C). In 5 of them, the symptoms worsened with manifestation of subcutaneous emphysema and pneumothorax. In particular two four months pregnant lactating cows (about 4 years old) began to show mild respiratory symptoms which rapidly aggravated becoming severe and one died in 24 h. The other one died the next day. Initially, only symptomatic treatments (ensure clean water and add dry feed) were prescribed but, after the death of the first cow, antibiotics and corticosteroids were administered to the other animals. Despite the pharmaceutical treatments, 3 more animals, (about 7 years old), died after the appearance of the same respiratory symptoms. About ten days later, respiratory and gastrointestinal symptoms of the other animals started to regress. Dead animals underwent necropsy to investigate the cause of death and organs, together with fecal material, were analyzed for the presence of bacterial, viral and parasite pathogens.

2.2. Histopathological Analysis

Tissues of the organs were fixed in 10% neutral phosphate-buffered formalin and processed by routine methods into paraffin blocks which were cut into 3–4 μm thick sections and stained with hematoxylin and eosin.

2.3. Bacteriological and Parasitological Analysis

Lungs, liver, kidneys, spleen, meseraic and supramammary lymphnodes as well as cephalorachid fluid of the first two dead cows were tested by bacterial culture methods to investigate the presence of bacterial pathogens possibly associated with the disease and the death. Briefly, samples were inoculated on both MacConkey agar no. 3 (CM0115 Oxoid, Thermo Fisher Scientific, Waltham, MA, USA) plates and blood agar (7% *v*/*v* ovine blood in blood agar base, CM0271 Oxoid, Thermo Fisher Scientific, Waltham, MA, USA) plates. MacConkey agar plates were incubated at 37 °C for 48 h, while blood agar plates were incubated at 37 °C for up to 72 h in presence/absence of 5% CO_2. The presence of *Mycoplasma* spp. was investigated in lungs and kidneys following OIE terrestrial manual 2018 (Chapter 3.4.8) protocol. In brief: samples were grinded in broth and inoculated both undiluted onto five solid media plates (*Mycoplasma* agar) and diluted 1:10 into five tubesof broth (*Mycoplasma* broth). Plates and tubes were incubated at 37 °C in a 5%CO_2 atmosphere and were inspected daily for 21 days. All the suspected colonies, isolated by microbiological methods as above described, underwent species confirmation by taxonomic identification through MicroSEQ® rapid microbial identification system (Thermo Fisher Scientific, Waltham, MA, USA), which is based on the 16s rRNA gene sequencing.

Fecal material collected during the disease state was analyzed for the presence of helminth eggs and coccidia oocysts by routine methods.

2.4. Viral Nucleic Acids Extraction Procedures

Samples (25 mg of tissue in 1 mL Phosphate buffered saline solution) from lungs, liver, kidneys, spleen, mediastinal lymphnodes, placenta, foetus and intestine content of the two animals were homogenated by Tissue Lyser (Qiagen GmbH—Hilden, Germany). Each organ was analyzed in triplicate, by sampling three different parts of the whole tissue, each one in turn analyzed in triplicate. In particular for the lungs we analyzed three samples from the left cranial lobe. Nucleic acid extraction was carried out from 200 μL of each organ homogenate by using QIAsymphony automated extraction system (Qiagen GmbH, Hilden, Germany) with the DSP Virus/Pathogen Mini kit (Qiagen GmbH, Hilden, Germany) according to the manufacturer's instructions. Nucleic acids were eluted in 60 μL of elution buffer containing 40 unit/μL RNase inhibitor (Promega Corporation, Madison, Wisconsin, USA) and immediately analyzed by Real-time PCR.

2.5. Real Time Virus Identification

DNA viruses like bovine alphaherpesvirus 1 (BoHV-1), bovine alphaherpesvirus 2 (BoHV2), bovine alphaherpesvirus 4 (BoHV4) were investigated by Real-time polymerase chain reaction using Quantitect Real time PCR detection kit (Qiagen GmbH). RNA viruses: bovine coronavirus, (BCoV), bovine viral diarrhea virus (BVDV), border disease virus (BDV), parainfluenza virus 3 (PI3) and respiratory syncytial virus (RSV) were analyzed by Real-time reverse transcription polymerase chain reaction using AGPATH reaction kit (Thermo Fisher Scientific). All the reactions were carried out with primers (Tema Ricerca srl, Castenaso, Bologna, Italy) and probes (Thermo Fisher Scientific) specific for the tested virus on a Quantstudio5 system (Thermo Fisher Scientific) with protocols routinely used in our laboratory. In particular BCoV was identified as described in literature [12], and BCoV positive control was kindly given by Friederich institute (Greifswald, Insel Riems, Germany). Organs were considered positive when at least one sample exhibited a mean threshold cycle (C_t) < 40. Threshold cycle of the positive organ was calculated as an average of the 3 replicates analyzed.

2.6. BCoV Sequencing and Strain Characterization

All the samples positive for bovine coronavirus, as well as the strain isolated by tissue culture were further processed by sequencing analysis to characterize the identified strains. In details, 5 uL of nucleic acids were amplified by a RT-PCR reaction targeting the partial sequence of two genes: a 456 bp fragment of the RNA-dependent RNA polymerase (*RdRp*) gene and a 454 bp fragment of the Nucleocapsid protein gene (*N*). In details RdRp PCR reaction was carried out as indicated in literature [13] with AGPATH reaction kit (Thermo Fisher Scientific), using 1.25 μL of each primer (10 μM) with the following thermal profile: 50 °C for 30 min, 95 °C for 15 min, 45 cycles of 94 °C for 30 s, 50 °C for 30 s, 68 °C for 30 s and a final elongation step of 72 °C for 10 min. RT-PCR reaction for the *N* gene was carried out as reported [14] with 5 uL of nucleic acids using the AGPATH reaction kit (Thermo Fisher Scientific) and 2 μL of each primer (10 μM).The thermal profile was: 42 °C for 30 min, 95 °C for 10 min, 40 cycles of 94 °C for 1 min, 55 °C for 1 min, 72 °C for 1 min and a final elongation step of 72 °C for 7 min. PCR products were analyzed by Tape station (Agilent Technologies—Santa Clara, CA, USA) using the D 1000 kit. Amplicons were sequenced by capillary electrophoresis as previously described [15]. The nucleotide sequence similarity searches were performed using the BLAST server (http://www.ncbi.nlm.nih.gov/genbank/index.html) and phylogenetic analysis was carried out using the Jalview vs. 2.10.5 (www.jalview.org) and MEGA vs. 7.0.26 (www.megasoftware.net) softwares.

2.7. Virus Isolation

Virus isolation was attemptedinHRT18 cells, Vero cells and A72 cells. HRT-18 cells were grown in Dulbecco's modified Eagle's Medium (D-MEM, Gibco, Thermo Fisher Scientific, Waltham, MA, USA), supplemented with 10% fetal bovine serum (FBS, Gibco, Thermo Fisher Scientific, Waltham, MA, USA), 1% antibiotic/antimicotic (Gibco, Thermo Fisher Scientific, Waltham, MA, USA), 1% L-glutamine (Gibco, Thermo Fisher Scientific, Waltham, MA, USA). Vero cells and A72 cells were cultured as above indicated but in MEM. BCoV isolation was carried out in cells cultured in 2% FBS medium. One ml of each organ (positive to BCoV) homogenate was diluted 1:10, filtered and inoculated in cell monolayers. After one hour of adsorption at 37 °C the inoculum was discarded. Cells were incubated at 37 °C and cytopathic effect was daily observed until 5 days after inoculation.

3. Results

3.1. Necroscopy Findings

Of the 52 cows present in the breeding farm, 5 (9.6% of the animals, 17.2% of the lactating cows) died with severe respiratory distress, death occurring 1–4 days after the appearance of the respiratory signs (caught and gasping breath). Anatomo-pathological inspection of the dead cows showed similar lesions in all animals as herein described. We first observed congested explorable mucous membranes and hemorrhagic lymphadenitis of the supra-mammary glands. Jejunum was affected by hemorrhagic enteritis with the rectal ampoule containing little hemorrhagic diarrhoea. There was catarrhal lymphadenitis of the mesenterics. Liver showed increased volume and was characterized by sub-capsular hemorrhages and diffuse centro-lobular necrosis. Moderate splenomegaly with sub capsular extravasations at the visceral surface was observed. Kidneys showed red infarcts involving cortical and medullar tissues (Figure 1A). Foetus of around 4 months old was characterized by diffuse subcutaneous hemorrhages. With respect to thoracic cavity we observed diffuse fibrinous-hemorrhagic pleurisy; thymus was studded with hemorrhages. Respiratory apparatus showed severe tracheo-bronchitis and muco-hemorrhagic bronchiolitis with the deposition of fibrin casts. Lungs (Figure 1B) were characterized by diffuse fibrinous pleurisy, emphysematous interstitial pneumonia and hemorrhagic mediastinal lymphadenitis. The heart, in diastole, revealed hemorrhages of the epicardium along the coronary and ventricular endocardium, thinning of the right ventricular wall and thickening of the left, with heart basis showing fibrinous epicarditis.

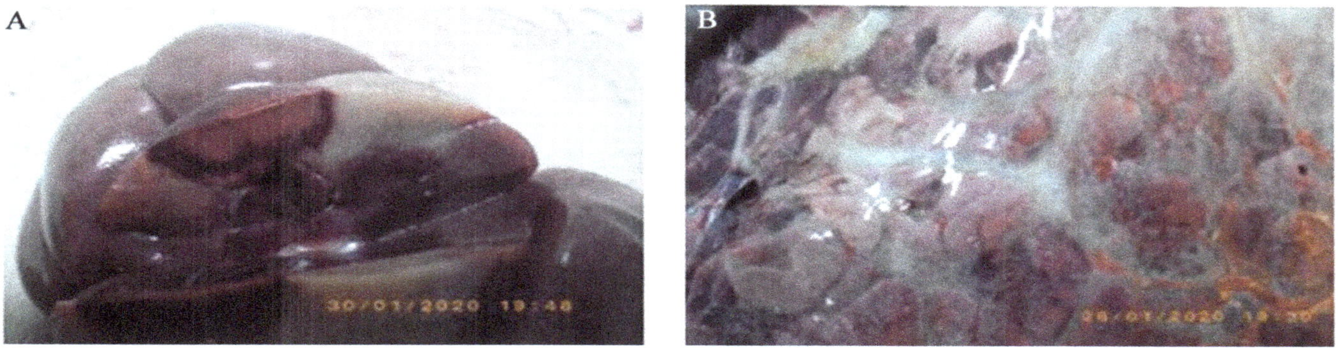

Figure 1. (**A**) Kidney showing infarcts involving cortical and medullary tissue. (**B**) Lung with diffuse fibrinous pleurisy and emphysematous interstitial pneumonia.

3.2. Histopathology

Microscopic examination of the lungs (Figure 2A,B) demonstrated pleural thickening and fibrin mixed with extra-pleural exudates with prevalent inflammatory population of neutrophils. It was observed the presence of areas of sub-pleural emphysema and alveolar rupture with accumulation of dense eosinophilic material as well as multifocal inflammatory thickening of the pulmonary interstitium with a clear prevalence of foamy macrophages, lymphocytes and plasma cells. Lympho-plasmacellular vasculitis and thrombosis were also described. The bronchial and bronchiolar lumen showed accumulation of dense material and cellular debris mixed with macrophages and lymphocytes. Moderate hyperplasia of the bronchiole-associated lymphoid tissue (BALT) was visible.

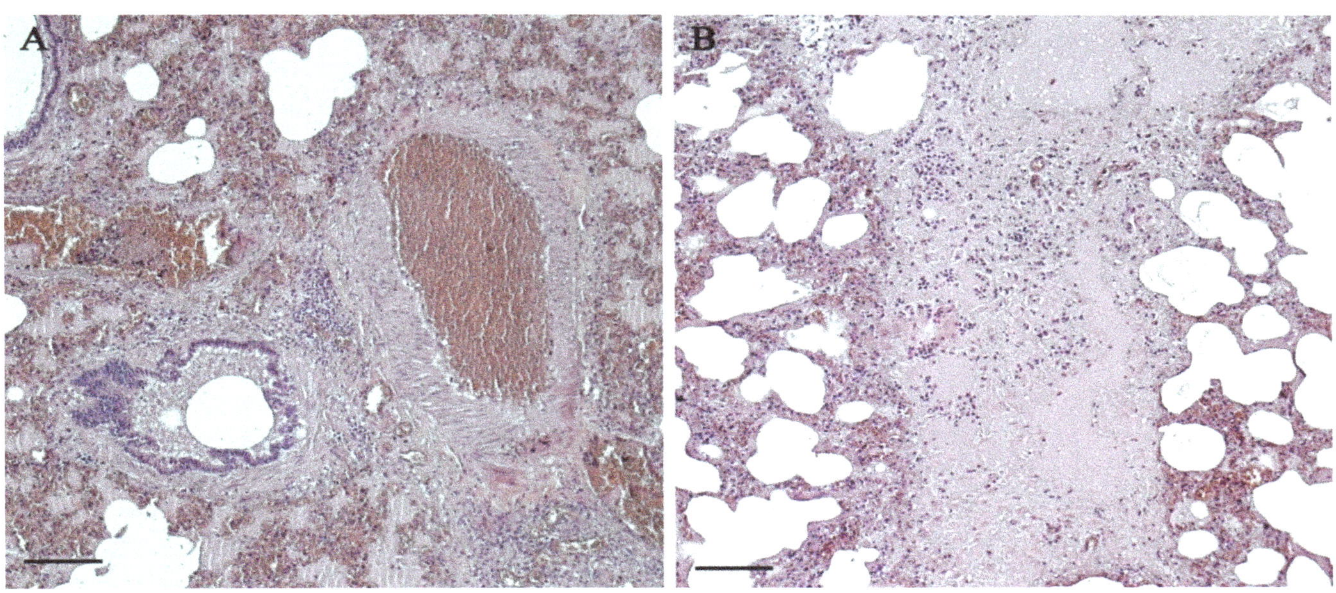

Figure 2. Histopathological observation of the lungs (10× magnification field). (**A**): vascular thrombosis, lympho-plasmacellular vasculitis and oedema. (**B**): interstitial pneumonia, oedema, fibrosis.

Sporadic multinucleated syncytial cells in the peri-bronchial site were identified. Ischemic necrosis of a thrombotic nature from vasculitis, characterized by the presence of fibrin, lymphocytes, plasma cells and rare granulocytes, was found in the liver, spleen, kidney (Figure 3A), thymus (Figure 3B) and skin of the fetus. Jejunum presented tissue disruption and morpho-structural alteration of the villi. Lymphocytes and granulocytes with a clear prevalence of eosinophils were mainly represented to mediate the inflammatory process into lamina propria and interstitium of mucosa.

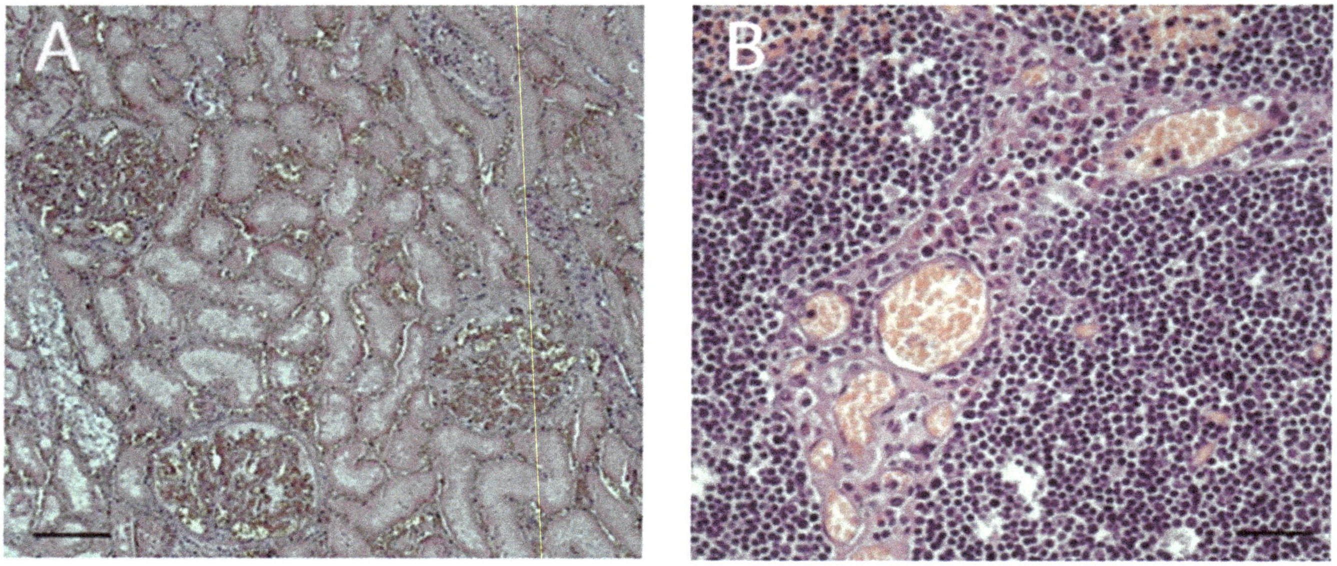

Figure 3. Histopathological observation of (**A**): kidney (10× magnification field) with glomerular thrombosis, tubular ischemic necrosis and interstitial congestion; (**B**) thymus (40× magnification field) characterized by vasculitis and ischemic necrosis.

3.3. Microbiology and Virology

Microbiological analysis revealed absence of pathogenic bacteria in all the analyzed organs. No parasites were recognized in the fecal material. Real time PCR carried out on the organs of the animals gave negative results for all the herpesviruses investigated as well for: BVDV, BDV and PI3. The only pathogen identified was BCoV, that was detected in: lungs, small intestine (jejunum), mediastinal lymph nodes, liver and placenta. Foetal thymus, kidney and spleen were negative for the virus. Among the positive organs, lungs showed a very high signal of fluorescence in both the cows analyzed, with a mean threshold cycle (C_t) of 19.8 and 20.2, respectively. The other organs displayed instead a mean C_t value ranging from 25 to 32. Virus was successfully isolated from lungs and jejunum on both A72 and Vero cells. Cells showed cytopatic effect after 4 days of culturing and isolates were considered positive when presenting the effect until the fourth serial passage. Isolated strains were confirmed as BCoV by both Real time PCR and sequencing.

3.4. Sequencing Analysis of BCoV

All the bovine coronavirus sequences directly obtained from the positive organs (lungs, jejunum, lymphnodes, liver and placenta) as well as those obtained from the virus isolated in cell culture were aligned and compared by Jaleview analysis software. All the sequences resulted identical to each other with respect to the two gene fragments investigated. Further phylogenetic analysis of the BCoV identified (partial *RdRp* gene, Genbank accession number, AC: MT602514) revealed (Figure 4), the highest homology (99%) with only one base substitution (C instead of A), with two bovine strains isolated in France from diarrheic fecal samples in 2013 (AC: KT318104) and 2014 (AC: KX982264), respectively. Among the bovine coronaviruses, our strain was also closely related (two nucleotides of difference) to a BCoV identified from a nasal swab pool in France in 2014 (MG757141.1), a BCoV isolated in India in 2015 from feces, and two BCoVs (one respiratory and one enteric) isolated in USA in 1996 and 2002, respectively. Among the non-bovine CoVs, the highest homology was shown with a bovine-like CoV isolated from an alpaca in USA in 2007, with a CoV isolated in a camel in the United

Arab Emirates in 2017 and with a human enteric coronavirus 4408 (FJ415324) collected in 1988 from a patient in Germany.

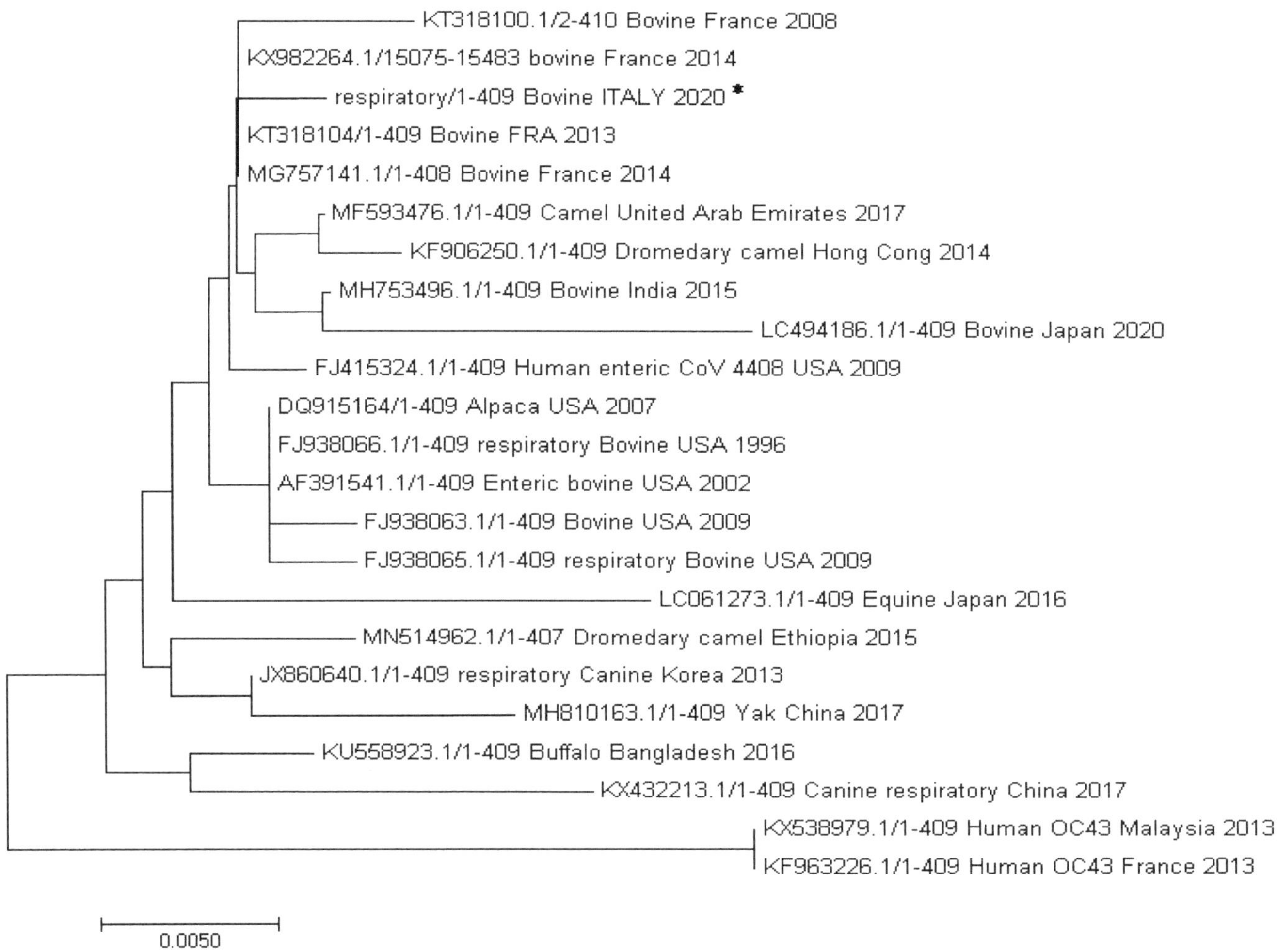

Figure 4. Analysis of a part of the *RdRp* gene (409 bp). The evolutionary history was inferred using the Neighbor-Joining method [16]. The optimal tree with the sum of branch length = 0.10942734 is shown. The evolutionary distances were computed using the Poisson correction method and are in the units of the number of amino acid substitutions per site. Evolutionary analyses were conducted in MEGA7 [17]. Sequence obtained in the present study (Bovine ITALY 2020) is indicated with an asterisk.

With respect to gene N (Figure 5), our sequence (GenBank accession MW074864) showed the highest homology (99%), with an enteric strain isolated from a bovine in France in 2013 (AC: KT318090.1), with only one base substitution (A instead of C).Among the bovine coronaviruses, our BCoV was also closely related (two nucleotides of difference) to two BCoVs identified in cows in France in 2014 respectively from deep nasal swabs and from bronchoalveolar lavages [18]. These samples were collected from herds affected with respiratory disease in the south-east of France from calves with acute signs of pneumonia. Among the non-bovine CoVs, the highest homology was shown with a dromedary camel CoV isolated in Ethiopia in 2015 and, like for the *RdRp* gene, with a human enteric coronavirus 4408 (FJ415324) collected in 1988 from a patient in Germany from which our sequence differs for 3 nucleotides.

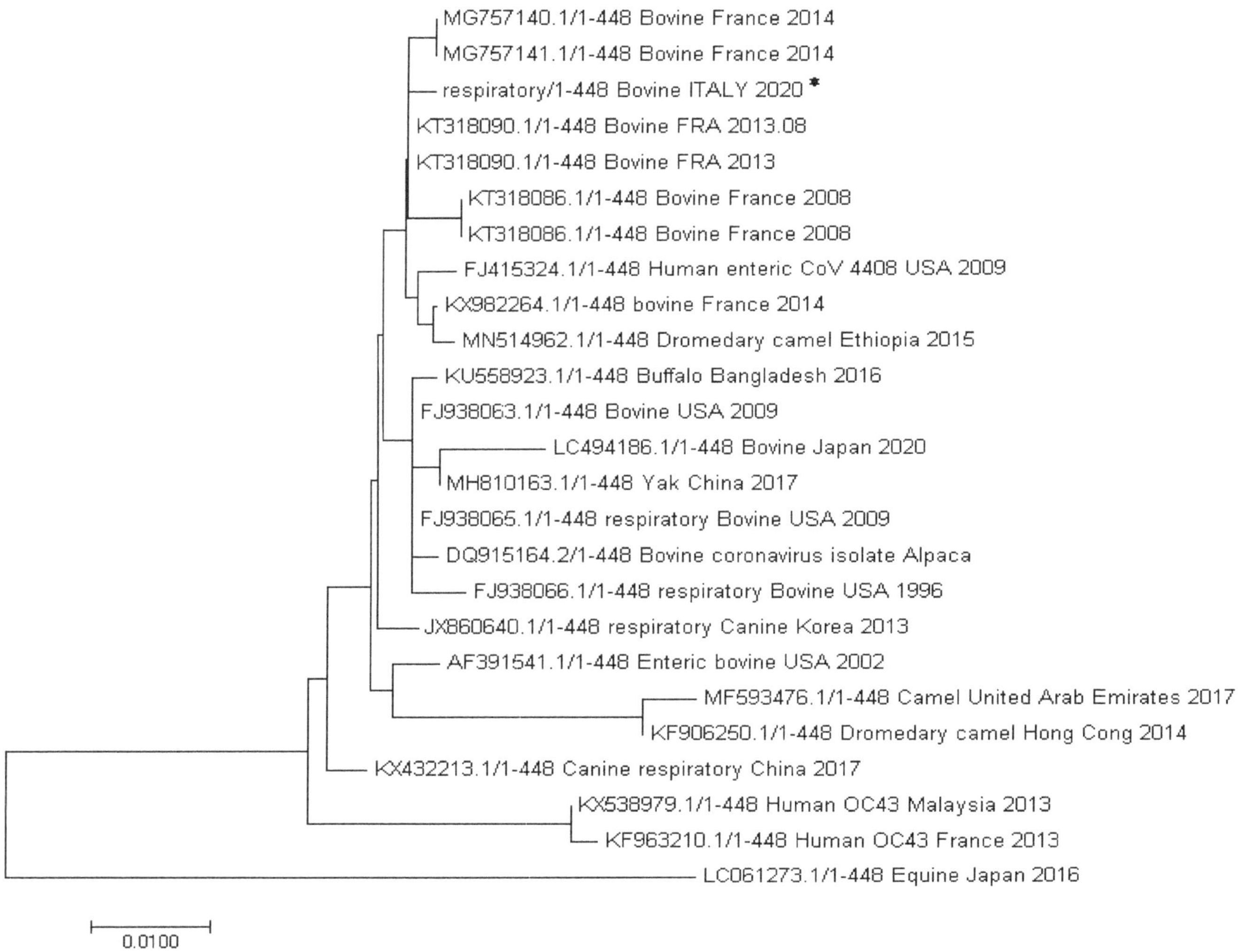

Figure 5. Phylogenetic analysis of a part of the *N* gene (454 bp). The evolutionary history was inferred using the Neighbor-Joining method [16]. The optimal tree with the sum of branch length = 0.10942734 is shown. The evolutionary distances were computed using the Poisson correction method and are in the units of the number of amino acid substitutions per site. Evolutionary analyses were conducted in MEGA7 [17]. Sequence obtained in the present study (Bovine ITALY 2020) is indicated with an asterisk.

4. Discussion

In our study we described a severe pulmonary infection, causing death in 5 animals from a high genealogy Friesian dairy cows breeding. The infection involved 48% of the animals (almost all the lactating cows), mostly exhibiting gastrointestinal and mild respiratory symptoms. Among infected animals, 20% (5 out of 25) experienced a stronger form of the disease, leading to death in a few days after the beginning of respiratory symptoms. In the samples analyzed we failed to identify any bacteria and virus typically responsible for pneumonia in bovines. The only pathogen found was BCoV. For this reason, the involvement of this virus in the fatal pneumonia was hypothesized, even though it was not possible to definitively conclude whether it was the primary cause of the disease or represented a secondary infection aggravating the symptoms.

With respect to BCoV role in the pneumonia herein described, as a matter of fact while the involvement of BCoV in enteric infections is well known, its role in bovine respiratory disease is controversial and principally related to mild respiratory symptoms. The virus has been indeed found in respiratory samples from both healthy and sick cattle [11,19–23] and more frequently identified in association with other respiratory pathogens [11,20,24–26]. Only few papers reported instead BCoVas the only recognized cause of the disease [9,24,27]. Furthermore, there are various studies in literature describing attempts to induce clinical respiratory symptoms by infecting healthy cattle with BCoV. Most experiments reported no respiratory symptoms development, with, in some cases the occurrence of gastrointestinal disease [28–31], while only few studies describe slight respiratory problems [32,33]. Our results seem to corroborate the role of this virus in respiratory outbreaks and to point out the ability of the virus to induce, in the same animal or within the same outbreak, both enteric and respiratory symptoms, confirming what already reported by Choulienko et al. [34]. With respect to the 5 fatal pneumonia cases, the observed exacerbation of the respiratory disease in these animals, resembling what happens for other severe coronavirus syndromes (like those caused by SARS, MERS, COVID-19), could be related to various co-factors including: immunosuppression (due to corticosteroids treatment), individual host susceptibility, co-morbidities, physical stresses [5]. Moreover, since through recombination events CoVs are able to gain novel biological properties, including an increased pathogenicity [1] we could also hypothesize the identification of a more pathogenic variant of bovine coronavirus, with acquired ability to cause fatal pneumonia in susceptible hosts. Interestingly, among the BCoV nucleotide sequence data available in GenBank to which our strain was compared, we observed close similarity, (with respect to *RdRp* and *N* genes) to sequences obtained from cows in France in 2014 [18].

These animals all exhibited acute signs of pneumonia but for all of them it was described a co-infecting bacterial or viral agent. In our case we failed to detect any other pathogen and could thus address the disease only to BCoV. With respect to bacteria, isolation can be compromised by antibiotic treatments which are usually prescribed too fast (at first respiratory symptoms appearance) by veterinarians. In our case, since the farm veterinary diagnosed the outbreak as WD, animals were not treated with antibiotics until the first death. We cannot completely exclude however that the breeder was autonomously already giving drugs to the symptomatic cows. Further studies including full genome sequencing and experimental infections should be done to better characterize the strain of BCoV and to shed light on its likely real ability to cause severe pneumonia like the one we herein described.

Many bovine-like CoVs have been indeed identified as enteric and/or respiratory pathogens in both livestock and wildlife species (wild ruminants, captive ruminants as well as water buffalo, camelids) [5,10,35–39]. With respect to the possibility of BCoV-like viruses to infect humans, in literature it has been described a case of child acute enteritis caused by a human CoV found genetically and antigenetically more closely related to BCoV than to HCoV-OC43 [40]. Moreover HCoV-OC43 has been supposed to derive from an ancestral BCoV strain (considering their close genetic and antigenic similarity) which skipped the species barrier and passed from rodents to humans through cattle [41–43]. Interestingly, phylogenetic analysis showed that our strain, with respect to the analyzed part of *RdRp* gene, was very closely related to an enteric HCoV-4408 described in a patient in Germany (see Figures 4 and 5). Interspecies transmission via wildlife and livestock host animals are key factors for the emerging of new, highly pathogenic, human coronaviruses. For this reason, it is of utmost importance to focus on and carefully investigate the outbreaks in which animal coronaviruses are involved, with particular regard to clinical symptoms and genetic classification. Finally, in the case of BCoVs, it is necessary to recommend the farmers to strictly follow all the protection and prevention biosafety measures necessary to limit the spread of such viruses among animals and to avoid any possible human contamination.

Author Contributions: Conceptualization, M.G.A., G.L., A.D.D., G.G. and G.F.; data curation, G.L. and G.B.; formal analysis, G.L., B.D.U., F.S., G.D.L., A.D.D., S.B., M.C.C., F.B. and M.G.R.; funding acquisition, G.F.; investigation, M.G.A. and G.F.; methodology, M.G.A. and G.B.; supervision, M.G.A, G.L., G.G. and G.F.; writing—original draft, M.G.A., G.L., B.D.U. and G.G. All authors have read and agreed to the published version of the manuscript.

References

1. Decaro, N.; Lorusso, A. Novel Human Coronavirus (SARS-CoV-2): A Lesson from Animal Coronaviruses. *Vet. Microbiol.* **2020**, *244*, 108693. [CrossRef] [PubMed]
2. Amer, H.M. Bovine-Like Coronaviruses in Domestic and Wild Ruminants. *Anim. Health Res. Rev.* **2018**, *19*, 113–124. [CrossRef] [PubMed]
3. Abdel-Moneim, A.S.; Abdelwhab, E.M. Evidence for SARS-CoV-2 Infection of Animal Hosts. *Pathogens* **2020**, *9*, 529. [CrossRef] [PubMed]
4. Saif, L.J. Animal Coronaviruses: What can they Teach Us about the Severe Acute Respiratory Syndrome? *Rev. Sci. Tech.* **2004**, *23*, 643–660. [CrossRef] [PubMed]
5. Saif, L.J.; Jung, K. Comparative Pathogenesis of Bovine and Porcine Respiratory Coronaviruses in the Animal Host Species and SARS-CoV-2 in Humans. *J. Clin. Microbiol.* **2020**, *58*. [CrossRef]
6. Stavrinides, J.; Guttman, D.S. Mosaic Evolution of the Severe Acute Respiratory Syndrome Coronavirus. *J. Virol.* **2004**, *78*, 76–82. [CrossRef]
7. Hon, C.C.; Lam, T.Y.; Shi, Z.L.; Drummond, A.J.; Yip, C.W.; Zeng, F.; Lam, P.Y.; Leung, F.C. Evidence of the Recombinant Origin of a Bat Severe Acute Respiratory Syndrome (SARS)-Like Coronavirus and its Implications on the Direct Ancestor of SARS Coronavirus. *J. Virol.* **2008**, *82*, 1819–1826. [CrossRef]
8. Corman, V.M.; Ithete, N.L.; Richards, L.R.; Schoeman, M.C.; Preiser, W.; Drosten, C.; Drexler, J.F. Rooting the Phylogenetic Tree of Middle East Respiratory Syndrome Coronavirus by Characterization of a Conspecific Virus from an African Bat. *J. Virol.* **2014**, *88*, 11297–11303. [CrossRef]
9. Decaro, N.; Campolo, M.; Desario, C.; Cirone, F.; D'Abramo, M.; Lorusso, E.; Greco, G.; Mari, V.; Colaianni, M.L.; Elia, G.; et al. Respiratory Disease Associated with Bovine Coronavirus Infection in Cattle Herds in Southern Italy. *J. Vet. Diagn. Investig.* **2008**, *20*, 28–32. [CrossRef]
10. Decaro, N.; Martella, V.; Elia, G.; Campolo, M.; Mari, V.; Desario, C.; Lucente, M.S.; Lorusso, A.; Greco, G.; Corrente, M.; et al. Biological and Genetic Analysis of a Bovine-Like Coronavirus Isolated from Water Buffalo (Bubalus Bubalis) Calves. *Virology* **2008**, *370*, 213–222. [CrossRef]
11. Ellis, J. What is the Evidence that Bovine Coronavirus is a Biologically Significant Respiratory Pathogen in Cattle? *Can. Vet. J.* **2019**, *60*, 147–152. [PubMed]
12. Decaro, N.; Elia, G.; Campolo, M.; Desario, C.; Mari, V.; Radogna, A.; Colaianni, M.L.; Cirone, F.; Tempesta, M.; Buonavoglia, C. Detection of Bovine Coronavirus using a TaqMan-Based Real-Time RT-PCR Assay. *J. Virol. Methods* **2008**, *151*, 167–171. [CrossRef] [PubMed]
13. Drosten, C.; Gunther, S.; Preiser, W.; van der Werf, S.; Brodt, H.R.; Becker, S.; Rabenau, H.; Panning, M.; Kolesnikova, L.; Fouchier, R.A.; et al. Identification of a Novel Coronavirus in Patients with Severe Acute Respiratory Syndrome. *N. Engl. J. Med.* **2003**, *348*, 1967–1976. [CrossRef] [PubMed]
14. Takiuchi, E.; Stipp, D.T.; Alfieri, A.F.; Alfieri, A.A. Improved detection of bovine coronavirus N gene in faeces of calves infected naturally by a semi-nested PCR assay and an internal control. *J. Virol. Methods* **2006**, *131*, 148–154. [CrossRef]
15. Amoroso, M.G.; Corrado, F.; De Carlo, E.; Lucibelli, M.G.; Martucciello, A.; Guarino, A.; Galiero, G. Bubaline Herpesvirus 1 Associated with Abortion in a Mediterranean Water Buffalo. *Res. Vet. Sci.* **2013**, *94*, 813–816. [CrossRef]
16. Saitou, N.; Nei, M. The Neighbor-Joining Method: A New Method for Reconstructing Phylogenetic Trees. *Mol. Biol. Evol.* **1987**, *4*, 406–425.
17. Kumar, S.; Stecher, G.; Tamura, K. MEGA7: Molecular Evolutionary Genetics Analysis Version 7.0 for Bigger Datasets. *Mol. Biol. Evol.* **2016**, *33*, 1870–1874. [CrossRef]
18. Salem, E.; Dhanasekaran, V.; Cassard, H.; Hause, B.; Maman, S.; Meyer, G.; Ducatez, M.F. Global transmission, spatial segregation, and recombination determine the long-term evolution and epidemiology of bovine coronaviruses. *Viruses* **2020**, *12*, 534. [CrossRef]
19. Hasoksuz, M.; Lathrop, S.L.; Gadfield, K.L.; Saif, L.J. Isolation of Bovine Respiratory Coronaviruses from Feedlot Cattle and Comparison of their Biological and Antigenic Properties with Bovine Enteric Coronaviruses. *Am. J. Vet. Res.* **1999**, *60*, 1227–1233.

20. Fulton, R.W.; Blood, K.S.; Panciera, R.J.; Payton, M.E.; Ridpath, J.F.; Confer, A.W.; Saliki, J.T.; Burge, L.T.; Welsh, R.D.; Johnson, B.J.; et al. Lung Pathology and Infectious Agents in Fatal Feedlot Pneumonias and Relationship with Mortality, Disease Onset, and Treatments. *J. Vet. Diagn. Investig.* **2009**, *21*, 464–477. [CrossRef]
21. Francoz, D.; Buczinski, S.; Bélanger, A.; Forté, G.; Labrecque, O.; Tremblay, D.; Wellemans, V.; Dubuc, J. Respiratory Pathogens in Quebec Dairy Calves and their Relationship with Clinical Status, Lung Consolidation, and Average Daily Gain. *J. Vet. Intern. Med.* **2015**, *29*, 381–387. [CrossRef] [PubMed]
22. Mitra, N.; Cernicchiaro, N.; Torres, S.; Li, F.; Hause, B.M. Metagenomic Characterization of the Virome Associated with Bovine Respiratory Disease in Feedlot Cattle Identified Novel Viruses and Suggests an Etiologic Role for Influenza D Virus. *J. Gen. Virol.* **2016**, *97*, 1771–1784. [CrossRef] [PubMed]
23. Workman, A.M.; Kuehn, L.A.; McDaneld, T.G.; Clawson, M.L.; Chitko-McKown, C.G.; Loy, J.D. Evaluation of the Effect of Serum Antibody Abundance Against Bovine Coronavirus on Bovine Coronavirus Shedding and Risk of Respiratory Tract Disease in Beef Calves from Birth through the First Five Weeks in a Feedlot. *Am. J. Vet. Res.* **2017**, *78*, 1065–1076. [CrossRef] [PubMed]
24. Storz, J.; Purdy, C.W.; Lin, X.; Burrell, M.; Truax, R.E.; Briggs, R.E.; Frank, G.H.; Loan, R.W. Isolation of Respiratory Bovine Coronavirus, Other Cytocidal Viruses, and Pasteurella Spp from Cattle Involved in Two Natural Outbreaks of Shipping Fever. *J. Am. Vet. Med. Assoc.* **2000**, *216*, 1599–1604. [CrossRef] [PubMed]
25. Cho, K.O.; Hoet, A.E.; Loerch, S.C.; Wittum, T.E.; Saif, L.J. Evaluation of Concurrent Shedding of Bovine Coronavirus Via the Respiratory Tract and Enteric Route in Feedlot Cattle. *Am. J. Vet. Res.* **2001**, *62*, 1436–1441. [CrossRef]
26. Fulton, R.W.; d'Offay, J.M.; Landis, C.; Miles, D.G.; Smith, R.A.; Saliki, J.T.; Ridpath, J.F.; Confer, A.W.; Neill, J.D.; Eberle, R.; et al. Detection and Characterization of Viruses as Field and Vaccine Strains in Feedlot Cattle with Bovine Respiratory Disease. *Vaccine* **2016**, *34*, 3478–3492. [CrossRef]
27. Fulton, R.W.; Step, D.L.; Wahrmund, J.; Burge, L.J.; Payton, M.E.; Cook, B.J.; Burken, D.; Richards, C.J.; Confer, A.W. Bovine Coronavirus (BCV) Infections in Transported Commingled Beef Cattle and Sole-Source Ranch Calves. *Can. J. Vet. Res.* **2011**, *75*, 191–199.
28. Reynolds, D.J.; Debney, T.G.; Hall, G.A.; Thomas, L.H.; Parsons, K.R. Studies on the Relationship between Coronaviruses from the Intestinal and Respiratory Tracts of Calves. *Arch. Virol.* **1985**, *85*, 71–83. [CrossRef]
29. Saif, L.J.; Redman, D.R.; Moorhead, P.D.; Theil, K.W. Experimentally Induced Coronavirus Infections in Calves: Viral Replication in the Respiratory and Intestinal Tracts. *Am. J. Vet. Res.* **1986**, *47*, 1426–1432.
30. Cho, K.O.; Hasoksuz, M.; Nielsen, P.R.; Chang, K.O.; Lathrop, S.; Saif, L.J. Cross-Protection Studies between Respiratory and Calf Diarrhea and Winter Dysentery Coronavirus Strains in Calves and RT-PCR and Nested PCR for their Detection. *Arch. Virol.* **2001**, *146*, 2401–2419. [CrossRef]
31. Park, S.J.; Kim, G.Y.; Choy, H.E.; Hong, Y.J.; Saif, L.J.; Jeong, J.H.; Park, S.I.; Kim, H.H.; Kim, S.K.; Shin, S.S.; et al. Dual Enteric and Respiratory Tropisms of Winter Dysentery Bovine Coronavirus in Calves. *Arch. Virol.* **2007**, *152*, 1885–1900. [CrossRef] [PubMed]
32. McNulty, M.S.; Bryson, D.G.; Allan, G.M.; Logan, E.F. Coronavirus Infection of the Bovine Respiratory Tract. *Vet. Microbiol.* **1984**, *9*, 425–434. [CrossRef]
33. Kapil, S.; Trent, A.M.; Goyal, S.M. Excretion and Persistence of Bovine Coronavirus in Neonatal Calves. *Arch. Virol.* **1990**, *115*, 127–132. [CrossRef] [PubMed]
34. Chouljenko, V.N.; Lin, X.Q.; Storz, J.; Kousoulas, K.G.; Gorbalenya, A.E. Comparison of Genomic and Predicted Amino Acid Sequences of Respiratory and Enteric Bovine Coronaviruses Isolated from the Same Animal with Fatal Shipping Pneumonia. *J. Gen. Virol.* **2001**, *82*, 2927–2933. [CrossRef]
35. Tsunemitsu, H.; el-Kanawati, Z.R.; Smith, D.R.; Reed, H.H.; Saif, L.J. Isolation of Coronaviruses Antigenically Indistinguishable from Bovine Coronavirus from Wild Ruminants with Diarrhea. *J. Clin. Microbiol.* **1995**, *33*, 3264–3269. [CrossRef]
36. Zhong, N.S.; Wong, G.W. Epidemiology of Severe Acute Respiratory Syndrome (SARS): Adults and Children. *Paediatr. Respir. Rev.* **2004**, *5*, 270–274. [CrossRef]
37. Decaro, N.; Desario, C.; Elia, G.; Mari, V.; Lucente, M.S.; Cordioli, P.; Colaianni, M.L.; Martella, V.; Buonavoglia, C. Serological and Molecular Evidence that Canine Respiratory Coronavirus is Circulating in Italy. *Vet. Microbiol.* **2007**, *121*, 225–230. [CrossRef]

38. Lorusso, A.; Desario, C.; Mari, V.; Campolo, M.; Lorusso, E.; Elia, G.; Martella, V.; Buonavoglia, C.; Decaro, N. Molecular Characterization of a Canine Respiratory Coronavirus Strain Detected in Italy. *Virus Res.* **2009**, *141*, 96–100. [CrossRef]
39. Woo, P.C.; Lau, S.K.; Wernery, U.; Wong, E.Y.; Tsang, A.K.; Johnson, B.; Yip, C.C.; Lau, C.C.; Sivakumar, S.; Cai, J.P.; et al. Novel Betacoronavirus in Dromedaries of the Middle East, 2013. *Emerg. Infect. Dis.* **2014**, *20*, 560–572. [CrossRef]
40. Zhang, X.M.; Herbst, W.; Kousoulas, K.G.; Storz, J. Biological and Genetic Characterization of a Hemagglutinating Coronavirus Isolated from a Diarrhoeic Child. *J. Med. Virol.* **1994**, *44*, 152–161. [CrossRef]
41. Vijgen, L.; Keyaerts, E.; Moes, E.; Thoelen, I.; Wollants, E.; Lemey, P.; Vandamme, A.M.; Van Ranst, M. Complete Genomic Sequence of Human Coronavirus OC43: Molecular Clock Analysis Suggests a Relatively Recent Zoonotic Coronavirus Transmission Event. *J. Virol.* **2005**, *79*, 1595–1604. [CrossRef] [PubMed]
42. Vijgen, L.; Keyaerts, E.; Lemey, P.; Maes, P.; Van Reeth, K.; Nauwynck, H.; Pensaert, M.; Van Ranst, M. Evolutionary History of the Closely Related Group 2 Coronaviruses: Porcine Hemagglutinating Encephalomyelitis Virus, Bovine Coronavirus, and Human Coronavirus OC43. *J. Virol.* **2006**, *80*, 7270–7274. [CrossRef] [PubMed]
43. Forni, D.; Cagliani, R.; Clerici, M.; Sironi, M. Molecular Evolution of Human Coronavirus Genomes. *Trends Microbiol.* **2017**, *25*, 35–48. [CrossRef] [PubMed]

4

Real Time Analysis of Bovine Viral Diarrhea Virus (BVDV) Infection and its Dependence on Bovine CD46

Christiane Riedel [1,*], Hann-Wei Chen [1], Ursula Reichart [2], Benjamin Lamp [3], Vibor Laketa [4,5] and Till Rümenapf [1]

1 Institute of Virology, Vetmeduni Vienna, 1210 Vienna, Austria; Hann-Wei.Chen@vetmeduni.ac.at (H.-W.C.); Till.Ruemenapf@vetmeduni.ac.at (T.R.)
2 VetCore Facility for Research, Vetmeduni Vienna, 1210 Vienna, Austria; ursula.reichart@vetmeduni.ac.at
3 Institute of Virology, Faculty of Veterinary Medicine, Justus-Liebig University, 35392 Gießen, Germany; Benjamin.J.Lamp@vetmed.uni-giessen.de
4 Department of Infectious Diseases, Virology, University of Heidelberg, 69120 Heidelberg, Germany; vibor.laketa@med.uni-heidelberg.de
5 German Center for Infection Research, 69120 Heidelberg, Germany
* Correspondence: christiane.riedel@vetmeduni.ac.at

Abstract: Virus attachment and entry is a complex interplay of viral and cellular interaction partners. Employing bovine viral diarrhea virus (BVDV) encoding an mCherry-E2 fusion protein ($BVDV_{E2\text{-}mCherry}$), being the first genetically labelled member of the family *Flaviviridae* applicable for the analysis of virus particles, the early events of infection—attachment, particle surface transport, and endocytosis—were monitored to better understand the mechanisms underlying virus entry and their dependence on the virus receptor, bovine CD46. The analysis of 801 tracks on the surface of SK6 cells inducibly expressing fluorophore labelled bovine CD46 ($CD46_{fluo}$) demonstrated the presence of directed, diffusive, and confined motion. 26 entry events could be identified, with the majority being associated with a $CD46_{fluo}$ positive structure during endocytosis and occurring more than 20 min after virus addition. Deletion of the $CD46_{fluo}$ E2 binding domain ($CD46_{fluo}\Delta$E2bind) did not affect the types of motions observed on the cell surface but resulted in a decreased number of observable entry events (2 out of 1081 tracks). Mean squared displacement analysis revealed a significantly increased velocity of particle transport for directed motions on $CD46_{fluo}\Delta$E2bind expressing cells in comparison to $CD46_{fluo}$. These results indicate that the presence of bovine CD46 is only affecting the speed of directed transport, but otherwise not influencing BVDV cell surface motility. Instead, bovine CD46 seems to be an important factor during uptake, suggesting the presence of additional cellular proteins interacting with the virus which are able to support its transport on the virus surface.

Keywords: *Pestivirus*; BVDV; CD46; life cell imaging; attachment; surface transport

---

1. Introduction

Before entering a host cell, viruses have to establish contact with the cell and travel to sites that are suitable for entry. This process of attachment can involve different receptor molecules and transport mechanisms, which can be classified into diffusion, drifts, and confinement [1]. Diffusive motion can be caused by interaction of viruses with a number of receptor molecules that is too low to cause confinement or can support the screening of the cell surface for suitable sites of endocytosis. Directed motion is the result of interaction of the virus with cellular proteins or lipid structures that are linked to F-actin. Understanding the extracellular movement of virus particles, as well as the kinetics of entry and protein expression, provides important insights into the key players involved in attachment and entry and in infection dynamics in general.

For the family *Retroviridae*—facilitated by the ease of generation of genetically labelled virus particles—attachment and entry dynamics have been studied excessively. Virus surfing—the directed, actin-dependent transport of virus particles on the outside of filopodia, cytonemes, and retraction fibres—was also discovered employing a member of the *Retroviridae*, namely murine leukemia virus (MLV) [2]. This mode of extracellular, directed transport has since been described for members of the *Adenoviridae* [1], *Herpesviridae* [3], and *Papillomaviridae* [4].

For the medically relevant family *Flaviviridae*, the lack of genetically labelled virus particles has been overcome by the utilization of lipophilic dyes or covalently linked fluorophores [5–8]. These studies demonstrated the diffusive movement of dengue virus along the cell surface to clathrin coated pits and the subsequent association with specific markers of endocytosis [8] and helped in the identification of T cell immunoglobulin mucin-1 as a dengue virus receptor [9]. Also, labelled hepatitis C virus (HCV) particles demonstrated the involvement of actin in cell surface and intracellular virus transport [7].

The genus *Pestivirus* is also part of the *Flaviviridae* and characterized by the presence of three viral surface glycoproteins—E^{rns}, E1, and E2—and an additional N-terminal protease, N^{pro}. Members of this genus are pathogens of cloven-hoofed animals, including the highly economically relevant pathogens bovine viral diarrhea virus (BVDV) and classical swine fever virus (CSFV). In recent years, genetically labelled BVDV and CSFV clones have been constructed based on N-terminal fusion of luciferase or fluorophores to either E^{rns} or E2 [10–13]. For a BVDV E2-fluorophore fusion protein, visualization of purified particles in fluorescence microscopy based on the specific fluorescence signal has been reported [13]. BVDV enters host cells after initial interactions of E^{rns} with heparan sulphates [14] and subsequent binding of E2 to its cellular receptor, bovine CD46 [15,16], by clathrin mediated endocytosis [17,18] and fusion occurs after endosomal acidification [18,19]. Interestingly, recent evidence implies that BVDV is preferably transmitted by direct cell-to-cell spread in a CD46 independent manner [12], indicating the involvement of additional factors in BVDV spread. The BVDV-1 clone employed in [12] also encodes for an mCherry-E2 fusion protein, in the backbone of strain NADL, demonstrating the utilization of different transmission modes in the presence of an E2-fusion protein.

Bovine CD46 is an ubiquitously expressed, type I transmembrane glycoprotein and exists as different splice variants, affecting the length of its heavily O-glycosylated, membrane proximal regions (STP) and its cytoplasmic C-terminus. The membrane distal, extracellular part of the protein consists of four complement control protein modules (CCP) which have been implicated in the binding of a variety of pathogens, leading to its description as a "pathogens magnet" [20]. Physiologically, CD46 is a cofactor of the inactivation of complement components C3b and C4b and also involved in T cell regulation, modulation of autophagy and reproductive biology (reviewed in [21]). Its surface levels are regulated by clathrin-dependent endocytosis [21] or micropinocytosis after cross-linking [22]. BVDV E2 binding to CD46 is mediated by the 30 C-terminal amino acids of CCP-1 [16]. Interestingly, CD46's physiological ligands mainly interact with the membrane proximal CCPs 3–4, while pathogens mostly interact with the membrane distal CCPs 1–2 [23].

While the function of bovine CD46 as a receptor for BVDV is well documented in the literature, it is currently unclear what its exact functions are during virus attachment and entry. Also, it has been shown that bovine CD46 is not sufficient for entry. To determine which stages of the entry process—attachment, surface motion, or uptake—are affected by CD46, we conducted life cell imaging experiments employing purified, fluorophore-E2 labelled BVDV particles and SK6 cell lines inducibly expressing fluorophore labelled CD46 with and without the virus interacting CCP-1 module [16].

2. Materials and Methods

2.1. Viruses and Cells

For propagation, cells were cultured in DMEM (Capricorn, Ebsdorfergrund, Germany) supplemented with 10% FCS (Bio & Sell, Feucht/Nürnberg, Germany) and penicillin/streptomycin (Merck, Darmstadt, Germany) at 37 °C, 5% CO_2. SK6 tet-on cells inducibly expressing bovine CD46 labelled with mCherry or mClover ($CD46_{fluo}$) have been described in [13]. The E2 binding CCP of CD46—as reported by [16]—was deleted by PCR (Vazyme Biotech, Nanjing, China) in the previously described $CD46_{fluo}$-encoding construct employing the following primers (Eurofins, Ebersberg, Germany): forward: cgaCGGTGTCCTACCCTAGCTGATC; reverse: GGCATCGGAGGACGTGGGCAG, resulting in $CD46_{fluo}\Delta$E2bind. SK6 tet-on cells were transfected with $CD46_{fluo}\Delta$E2bind by electroporation and clonally selected as described in [13].

For the determination of susceptibility of SK6 $CD46_{fluo}$ or $CD46_{fluo}\Delta$E2bind cells to $BVDV_{E2\text{-}mCherry}$, 2×10^5 MDBK, SK6 $CD46_{fluo}$ or $CD46_{fluo}\Delta$E2bind cells or SK6 cells inducibly expressing GFP were seeded in each well of a 24-well plate 24 h before the start of the experiment. SK6 cells are of porcine origin and porcine CD46 is not a receptor for BVDV [16]. Cells were induced 16 h before infection with 2.5 μg/mL doxycycline (Merck, Darmstadt, Germany). Cells were infected with ten-fold dilutions of a BVDV-1 strain expressing mCherry fused to the N-terminus of E2 ($BVDV_{E2\text{-}mCherry}$) [13] for 4h. Thereafter, medium was exchanged to medium containing 1% carboxymethylcellulose to prevent virus transfer via the culture medium. 48 h after infection, infected foci were quantified by fluorescence microscopy (Olympus IX-70, Tokyo, Japan) to determine the titer and the susceptibility was calculated in % by dividing the titer determined on a given cell line through the titer determined on MDBK cells. $BVDV_{E2\text{-}mCherry}$ was propagated on MDBK cells in 5-layer tissue culture flasks (Corning, Corning, NY, USA) and purified and concentrated as described in [13]. The sequence of the plasmid encoding the full sequence of $BVDV_{E2\text{-}mCherry}$ is provided as supplementary data.

For life cell imaging, 2×10^4 SK6 $CD46_{fluo}$ or $CD46_{fluo}\Delta$E2bind cells were seeded in each well of an IBIDI μ slide 8 well chamber slide 24 h before the start of the experiment in medium devoid of phenol red. 16 h before the start of the experiment, expression of $CD46_{fluo}$ or $CD46_{fluo}\Delta$E2bind was induced by addition of 2.5 μg/mL doxycycline (Merck, Darmstadt, Germany).

2.2. Life Cell Imaging

All data was acquired on an Andor Revolution spinning disk confocal microscope (Oxford Instruments, Abingdon, UK) based on a Yokogawa CSU W1 with Nikon Ti2 stand equipped with two Andor DU-888 cameras. Imaging was performed in a humidified chamber at 37 °C and 5% CO_2. An APO TIRF NA 1.49 100× magnification oil immersion objective was used, resulting in a lateral pixel size of 0.13 μm. For the detection of $CD46_{fluo}$ and $CD46_{fluo}\Delta$E2bind, mClover was excited by a 515 nm laser for 0.1 s and the emitted signal was bandpass filtered with a 540/30 nm filter. E2-mCherry was excited by a 594 nm laser for 0.1 s and the emitted light was bandpass filtered with a 647/57 nm filter before detection. Excitation and detection of each fluorophore was performed consecutively.

For the examination of virus attachment, cell surface transport, and entry, one frame/10 s was recorded starting directly, 5, 10, 15, 20, or 25 min after virus addition (multiplicity of infection (MOI) = 10) and data was acquired for 5 or 10 min. Three focal planes (Z-step size = 0.8 μm) were acquired for each time point to compensate for potential focusing errors and to increase the area accessible for analysis. The z-level was chosen close to the cover slip to allow imaging of filopodia, retraction fibers, lamellipodia, and the lamella. In order to judge intracellular background levels during E2-mCherry excitation, one z-stack was acquired of each field of view to be employed in the experiment before addition of virus.

To follow the time course of infection, cells were imaged at one z-level every 10 min starting 60 min after infection until 16 h after infection. Two different MOIs (1 and 10) were employed to assess the effect of different MOIs on the development of E2-mCherry signal. Due to phototoxicity, it was not possible to acquire several z-levels.

2.3. Image Processing and Analysis

All image processing and particle tracking was performed in ImageJ [24]. Raw frames were filtered with a Gaussian filter (sigma = 1.4) to improve data visualization. For initial particle tracking, maximum intensity projections along the z-axis were generated and particles tracked employing ImageJ's [24] manual tracking plug-in. Subsequently, tracks were verified on the full z-stack and their localization (lamellipodium, lamella, cell body) as well as their direction of movement (towards, tangential, away, random, with reference to the cell body) and the association with $CD46_{fluo}$ or $CD46_{fluo}\Delta$E2bind was documented. A python script (supplementary information) was used to analyze the output of the manual tracking plug-in with regard to direct and relative distance covered by a given particle, directionality (ratio direct to relative distance), average, minimum and maximum speed as well as the standard deviation of speed for a given track. The mean squared displacement (MSD) was calculated in R employing a customized script based on the code developed by [25]. Fits of the MSD curves were employed to calculate the velocity (V) of directed movement in case of an exponential slope using the following formula: $y = V^2x^2 + D_0x + a$ and the diffusion coefficient (D_0) was calculated using $y = 4D_0x + a$ in case of a linear slope. A two-tailed Student's t-test was performed to assess the likelihood of significant differences.

3. Results

3.1. BVDV Entry Is a Slow Process

To assess the infection cycle of BVDV in real time, we employed a previously described labelling strategy of the viral E2 surface glycoprotein [12,13]. SK6 cells inducibly expressing the fluorophore labelled, cellular surface receptor, bovine CD46 were chosen as system to study the infection cycle, as these cells demonstrated a high susceptibility to infection with BVDV after induction. SK6 cells not expressing bovine CD46 display a low susceptibility to BVDV infection, which is not mediated by porcine CD46, as porcine CD46 has previously been shown not to be involved in BVDV invasion [16]. After initial experiments employing either a system of mClover labelled BVDV and mCherry labelled CD46 or vice versa, we decided to employ mCherry labelled BVDV ($BVDV_{E2\text{-}mCherry}$) and mClover labelled CD46 ($CD46_{fluo}$), as strong photobleaching of mClover labelled BVDV rendered it inapplicable for life cell imaging.

Time series of 5 or 10 min duration with a frame rate of one frame/10 s were acquired at different time points (0–25 min in 5 min steps) after addition of $BVDV_{E2\text{-}mCherry}$ (MOI 10). Association of mCherry positive particles with the surface of SK6 $CD46_{fluo}$ cells could readily be observed and 801 particles were tracked by hand (n cells = 160). Due to the low signal to noise ratio, automatic tracking approaches did not improve the ease of analysis and were therefore not utilized. Entry events were rarely observed (n = 26, 2.8% of total particles tracked) and the majority occurred more than 20 min after virus addition (Figure 1A). In 65.5% of these entry events, the signal of the virus was associated with a $CD46_{fluo}$ positive vesicular structure. Association with such a vesicle was maintained after endocytosis in 76% of events. After endocytosis, particles could on average be tracked for 2.8 min and migrated on average 3 μm inside the cell (Figure 1A). Two examples of mCherry positive particles entering a cell are shown in Figure 1B,C and movies 1 and 2.

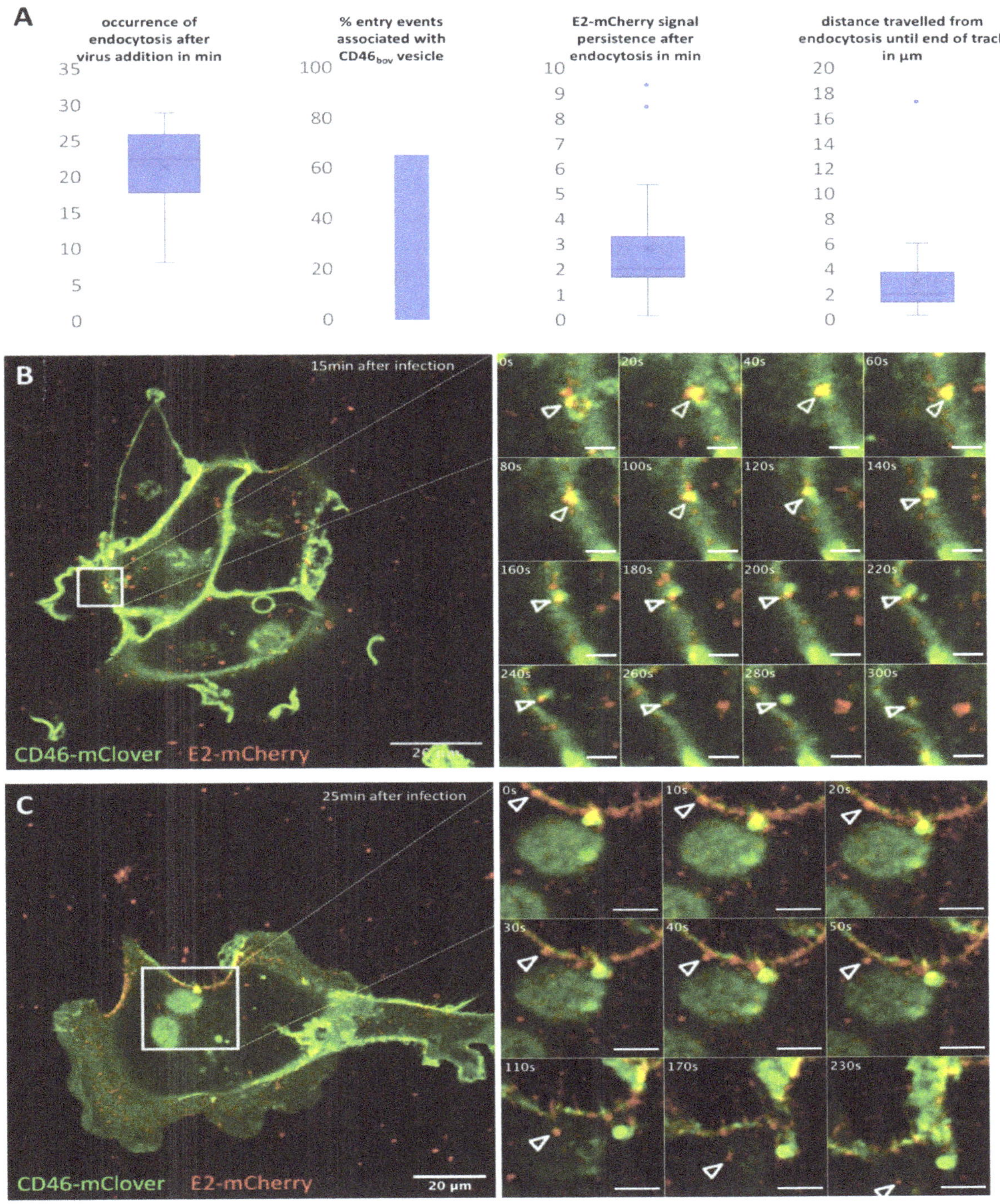

Figure 1. Characterization of $BVDV_{E2\text{-}mCherry}$ entry into SK6 $CD46_{fluo}$ cells. (**A**) Characterization of 26 entry events of $BVDV_{E2\text{-}mCherry}$ in SK6 $CD46_{fluo}$ cells with regard to occurrence after virus addition, association with $CD46_{fluo}$ signal, intracellular persistence of the E2-mCherry signal and intracellular distance travelled. Outliers (Q3 + 1.5-times interquartile range) are indicated by dots. (**B**,**C**) Examples of entry events of $BVDV_{E2\text{-}mCherry}$ (red) into SK6 $CD46_{bov}$ (green) cells. The full field of view at the time of the start of acquisition (time after virus addition is specified in the top right corner) is shown and the area of interest is indicated by grey squares. Frames as depicted in the detail images were acquired every 10 s for up to 10 min after the start of acquisition. Times indicated in s refer to the start of acquisition. The length of the scale bar in the detail images in (**B**) = 2.5 µm and in (**C**) = 5 µm.

Due to the intracellular background level in the mCherry emission range, the amount of intracellular, mCherry positive foci and their migration behavior was not analyzed as an unambiguous differentiation between background and specific signal was not possible.

Particles travelled with an average speed of 0.062 µm/s (s.d. 0.036 µm/s), an average maximum speed of 0.147 µm/s (s.d. 0.15) and an average directionality—defined as the ratio of direct distance versus real distance covered by a particle—of 0.34 (s.d. 0.22) on SK6 $CD46_{fluo}$ cells.

Directed transport of viruses along the outside of filopodia, cytonemes, and retraction fibers has been described for enveloped and non-enveloped viruses. The potential usurpation of this transport route was hence also examined in the context of $BVDV_{E2\text{-}mCherry}$. Virus surfing could be observed for 16 particles (2.0% of total tracks, movie 3). These particles migrated with an average velocity of 0.070 µm/s and an average directionality of 0.446, indicating an advantage of this type of transport regarding movement in a given direction. The average maximum speed of these particles was 0.176 µm/s, indicating a potential coupling to retrograde actin flow [2,26].

3.2. First Detection of BVDV E2-mCherry Signal Is Depending on MOI

In order to further analyze the progression of infection and to visualize the intracellular distribution of E2-mCherry over time, time series starting 60 min after virus addition and running for 16 h (1 frame every 10 min) were recorded. In all cells observed, an evenly distributed, slightly granular E2-mCherry signal was present from the initial detection of a specific signal (movies 4 and 5). This intracellular distribution pattern was reminiscent of an ER staining pattern, which is in good accordance with the localization of E2 in the ER lumen as already reported by [27,28]. Interestingly, the time after which an E2-mCherry signal could be resolved correlated with the MOI employed in a given experiment. For an MOI of 1, E2-mCherry could be detected on average 645 min after virus addition (n = 13) (Figure 2A, movie 4), whereas E2-mCherry could already be resolved on average 195 min (n = 16, movie 5) after infection if an MOI of 10 was used.

To gain further insights into the dynamics of E2-mCherry trafficking 20 h after infection, cells were imaged for 5 min with a frame rate of 1 frame/10 s. In addition to the diffuse, granular staining pattern of E2-mCherry, point-shaped, high signal intensities could be observed (Figure 2B, movie 6). They were partially associated with high $CD46_{fluo}$ signal intensities and this association was maintained during the whole course of the experiment. High intensity E2-mCherry foci could both be stationary or highly mobile (up to 0.5 µm/s), especially in the cell periphery (movie 6).

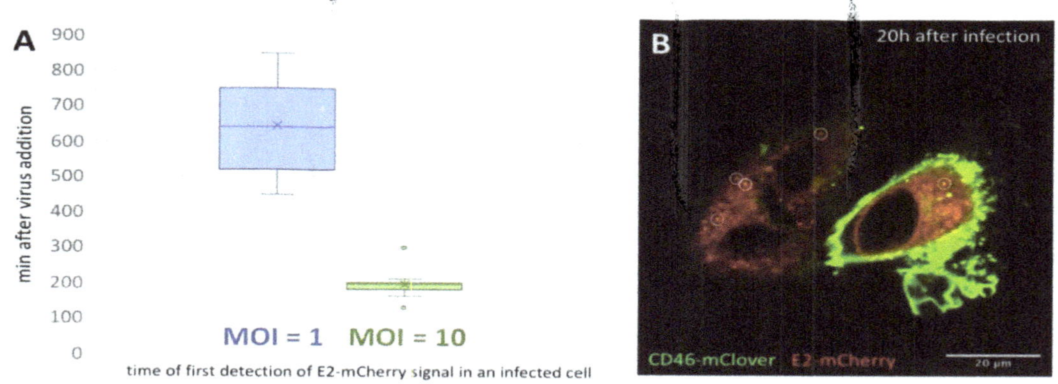

Figure 2. E2-mCherry signal development but not signal distribution is depending on the MOI. (**A**) Occurrence of E2-mCherry signal in min after addition of $BVDV_{E2\text{-}mCherry}$ at an MOI of 1 (blue) or 10 (green) to SK6 $CD46_{fluo}$ cells. SK6 $CD46_{fluo}$ cells were imaged recording one frame every 10 min at one z-level for 16 h. The mean is indicated by x and outliers (Q3 + 1.5-times interquartile range) are indicated by dots. (**B**) Distribution of E2-mCherry (red) and $CD46_{fluo}$ (green) signal 20 h after infection with $BVDV_{E2\text{-}mCherry}$ in SK6 $CD46_{fluo}$ cells. SK6 $CD46_{fluo}$ cells were imaged for 10 min recording 3 z-levels (0.8 µm) every 10 s (movie 6). Points of high E2-mCherry intensity that are colocalizing with $CD46_{fluo}$ are indicated by white circles.

3.3. $CD46_{fluo}$ Decreases the Speed of Directed Surface Motion of $BVDV_{E2\text{-}mCherry}$

In order to elucidate the effect of specific receptor binding on virus entry, SK6 cells inducibly expressing fluorophore-labelled CD46 with a deleted E2-binding domain ($CD46_{fluo}\Delta$E2bind) were generated based on previous results by [16], reporting the CCP-1 as interaction partner. These cells showed a susceptibility to BVDV comparable to the susceptibility of SK6 cells inducibly expressing GFP (Figure 3). GFP expressing cells were chosen as control to account for a potential effect of induced expression on virus replication. The susceptibility of SK6 $CD46_{fluo}\Delta$E2bind cells was more than 250-fold reduced in comparison to SK6 cells expressing unmodified $CD46_{fluo}$ after induction of expression.

This system was chosen over experiments employing inhibition of virus attachment by antibodies targeting neutralizing epitopes of E2 or functionally important domains of CD46 as it—in our opinion—provided the most direct and defined system to study the role of E2-CD46 interaction in the viral life cycle by life cell imaging. An inhibition of infection by BVDV tagged with a fluorophore at the E2 N-terminus employing before mentioned antibodies has already been demonstrated by [12] and this inhibition is comparable to BVDVs not bearing a tag at the E2 N-terminus. This clearly demonstrates the importance of the same domains in CD46-E2 interactions.

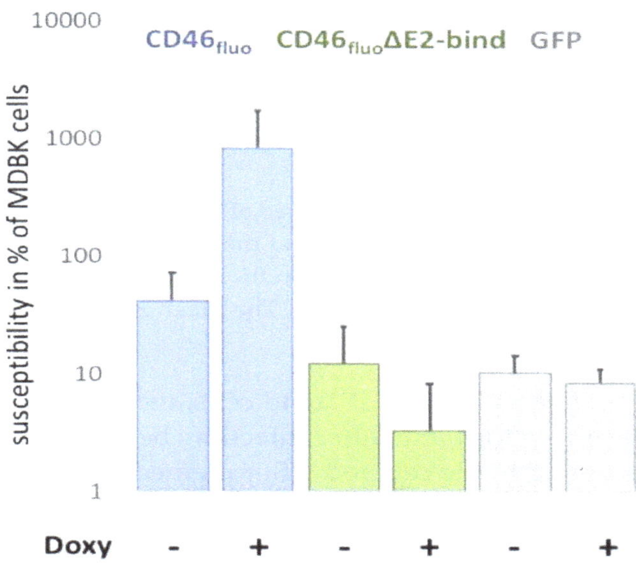

Figure 3. Deletion of CCP-1 reduces $CD46_{fluo}$ effect of the susceptibility of SK6 cells to the level of GFP-expressing controls. Susceptibility of SK6 $CD46_{fluo}$ (blue), $CD46_{fluo}\Delta$E2bind (green) and GFP-expressing (grey) SK6 cells to infection with $BVDV_{E2\text{-}mCherry}$ in % of MDBK cells (=100%) with and without the induction of expression by the addition of doxycycline (Doxy) (n = 6). Cells were infected with serial dilutions of $BVDV_{E2\text{-}mCherry}$ for 4 h. Subsequently, medium was exchanged to medium containing 1% carboxymethycellulose and E2-mCherry positive foci were detected 48 h after infection by fluorescence microscopy to determine the focus forming units (ffu)/mL. Susceptibility of a given cell line was calculated as the percentage of ffu/mL determined for MDBK cells, which was set to 100%.

To assess the effect of receptor binding on the surface movement of $BVDV_{E2\text{-}mCherry}$, 1081 mCherry-positive particles were tracked on SK6 $CD46_{fluo}\Delta$E2bind cells (n cells = 297). Of those 1081 particles, only 2 particles (0.2%) could be observed entering a cell, which is 7% of the entry events found for SK6 $CD46_{fluo}$ cells. One of these events was associated with a $CD46_{fluo}\Delta$E2bind after uptake.

In order to better understand the movement of particles on the surface of SK6 $CD46_{fluo}$ and SK6 $CD46_{fluo}\Delta$E2bind cells, particle trajectories were further analyzed. The average direct distance covered on the cell surface during a given observation period was 3.15 μm (s.d. 2.71 μm) for SK6 $CD46_{fluo}$ and 2.83 μm (s.d. 2.18 μm) for SK6 $CD46_{fluo}\Delta$E2bind cells (Figure 4), while the average real distance covered was 10.9 µm (s.d. 8.64 µm) for $CD46_{bov}$ and 9.14 µm (s.d. 6.06 µm) for $CD46_{bov}\Delta$E2bind. The average directionality—defined as the quotient of direct versus real distance—was 0.34 (s.d. 0.22) for SK6 $CD46_{bov}$ and 0.37 (s.d. 0.23) for SK6 $CD46_{bov}\Delta$E2bind cells and therefore seems unaffected by CD46 binding. Particles on SK6 $CD46_{fluo}$ cells travelled with an average velocity of 0.062 µm/s (s.d. 0.036 µm/s) and an average maximum speed of 0.147 µm/s (s.d. 0.15). Particles on SK6 $CD46_{fluo}\Delta$E2bind cells were characterized by an average velocity of 0.063 µm/s (s.d. 0.028 µm/s) and an average maximum speed of 0.136 µm/s (s.d. 0.063 µm/s), indicating no effect of CD46 binding on observed velocities.

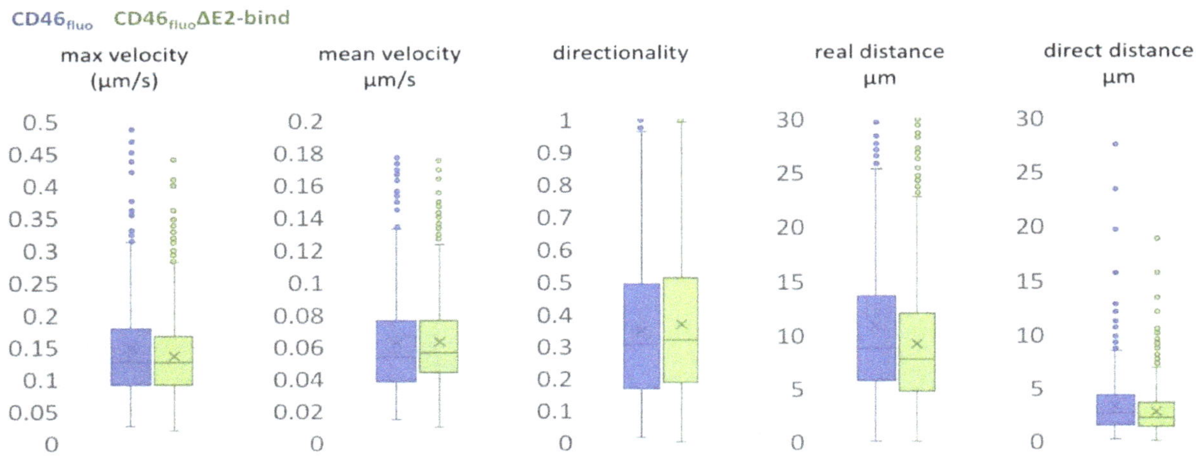

Figure 4. Movements of $BVDV_{E2\text{-}mCherry}$ on the surface of SK6 $CD46_{fluo}$ (blue) or $CD46_{fluo}\Delta$E2bind cells (green) are comparable. Box and Whisker blots of maximum and mean velocity, directionality, real distance and direct distance of particles tracked on the surface of SK6 $CD46_{fluo}$ (blue, $n = 801$) or $CD46_{fluo}\Delta$E2bind cells (green, $n = 1081$), respectively. The mean is indicated by x and outliers (Q3 + 1.5-times interquartile range) are indicated by dots.

On both, SK6 $CD46_{fluo}$ and SK6 $CD46_{fluo}\Delta$E2bind cells, the majority of particles was localized on the lamella or lamellipodium up to 10 min after infection; beginning with 15 min after infection, the majority of particles was bound to the cell body (Supplementary Figure S1). On average 51% of the particles on SK6 $CD46_{fluo}$ cells were associated with an increased CD46 signal intensity for at least 3 consecutive frames. On SK6 $CD46_{fluo}\Delta$E2bind cells, this percentage increased to an average of 74%. To assess potential differences in particle travelling directions, the overall direction of movement of a given particle was described as moving random or away from, tangential to or towards the cell body. Such a direction could unambiguously be assigned to 423 tracks on SK6 $CD46_{fluo}$ cells and 705 tracks on SK6 $CD46_{fluo}\Delta$E2bind cells (Supplementary Figure S2). 3% of particles tracked on SK6 $CD46_{fluo}$ cells and 12% of particles tracked on SK6 $CD46_{fluo}\Delta$E2bind cells showed a movement away from the cell body, whereas 57% and 42% respectively exhibited random movement. Tangential movement was observed for 17% of particles on SK6 $CD46_{fluo}$ cells and 18% of SK6 $CD46_{fluo}\Delta$E2bind cells. 23% and 29% of particles exhibited movement towards the cell body on SK6 $CD46_{fluo}$ cells and SK6 $CD46_{fluo}\Delta$E2bind cells, respectively. These results indicate that the major difference in the direction of particle transport is a four times reduced number of particles moving away from the cell body if CD46 is functional.

To further characterize the number of tracks following a certain type of motion on the cell surface and to determine transport velocities and the diffusion coefficients (D_0), MSD analysis was performed. Within both datasets, tracks exhibiting characteristics of directed motion, as well as limited diffusion or purely diffusive motility, could be identified. For SK6 $CD46_{fluo}$ cells, 86 tracks (10.7% of total tracks, 47.5% of tracks in MSD analysis) exhibited linear slopes, indicative of purely diffusive motion, while 46 tracks (4.3% of total tracks, 31.7% of tracks in MSD analysis) were identified for SK6 $CD46_{fluo}\Delta$E2bind cells (Figure 5A). The calculated diffusion coefficients were 0.020 µm²/s (s.d.

0.017 $\mu m^2/s$) for SK6 $CD46_{bov}$ cells and 0.015 $\mu m^2/s$ (s.d. 0.019 $\mu m^2/s$) for SK6 $CD46_{fluo}\Delta$E2bind cells and were not significantly different ($p = 0.103$). 70 tracks exhibiting an exponential slope could be identified for SK6 $CD46_{bov}$ cells (8.7% of total tracks, 38.7% of tracks in MSD analysis) and 61 for SK6 $CD46_{bov}\Delta$E2bind cells (5.6% of total tracks, 42.1% of tracks in MSD analysis) (Figure 5B). The calculated average particle velocity was 0.028 µm/s (s.d. 0.014 µm/s) for SK6 $CD46_{fluo}$ cells and 0.039 µm/s (s.d. 0.018 µm/s) for SK6 $CD46_{fluo}\Delta$E2bind cells, suggesting a significantly increased directional transport speed on SK6 $CD46_{fluo}\Delta$E2bind cells ($p < 0.001$). Twenty-five tracks on SK6 $CD46_{fluo}$ cells (3.1% of total tracks, 13.8% of tracks in MSD analysis) and 38 tracks on SK6 $CD46_{fluo}\Delta$E2bind cells (3.5% of total tracks, 26.2% of tracks in MSD analysis) showed characteristics indicative of limited diffusion in MSD analysis.

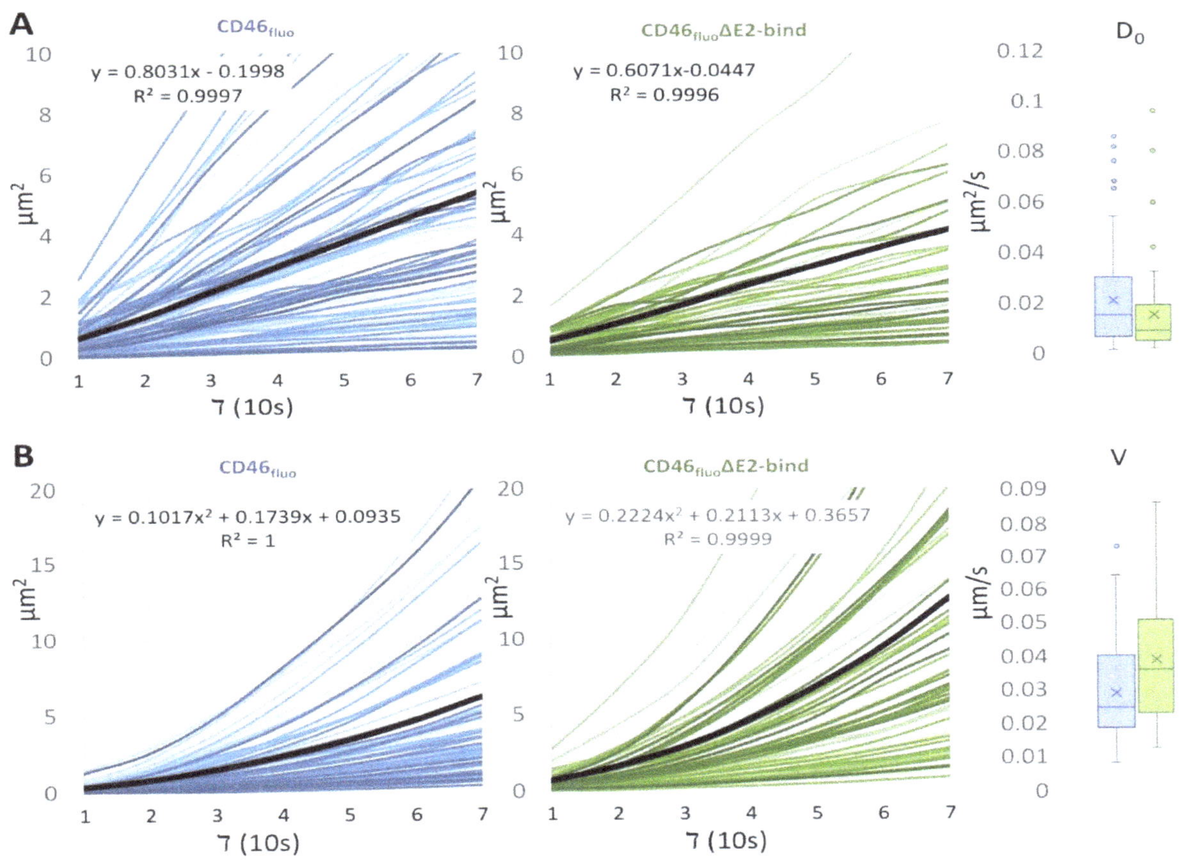

Figure 5. The average velocity of directed motion of $BVDV_{E2\text{-}mCherry}$ particles is increased on the surface of SK6 $CD46_{fluo}\Delta$E2bind cells. MSD analysis of particle movement on SK6 $CD46_{fluo}$ and $CD46_{fluo}\Delta$E2bind cells. (**A**) Slopes of tracks on SK6 $CD46_{fluo}$ (blue) and $CD46_{fluo}\Delta$E2bind (green) cells displaying a linear increase and distribution of the calculated diffusion coefficient D_0 depicted as box and whisker blot. The mean is indicated by x and outliers (Q3 + 1.5 times interquartile range) are depicted as dots. Average slopes are depicted as thick black lines. (**B**) Slopes of tracks on SK6 $CD46_{fluo}$ (blue) and $CD46_{fluo}\Delta$E2bind (green) cells displaying an exponential increase and distribution of the calculated particle velocities V, depicted as box and whisker blot. The mean is indicated by x and outliers (Q3 + 1.5 times interquartile range) are depicted as dots. Average slopes are depicted as thick black lines.

4. Discussion

Virus attachment and entry are governed by various affinities and highly dynamic processes. For BVDV, our findings suggest the presence of different types of motility on the cell surface, being diffusion, directed motion, and confined diffusion. This is different from observations of Dengue virus, as the main motion type until the association with a clathrin-coated pit is diffusion [8]. Virus surfing, as a movement frequently utilized by other viruses (e.g., MLV), was rarely observed, albeit the presence of filopodia, cytonemes, and retraction fibers, implying a minor role of this transport mechanism for BVDV, at least in this experimental setup. All motion types could be observed independent of the presence or absence of the BVDV-binding competent cellular receptor, CD46 and track properties were comparable. Similarly, the proportions of cellular compartments—lamellipodium, lamella, and cell body—with associated virus particles were not affected by CD46's ability to bind E2 when comparing different time points after infection. However, when analyzing directed motion in more detail by MSD analysis, track velocities were significantly increased if CD46 was not able to interact with E2. This might suggest that another interaction partner on the cellular surface—for example heparan sulphate or an as of yet unidentified attachment factor—might be responsible for coupling to the underlying actin network and that CD46 is rather involved in deceleration of particle transport on the cell surface or the anchoring of particles at potential sites of endocytosis. The importance of attachment factors such as heparan sulphate has also been demonstrated for other members of the *Flaviviridae* (reviewed in [29]). Also, CD46 is not sufficient to render cell lines derived from non-cloven-hoofed animals or humans susceptible to infection with BVDV. Instead, it increases the amount of cell-associated virus [15]. This indicates that additional cellular factors are required for successful virus infection after binding to CD46. Interestingly, overexpression of $CD46_{fluo}\Delta E2bind$ resulted in a further drop of susceptibility to BVDV, which might indicate the sequestration of a potential additional entry factor by $CD46_{fluo}\Delta E2bind$.

In general, the number of observable entry events into SK6 $CD46_{fluo}$ was very low (2.8% of tracked particles). This might indicate that cellular uptake of BVDV is a rather inefficient process. However, during data acquisition, we were not able to sample the whole cellular surface due to the short frame interval and phototoxicity. The focus of acquisition was on the cellular surface in contact with the growth support, to clearly depict cellular protrusions, the lamellipodium and the lamella. Particles could frequently be observed exiting the acquisition planes to regions of the cell body that were inaccessible in the chosen acquisition scheme. It is therefore possible that the low amount of observed entry events is—at least partially—due to a preference of BVDV to enter cells at specific areas of the cell body. Also, the specific infectivity of $BVDV_{E2\text{-}mCherry}$ is below 1:10, meaning that more than 10 genome equivalents are needed for successful establishment of infection. It is currently unclear what particle defects are responsible for this phenomenon, but it has to be taken into consideration that a certain number of particles are already unable to evoke cellular uptake. In order to clarify these open questions and to also examine the entry process of BVDV into primary host cells, MDBK CD46 knock-out cell lines would be a valuable tool for future elucidation of the entry process.

Contrasting the increased speed of particle transport, cell entry events were very rare if CD46 was E2-binding incompetent. This, in combination with the rather rare CD46—virus co-migration on the cell surface, might implicate that CD46 is important for the signaling to evoke endocytosis, but not for surface movements towards potential sites of endocytosis. The frequently observed association of virus particles with CD46 positive vesicles after endocytosis and their comigration for several frames further supports this hypothesis, but additional experiments will be required for verification. Still, $BVDV_{E2\text{-}mCherry}$ is able to enter host cells independent of a functional CD46 molecule. This strongly indicates the potential to use other entry receptors, but with much lower efficiency. The importance of factors different from CD46 in BVDV propagation is also highlighted by recent results reporting that BVDV cell-to-cell spread is independent of CD46 [12].

The CD46 splice variant employed in this study is identical to the bovine CD46 variant initially reported by [15]. Unfortunately, we were not able to elucidate the effects of different allelic versions of CCP-1 and different CD46 splice variants on the dynamics of BVDV entry due to the huge efforts of data analysis. A different permissiveness to infection of these different allelic and splice variants has however already been demonstrated [30] and their effect on the dynamics of BVDV entry will be an interesting topic of future studies.

Taking advantage of the easy tracking of virus protein production in infected cells, the effect of different MOIs on the earliest time point of specific fluorescence detection was examined. The highly significant difference observed leads to the conclusion that signal development is depending on the virus dose applied and that superinfection exclusion is not acting fast enough to prevent the infection of one cell with several particles in the context of this experimental setup [31]. Surveillance of the signal development of $BVDV_{E2\text{-}mCherry}$ after infection revealed an initially finely granular, likely ER-associated [27,28] distribution throughout the whole cell, which intensified over time and finally also developed strong signal foci. Therefore, it seems likely that E2 is quickly distributed throughout the cell and not restricted to and radially expanding from a potential initial replication site. To better understand viral replication sites, additional studies are warranted to elucidate how the intracellular distribution of E2 is reflecting the overall distribution of non-structural proteins like NS3 and NS5B as part of the replication complex. This, in combination with ultrastructural studies, will provide further insights into the morphology of replication sites and allow comparison to the detailed morphological studies already performed on the membranous replication compartments of HCV [32] and flaviviruses [33,34]. The occasional association of CD46 positive intracellular foci with E2 mCherry positive foci suggests that CD46 is usually excluded from E2 mCherry containing compartments or only present in amounts below the detection limit of this experimental setup. Whether this association is unfavorable for the virus or serves an as of yet unknown purpose—like facilitation of exocytosis by taking advantage of CD46 transport to the cell surface—will need to be elucidated in the future.

In the presented study a large variety of BVDV surface motions has been documented. Interestingly, apart from a decrease in the velocity of directed motion, no effect of $CD46_{fluo}$ on the surface transport of BVDV could be identified, indicating a minor role during this process. First insights into the progression of virus infection indicate the quick distribution of BVDV protein throughout the ER in an initial virus dose dependent manner. It will be highly interesting to identify and characterize the additional factors orchestrating BVDV entry to develop a clear picture of this process.

Supplementary Materials:
Figure S1: Particle localization on the cell surface depending on the time after virus addition, Figure S2: Directions of movements of virus particles on the cell surface with reference to the cell body. supplementary information: python script used for track analysis, legend of the movie files, nucleotide sequence of the plasmid encoding the genome of $BVDV_{E2\text{-}mCherry}$; Movie 1: Example 1 of an mCherry positive particle entering a cell, Movie 2: Example 2 of an mCherry positive particle entering a cell, Movie 3: Surfing of a $BVDV_{E2\text{-}mCherry}$ particle on the surface of a retraction fibre., Movie 4: Development of E2-mCherry (red) signal after infection of SK6 TO CD46fluo cells with an MOI of 1, Movie 5: Development of E2-mCherry (red) signal after infection of SK6 TO CD46fluo cells with an MOI of 10, Movie 6: Colocalization of E2-mCherry and $CD46_{fluo}$ inside the cell.

Author Contributions: C.R. designed the study. B.L., C.R., H.-W.C. and V.L. performed the experiments. C.R., T.R., U.R. and V.L. analysed the data. C.R. wrote the manuscript and all authors commented on it. All authors have read and agreed to the published version of the manuscript.

Acknowledgments: We would like to acknowledge the microscopy support from the Infectious Diseases Imaging Platform (IDIP) at the Center for Integrative Infectious Disease Research, Heidelberg, Germany. The authors thank Tobias Rasse and Christian Tischer for their support and the fruitful discussions. We would like to thank the University of Veterinary Medicine Vienna for Open Access Funding.

References

1. Burckhardt, C.J.; Greber, U.F. Virus movements on the plasma membrane support infection and transmission between cells. *PLoS Pathog.* **2009**, *5*, e1000621. [CrossRef] [PubMed]
2. Lehmann, M.J.; Sherer, N.M.; Marks, C.B.; Pypaert, M.; Mothes, W. Actin- and myosin-driven movement of viruses along filopodia precedes their entry into cells. *J. Cell Biol.* **2005**, *170*, 317–325. [CrossRef] [PubMed]
3. Oh, M.-J.; Akhtar, J.; Desai, P.; Shukla, D. A role for heparan sulfate in viral surfing. *Biochem. Biophys. Res. Commun.* **2010**, *391*, 176–181. [CrossRef] [PubMed]

4. Schelhaas, M.; Shah, B.; Holzer, M.; Blattmann, P.; Kühling, L.; Day, P.M.; Schiller, J.T.; Helenius, A. Entry of human papillomavirus type 16 by actin-dependent, clathrin- and lipid raft-independent endocytosis. *PLoS Pathog.* **2012**, *8*, e1002657. [CrossRef] [PubMed]
5. Ayala-Nuñez, N.V.; Wilschut, J.; Smit, J.M. Monitoring virus entry into living cells using DiD-labeled dengue virus particles. *Methods* **2011**, *55*, 137–143. [CrossRef]
6. Zhang, S.L.-X.; Tan, H.-C.; Hanson, B.J.; Ooi, E.E. A simple method for Alexa Fluor dye labelling of dengue virus. *J. Virol. Methods* **2010**, *167*, 172–177. [CrossRef]
7. Coller, K.E.; Berger, K.L.; Heaton, N.S.; Cooper, J.D.; Yoon, R.; Randall, G. RNA Interference and Single Particle Tracking Analysis of Hepatitis C Virus Endocytosis. *PLoS Pathog.* **2009**, *5*, e1000702. [CrossRef]
8. van der Schaar, H.M.; Rust, M.J.; Chen, C.; van der Ende-Metselaar, H.; Wilschut, J.; Zhuang, X.; Smit, J.M. Dissecting the cell entry pathway of dengue virus by single-particle tracking in living cells. *PLoS Pathog.* **2008**, *4*, e1000244. [CrossRef]
9. Dejarnac, O.; Hafirassou, M.L.; Chazal, M.; Versapuech, M.; Gaillard, J.; Perera-Lecoin, M.; Umana-Diaz, C.; Bonnet-Madin, L.; Carnec, X.; Tinevez, J.Y.; et al. TIM-1 Ubiquitination Mediates Dengue Virus Entry. *Cell Rep.* **2018**, *23*, 1779–1793. [CrossRef]
10. Tamura, T.; Fukuhara, T.; Uchida, T.; Ono, C.; Mori, H.; Sato, A.; Fauzyah, Y.; Okamoto, T.; Kurosu, T.; Setoh, Y.X.; et al. Characterization of Recombinant Flaviviridae Viruses Possessing a Small Reporter Tag. *J. Virol.* **2018**, *92*, e01582-17. [CrossRef]
11. Tamura, T.; Igarashi, M.; Enkhbold, B.; Suzuki, T.; Okamatsu, M.; Ono, C.; Mori, H.; Izumi, T.; Sato, A.; Fauzyah, Y.; et al. In vivo dynamics of reporter Flaviviridae viruses. *J. Virol.* **2019**. [CrossRef] [PubMed]
12. Merwaiss, F.; Czibener, C.; Alvarez, D.E. Cell-to-Cell Transmission Is the Main Mechanism Supporting Bovine Viral Diarrhea Virus Spread in Cell Culture. *J. Virol.* **2019**, *93*. [CrossRef] [PubMed]
13. Riedel, C.; Lamp, B.; Chen, H.-W.; Heimann, M.; Rümenapf, T. Fluorophore labelled BVDV: A novel tool for the analysis of infection dynamics. *Sci. Rep.* **2019**, *9*, 5972. [CrossRef]
14. Iqbal, M.; Flick-Smith, H.; McCauley, J.W. Interactions of bovine viral diarrhoea virus glycoprotein E(rns) with cell surface glycosaminoglycans. *J. Gen. Virol.* **2000**, *81*, 451–459. [CrossRef] [PubMed]
15. Maurer, K.; Krey, T.; Moennig, V.; Thiel, H.-J.; Rümenapf, T. CD46 is a cellular receptor for bovine viral diarrhea virus. *J. Virol.* **2004**, *78*, 1792–1799. [CrossRef] [PubMed]
16. Krey, T.; Himmelreich, A.; Heimann, M.; Menge, C.; Thiel, H.-J.; Maurer, K.; Rümenapf, T. Function of bovine CD46 as a cellular receptor for bovine viral diarrhea virus is determined by complement control protein 1. *J. Virol.* **2006**, *80*, 3912–3922. [CrossRef]
17. Grummer, B.; Grotha, S.; Greiser-Wilke, I. Bovine Viral Diarrhoea Virus is Internalized by Clathrin-dependent Receptor-mediated Endocytosis. *J. Vet. Med. Ser. B* **2004**, *51*, 427–432. [CrossRef]
18. Lecot, S.; Belouzard, S.; Dubuisson, J.; Rouillé, Y. Bovine viral diarrhea virus entry is dependent on clathrin-mediated endocytosis. *J. Virol.* **2005**, *79*, 10826–10829. [CrossRef]
19. Krey, T.; Thiel, H.-J.; Rümenapf, T. Acid-resistant bovine pestivirus requires activation for pH-triggered fusion during entry. *J. Virol.* **2005**, *79*, 4191–4200. [CrossRef]
20. Cattaneo, R. Four viruses, two bacteria, and one receptor: Membrane cofactor protein (CD46) as pathogens' magnet. *J. Virol.* **2004**, *78*, 4385–4388. [CrossRef]
21. Ni Choileain, S.; Astier, A.L. CD46 processing: A means of expression. *Immunobiology* **2012**, *217*, 169–175. [CrossRef]
22. Crimeen-Irwin, B.; Ellis, S.; Christiansen, D.; Ludford-Menting, M.J.; Milland, J.; Lanteri, M.; Loveland, B.E.; Gerlier, D.; Russell, S.M. Ligand binding determines whether CD46 is internalized by clathrin-coated pits or macropinocytosis. *J. Biol. Chem.* **2003**, *278*, 46927–46937. [CrossRef] [PubMed]
23. Persson, B.D.; Schmitz, N.B.; Santiago, C.; Zocher, G.; Larvie, M.; Scheu, U.; Casasnovas, J.M.; Stehle, T. Structure of the extracellular portion of CD46 provides insights into its interactions with complement proteins and pathogens. *PLoS Pathog.* **2010**, *6*, e1001122. [CrossRef] [PubMed]
24. Schneider, C.A.; Rasband, W.S.; Eliceiri, K.W. NIH Image to ImageJ: 25 years of image analysis. *Nat. Methods* **2012**, *9*, 671–675. [CrossRef] [PubMed]
25. Marini, F.; Mazur, J.; Binder, H. flowcatchR: A user-friendly workflow solution for the analysis of time-lapse cell flow imaging data. *F1000Research* **2015**, *4*. [CrossRef]
26. Kohler, F.; Rohrbach, A. Surfing along Filopodia: A Particle Transport Revealed by Molecular-Scale Fluctuation Analyses. *Biophys. J.* **2015**, *108*, 2114–2125. [CrossRef] [PubMed]

27. Schmeiser, S.; Mast, J.; Thiel, H.-J.; König, M. Morphogenesis of pestiviruses: New insights from ultrastructural studies of strain Giraffe-1. *J. Virol.* **2014**, *88*, 2717–2724. [CrossRef]
28. Gray, E.W.; Nettleton, P.F. The Ultrastructure of Cell Cultures Infected with Border Disease and Bovine Virus Diarrhoea Viruses. *J. Gen. Virol.* **1987**, *68*, 2339–2346. [CrossRef]
29. Gerold, G.; Bruening, J.; Weigel, B.; Pietschmann, T. Protein Interactions during the Flavivirus and Hepacivirus Life Cycle. *Mol. Cell. Proteomics* **2017**, *16*, S75–S91. [CrossRef]
30. Zezafoun, H.; Decreux, A.; Desmecht, D. Genetic and splice variations of Bos taurus CD46 shift cell permissivity to BVDV, the bovine pestivirus. *Vet. Microbiol.* **2011**, *152*, 315–327. [CrossRef]
31. Lee, Y.-M.; Tscherne, D.M.; Yun, S.-I.; Frolov, I.; Rice, C.M. Dual Mechanisms of Pestiviral Superinfection Exclusion at Entry and RNA Replication. *J. Virol.* **2005**, *79*, 3231–3242. [CrossRef] [PubMed]
32. Romero-Brey, I.; Merz, A.; Chiramel, A.; Lee, J.-Y.; Chlanda, P.; Haselman, U.; Santarella-Mellwig, R.; Habermann, A.; Hoppe, S.; Kallis, S.; et al. Three-Dimensional Architecture and Biogenesis of Membrane Structures Associated with Hepatitis C Virus Replication. *PLoS Pathog.* **2012**, *8*, e1003056. [CrossRef] [PubMed]
33. Welsch, S.; Miller, S.; Romero-Brey, I.; Merz, A.; Bleck, C.K.E.; Walther, P.; Fuller, S.D.; Antony, C.; Krijnse-Locker, J.; Bartenschlager, R. Composition and three-dimensional architecture of the dengue virus replication and assembly sites. *Cell Host Microbe* **2009**, *5*, 365–375. [CrossRef] [PubMed]
34. Cortese, M.; Goellner, S.; Acosta, E.G.; Neufeldt, C.J.; Oleksiuk, O.; Lampe, M.; Haselmann, U.; Funaya, C.; Schieber, N.; Ronchi, P.; et al. Ultrastructural Characterization of Zika Virus Replication Factories. *Cell Rep.* **2017**, *18*, 2113–2123. [CrossRef]

5

Bovine Viral Diarrhea Virus: Recent Findings about its Occurrence in Pigs

Luís Guilherme de Oliveira [1,*], Marina L. Mechler-Dreibi [1], Henrique M. S. Almeida [1] and Igor R. H. Gatto [2]

[1] School of Agricultural and Veterinarian Sciences, São Paulo State University (Unesp), Jaboticabal. Via de Acesso Prof. Paulo Donato Castelanne s/n, Jaboticabal - SP 14884-900, Brazil; mlopesvet@gmail.com (M.L.M.-D.); henri_almeida2003@yahoo.com.br (H.M.S.A.)

[2] Ourofino Animal Health Ltda. Rodovia Anhanguera SP 330, Km 298. Distrito Industrial, Cravinhos – SP 14140-000, Brazil; igatto_10@hotmail.com

* Correspondence: luis.guilherme@unesp.br

Abstract: Bovine viral diarrhea virus (BVDV) is an important pathogen belonging to the *Pestivirus* genus, *Flaviviridae* family, which comprises viral species that causes an economic impact in animal production. Cattle are the natural host of BVDV and the main source of infection for pigs and other animal species. Due to its antigenic and genetic similarity with other important pestiviruses such as Classical Swine Fever Virus (CSFV), several studies have been conducted to elucidate the real role of this virus in piglets, sows, and boars, not only in the field but also in experimental infections, which will be discussed in this paper. Although BVDV does not pose a threat to pigs as it does to ruminants, the occurrence of clinical signs is variable and may depend on several factors. Therefore, this study presents a survey of data on BVDV infection in pigs, comparing information on prevalence in different countries and the results of experimental infections to understand this type of infection in pigs better.

Keywords: BVDV; experimental infection; natural infection; pigs

---

1. Updates on BVDV Infection in Swine

Bovine viral diarrhea (BVD) is an infection caused by the bovine viral diarrhea virus (BVDV), belonging to the genus *Pestivirus*, family *Flaviviridae*, with single-stranded positive polarity RNA [1]. Viruses belonging to the *Pestivirus* genus infect hosts of several animal species and include viral agents of great impact for animal production [2,3]. The *Pestivirus* species have been recently named from A to K and, among them, the *Pestivirus* A (BVDV-1), *Pestivirus* B (BVDV-2), *Pestivirus* C (Classical Swine Fever Virus), and *Pestivirus* K (atypical porcine pestivirus) are the main viral species related to swine [4]. BVDV has two genotypes, type 1 and type 2, which are classified into sub-genotypes: BVDV-1 (1a to 1u), adding up to 21 sub-genotypes, and BVDV-2 (2a to 2d), with four sub-genotypes [5]. BVDV-1 is related to most reference strains, is commonly used for vaccine production, and was most frequently isolated from mild to moderate clinical cases in cattle. Conversely, BVDV-2 was isolated from acute disease outbreaks, also presenting strains of mild and moderate virulence [6].

Based on the effect of replication on cell culture, BVDV isolates can be divided into cytopathic (cp) and non-cytopathic (ncp), with the ncp isolates being responsible for most natural infections and persistent fetal infections, and cp isolates constituting a minority, which are isolated almost exclusively from cattle with mucosal disease [6].

Cattle are natural hosts of BVDV, considered the major source of infection for pigs and other animal species [7,8]. Usually, positive pig herds for BVDV occur when cattle and pigs are raised on the same farm, and the direct contact between these animal species is considered the main source of BVDV transmission for pigs [7]. Infection caused by BVDV in pigs has been reported in China [9], the Netherlands [10], Brazil [11–13], Austria [14], Germany [15], Norway [16], Ireland [17], Denmark [18] and others. These data were found not only in domestic pigs but also in wild boars [19], which raise concerns about risk factors involved in BVDV infection, the clinical form of the disease, and the existence of accurate diagnostic tests. In Brazil, BVDV-1d was frequently reported in cattle [20]. Mósena et al. [11] states that by the phylogenetic analysis of sequenced samples collected from backyard pigs, classified as BVDV-1d and BVDV-2a, it is possible that one of the obtained sequences originated from contact between cattle and pigs.

It is known that all pestiviruses are genetically and antigenically related, and BVDV infection in pigs may be presented with a great variability of clinical signs [21]. Even though BVDV infections in pigs are not as problematic as Classical Swine Fever Virus (CSFV) infections, it is believed that distinguishing these two diseases could be difficult due to the similar clinical signs when considering low pathogenicity strains [22]. Reports of clinical signs associated with the infection consisting of anemia, delayed development, rough hair, polyarthritis, congenital tremors (CT), petechiae on the skin, diarrhea, conjunctivitis, and cyanosis [23]. Clinical signs similar to CSF, and sudden death [24] were also observed when the BVDV strain was isolated from both pigs and cattle from the same farm [24]. On the other hand, several recent studies with experimental infection did not report the presence of clinical signs of infection [25–34]. This may occur due to an inadequate level of viremia or a low virulence strain, biotype of the virus, host adaptation and/or route of inoculation [31–35]. A possible explanation is that cases in which BVDV infection-induced large numbers of lesions in adult pigs have been caused by viral strains that passed along previous adaptations in this species [23].

BVDV has a predilection for replication in defense cells, mainly lymphocytes, but it also infects monocytes and dendritic cells. As antigen presenters, dendritic cells play an important role in cellular immunity by initiating the nonspecific immune response against various pathogens [35]. Its infection promotes lysis of monocytes as a mechanism for evading the immune system, affecting the recognition and subsequent development of a specific immune-humoral response [36].

BVDV can contaminate cell cultures and fetal calf serum [37]. In countries that promote CSFV vaccination, the BVDV prevalence found in swine herds has been associated with the widespread use of live vaccines for Classical Swine Fever (CSF), which were produced with bovine sera from positive Chinese bovine herds [9]. Batches of live CSFV vaccines used in China confirmed five BVDV-contaminated samples out of 23 collected for testing [38].

Serological diagnosis by enzyme-linked immunosorbent assay (ELISA) is more efficient, cheaper, and faster than molecular techniques [37]. The neutralizing antibody titers in the serum of animals previously exposed to a Pestivirus member are usually medium to high regarding the homologous viral species, and low (or non-reactive) regarding other species [6]. Anti-BVDV antibodies were shown to be able to protect pigs against CSFV infection and the manifestation of clinical signs, even though the anti-CSFV antibody titers were low, which could hinder CSFV outbreaks in herds with a high prevalence of anti-BVDV antibodies [22]. The same condition could occur in the presence of anti-Border Disease Virus (BDV) antibodies, as cross-reactions could affect the transmission of CSFV and should be evaluated for an accurate diagnosis of a CSFV infection and for implementing specific surveillance protocols in cases of outbreaks [10].

Reverse transcription-polymerase chain reaction (RT-PCR) is widely used for detecting the viral agent for differential diagnosis [39], since samples of blood, milk, saliva, and tissue can be successfully tested [40], and can be stored for a long time with minimal losses [41]. Researchers have adapted numerous variations of PCR methods for the detection of infectious agents, using DNA templates as well as RNA templates after an RT step [42], which has enabled more accurate, sensible and specific diagnostics. Direct sequencing of the RT-PCR product for fragments of 5′UTR and N-terminal autoprotease (N^{pro}) may also provide accurate differential diagnosis [19].

Given the antigenic and genetic similarity and the improvement in laboratory diagnostic methods, the comparison between results from recent and former studies should be cautious. Several studies that examine data collection in the field, as well as experimental infection with BVDV, have been conducted, and the results that contrast with the former data in the literature will be further discussed.

2. Data Collection from Backyard and Intensive Pig Herds

Aiming at collecting data on the occurrence of anti-BVDV antibodies in Brazilian swine herds, cross-sectional studies were carried out [12,13] in the backyard and intensive pig herds, respectively, located in the CSF-free zone of Brazil. For the first study, 56 pig herds from the northwest region of the state of São Paulo were evaluated, which are part of 11 municipalities. Blood samples were collected for serological testing by virus neutralization (VN), and titers higher than ten were considered positive. Out of the 360 serum samples, 4.72% (17/360) were reactive to BVDV in VN, which is 1.94% (7/360) reactive to BVDV-1 (Singer strain), with antibody titers ranging from 10 to 640, and 3.06% (11/360) reactive to BVDV-2 (VS-253 strain), with antibody titers ranging from 10 to 80, and only one reactive sample against both genotypes. Regarding herds, 27% (15/56) presented at least one animal positive to any of the genotypes. The prevalence of BVDV in bovine herds in the same region where this study was conducted was 56.49% [43], which may have resulted in the highest prevalence values of swine in the region when compared to previous reports [10]. Most of the farms evaluated in this study had cattle and pigs in close contact. As ruminants are the main source of BVDV infection for pigs [7,8], the prevalence of the disease in cattle herds is closely related to the presence of infections and influences the prevalence of the disease in pigs [9,10,44].

On the other hand, in a cross-sectional study carried out in 33 commercial pig herds, collected 1705 blood samples for analysis [13]. Samples were also tested by VN, and 5.34% (91/1705) of the samples were sero-reactive to BVDV with antibody titers ranging from 10 to 80. Of these, 3% (51/1075) were positive for reference strains of BVDV-1 (Singer strain) and 2.35% (40/1705) for reference strains of BVDV-2 (VS-253 strain), with 0.1% (2/1705) of samples with cross-reactions between both genotypes. Herds were sampled from 27 municipalities, located in seven Brazilian states, which are part of three different regions (South, Southeast, and Midwest). In 64% of herds (21/33), there was at least one positive sample for any of the BVDV genotypes in VN. As the presence of anti-BVDV antibodies in swine serum can lead to false-positive results in serological tests for the diagnosis of CSFV, the positive samples from both studies were sent for anti-CSFV antibodies detection, and were both negative. A survey carried out in The Netherlands [10] on commercial farm animals found a prevalence of 2.5% for gilts and 0.42% for finishing animals via ELISA. The difference in prevalence found in finishing animals from these two studies can be explained not only by the sensitivity of the techniques used but also by the different levels of biosecurity in the farms studied.

In a more recent study [11], swine sera were collected from 320 backyard pig herds in southern Brazil. Serum samples were tested by VN against BVDV-1a, -1b, and -2 strains, resulting in 4.2% (27/639) positive samples. Of those, 16 samples presented the highest titers against BVDV-1a (2 samples), BVDV-1b (5 samples), and BVDV-2 (9 samples). These studies confirm that ruminant Pestiviruses have been circulating in swine herds and must be considered in future Pestivirus control programs conducted in Brazil.

The low prevalence of BVDV in pigs was also found by other authors in Norway, Ireland, Denmark, and The Netherlands [16–18] (Table 1). Not only domestic pigs are a concern when it comes to Pestivirus infections since wild boar have been described as important reservoirs or transmitters of pathogens in nature due to their ability to reach long distances and transmit diseases to domestic swine. Other studies [45–47] have reported a low prevalence of BVDV in wild boar in Germany, the Czech Republic, and Eastern Serbia, respectively. Weber [19] was the first to detect BVDV RNA in wild boars' blood samples, and Gatto [48] first reported the presence of anti-BVDV antibodies in Thayasuids. In general, the low prevalence of anti-BVDV antibodies in pigs may be associated not only with the level of interaction between pigs and ruminants but also with the host-pathogen specificity, which seems to be lower in pigs compared to cattle. In intensive pig farming, biosecurity measures reduce or eliminate the presence of some infectious agents. Some researchers [10,44] attributed the low prevalence of BVDV in swine herds in their studies to the high specialization of agriculture, in which interspecific contact was reduced due to single zootechnical breeding on the property.

Table 1. Bovine viral diarrhea virus prevalence in intensive pig farming, backyard pig herds, and wild boars observed by several authors in different regions worldwide.

References	Type of Pig Production	Animal Category	Number of Samples/Number of Herds	Type of Sample	Diagnostic Tool	Region	BVDV Prevalence
Loken et al., 1991	-	Adult pigs	1317/887	Serum	Virus neutralization	Norway	2.2%
Graham et al., 2001	-	-	660/46	Serum	ELISA*	Northern Ireland	0.15%
Loeffen et al., 2009	Intensive pig farming	Finishing pigs	1890/189	Serum	ELISA and Virus neutralization	The Netherlands	0.42%
Loeffen et al., 2009	Intensive pig farming	Sows	6020/616	Serum	ELISA and Virus neutralization	The Netherlands	2.5%
Deng et al., 2012	-	Pigs with clinical signs	511/11	Serum and tissue homogenate	Nested-RT-PCR	China (herds from 11 provinces)	26.8%
Gatto et al., 2017	Intensive pig farming		1705/33	Serum	Virus neutralization	Brazil (herds from six states)	5.34%
Almeida et al., 2017		Piglets and adults	360/56	Serum	Virus neutralization	Northwestern region of São Paulo State, Brazil	4.72%
Mósena et al., 2020	Backyard pig herds	Male and female animals 6–72 mo old	639/320	Serum	RT-PCR and virus neutralization	Rio Grande do Sul, Brazil	4.2%
Dahle et al., 1993	Wild boars	-	841 samples	Serum	Direct Neutralizing Peroxidase linked antibody assay (NPLA)	Northern Germany	0.83%
Sedlak et al., 2008	Wild boars	-	352 samples	Serum	ELISA	Czech Republic	1%
Milicevik et al., 2018	Wild boars	-	50 samples	Spleen	qRT-PCR	Eastern Serbia	8%
Weber et al., 2016	Farmed wild boars	-	40 samples	Lung	RT-PCR	Rio Grande do Sul, Brazil	2.5%
Gatto et al., 2020	Farmed white-lipped peccaries	-	72 samples	Serum	Virus neutralization	Midwest Brazil	1.38%

*ELISA: enzyme-linked immunosorbent assay.

In China, swine samples with clinical signs such as diarrhea, miscarriage, and death, between 2007 and 2010, were tested for BVDV by nested RT-PCR. Unlike that heretofore described, the observed prevalence was 23.1% in 2007, 27.7% in 2008, 33.6% in 2009, and 23.6% in 2010, showing a high prevalence of BVDV-1 infection [9] when compared to the abovementioned study. These numbers should be analyzed carefully since only samples from clinical cases compatible with BVDV infection were analyzed. As stated by these authors, the use of live vaccines against CSFV may also be directly related to this higher prevalence of BVDV in pig herds from China, since, in general, the prevalence of BVDV in pig herds is low.

3. Experimental Infection with BVDV in Pigs: Routes of Transmission and Disease Development

The lack of studies concerning the routes of transmission of BVDV between piglets highlighted the need to develop researches clarifying this information (Table 2). Three studies were separately conducted with three groups of two weaned piglets separated by isolation cabinets: the challenged, sentinel, and control groups. The isolation cabinets were arranged to allow only a specific route of transmission, namely airborne, nose-to-nose [25], and by back pond water [26]. Although all challenged piglets shed the virus and seroconverted, only transmission by the back-pond water was confirmed since sentinel animals also shed the virus and seroconverted in this study. An interesting fact regarding the viral shedding observed in these studies was the intermittent pattern of nasal shedding. Challenged piglets shed the virus between 5- and 24-days post-inoculation, intermittently, detected by RT-PCR of nasal swabs. In the challenged groups, clinical signs such as diarrhea, rough hair, and oculo-nasal discharge were observed about 15 dpi, when the piglets started seroconversion. Despite other pathogens that have not been searched for, these clinical signs may be suggestive of BVDV infection since it was not observed in piglets from the control group.

Table 2. Results obtained in experimental inoculation studies of bovine viral diarrhea virus in swine.

References	BVDV Strain	Route of Inoculation	Animal Category	BVDV-Shedding	Viremia	Seroconversion (Dpi / % of Positive Pigs)	Consequences of Infection
Stewart et al., 1980	-	Intranasal-oral	Pregnant sows	-	7 dpi	21 dpi / 100%	Intrauterine infection in one litter, fewer fetuses than corpora lutea. Not observed in fetuses
Terpstra and Wensvoort, 1988	76/4 and 77/5 strains	Natural infection	Sows and piglets	-	-	35 dpi / (NA)	Piglets with clinical signs similar to CSF
Paton and Done, 1994	91/1 and 87/6 strains	Intrauterine	Pregnant sows	only congenital persistently infected fetus, for 2.5 years	4–6 dpi in fetuses	variable in piglets, but all sows seroconverted	Intrauterine infection, some fetuses with no clinical signs, some with persistent congenital infection
Terpstra and Wensvoort, 1997	Van Ee, Appel and Toering	Natural infection	Piglet	urine, oropharyngeal fluids, and semen of persistently infected boar	Observed	30 dpi - 8 mo / (NA)	Congenital persistent infection, leukopenia, viral replication in several organs, clinical signs resembling chronic CSF
Kulcsar et al., 2001	Oregon C24V strain	Intranasal and subcutaneous	Pregnant sows	Not observed	-	28 dpi / 100%	No clinical signs on sows, birth of weak piglets with ruffled hair coat, splay leg, trembling, myoclonia, diarrhea, fever, death
Makoschey et al., 2002	BVDV-2	-	Piglets	-	-	Observed / 100%	Inapparent infection with a slight increase in body temperature in some piglets, viral replication in cells/organs. Slight leukopenia and/or thrombocytopenia
Walz et al., 2004	BVDV-1 ncp	Intranasal inoculation	Pregnant gilts	-	5–7 dpi	21 dpi / 100%	No clinical signs observed in gilts or piglets; transplacental infection occurred in only one fetus from one gilt. No antibodies were found in piglets
Wieringa- Jelsma et al., 2006	St. Oedenrode strain	Intranasal inoculation	Weaned pigs	2–11 dpi	7 dpi	21 dpi / 100%	Not observed
Dos Santos et al., 2017	BVDV-1 (Singer) cp	Oronasal inoculation	Weaned piglets	10–25 dpi	Not observed	25 dpi / 62.5%	Diarrhea, rough hair, nasal discharge
Nascimento et al., 2017	BVDV-1 (Singer) cp	Oronasal inoculation	Weaned piglets	5–24 dpi	Not observed	25 dpi / 100%	Diarrhea, shivering, nasal discharge
Mechler et al., 2018	BVDV-2 (VS-260) ncp	Oronasal and intrauterine inoculation	Pregnant gilts	No	Not observed	20 dpi / 100%	Not observed
Pereira et al., 2018	BVDV-2 (VS-253) cp	Oronasal inoculation	Pregnant gilts	6–24 dpi	3–12 dpi	12–33 dpi / 70%	Thrombocytopenia
Gomes et al., 2019	BVDV-2 (VS 260) ncp	Oronasal inoculation	Pregnant gilts	No	Not observed	20 dpi / 100%	Not observed
Storino et al., 2020	BVDV-2 (LVB 16557/15) ncp	Oronasal, intramuscular and intravenous inoculation	Boars	No	Not observed	20–40 dpi / 12.5%	Lymphocytosis and monocytopenia

Dpi: days post-inoculation; cp: cytopathic; ncp: non-cytopathic.; NA = not applicable.

These studies proved that BVDV can infect weaned piglets, which shed the virus by the nasal route, presented clinical signs, and seroconverted. The presence of BVDV in nasal secretions indicates that pigs can be a source of infection for other animals, especially if piglets become infected by high virulent strains of BVDV. In the literature, BVDV shedding by a persistently infected boar has also been reported [49], with the detection of the virus in oropharyngeal fluid, urine, and semen.

Although BVDV infection in young pigs can occur without clinical manifestation of the disease [32], other authors have reported the appearance of reproductive problems in pregnant gilts, such as abortions, birth of small piglets, stillborn and congenital persistently infected animals (PI) [22]. In cattle, during acute infection, viremia and viral shedding are usually transient and at low titers, but even so, they can result in vertical transmission [50]. BVDV-2 infection can lead to the occurrence of fetal malformations in cattle; however, if the fetus survives the infection long enough, non-specific changes in maturation may occur in the lymphoid tissues [51]. In bovine herds infected by BVDV, several fetal malformations were described comprising cerebellar hypoplasia, poor myelinization of the spinal cord, hydrocephalus, microcephaly, retinal atrophy or dysplasia, and many others [6]. Diseases affecting myelin sheath formation or nerve synapses alter electrical impulses in neurons, which may lead to tremors [52].

Congenital infection of piglets born from gilts infected with BVDV has been reported in some studies [22,23], in which piglets died between the 2nd and the 16th week of life with signs similar to that of CSF, in addition to showing growth retardation. In a study in which pregnant sows were inoculated with BVDV on the 35th and 45th day of gestation by intrauterine and intranasal route, respectively, nine piglets born from females infected by the intrauterine route and five born from animals infected by intranasal route were born persistently infected [22]. Other studies have also shown transplacental infection, with the virus isolated in at least one of the fetuses [32,53,54].

Conversely, Pereira [27] inoculated BVDV-2 in groups of pregnant gilts at different stages of gestation and before artificial insemination (AI). Seroconversion and a transient viremia were detected, but reproductive losses and clinical signs of the disease in gilts and piglets were not observed. Other recent studies analyzed groups of gilts inoculated by BVDV-2 by oronasal [28,29] and intrauterine [28] routes on the 45th day of pregnancy, before the fetal immunocompetence period. No transplacental transmission was observed since piglets from oro-nasally inoculated gilts were born BVDV-free; no anti-BVDV antibodies were detected in piglets at birth but were acquired by colostral passive transfer. Congenital persistent infection was not observed since piglets did not shed BVDV at any moment. Rates of BVDV transmission between pigs under field conditions is very low, and under experimental conditions it would be even more limited [33].

Regarding intrauterine inoculation [28], piglets were born with no clinical signs of infection and no signs of hypomyelination or CT. Surprisingly, high anti-BVDV-2 antibody titers were found. Serological investigations in bovine fetuses experimentally inoculated with the virus also indicated the development of specific immune competence before the period already established in the literature [51]. The average period of seroconversion of the gilts challenged with the virus was 20 days [28], varying between 12 and 33 days [27]. Other studies have described BVDV inducing viremia seven days post-infection and seroconversion three weeks after experimental inoculation in pigs [55–57]. BVDV was discarded as an etiological agent of CT [28], differently from atypical porcine pestivirus (APPV), which was linked to CT-disease in experimental and natural infection conditions [58–61].

Understanding the role of BVDV in the reproductive system of boars is valuable information, considering that biotechnological procedures have the expressive potential of spreading diseases to free herds [62]. When it comes to boars, the presence of agents of the genus Pestivirus has been confirmed in porcine semen. Shedding of CSFV in porcine semen was the first to be reported under natural and experimental infection [63], as well as virus transmission to sows and fetuses by AI and transplacentally, respectively [64]. Recently, APPV was also detected in the semen and preputial fluid of naturally infected boars, with a high viral load in semen [65]. Experimental infection with BVDV-2 did not result in changes in the post-period of pre-inoculation in most of the seminal characteristics evaluated, and no viral shedding was detected in semen or preputial fluid, but lymphocytosis and monocytopenia were observed [30]. Considering a mild and transient viremia, the likelihood that the circulating virus in the blood reaches different organs was low. Also, the blood-testis barrier would decrease the chance of reaching semen, which may explain the absence of viral RNA detection in the reproductive tract of the inoculated boars [30]. A BVDV persistently infected boar presented viral shedding in the ejaculate, which contained no sperm cells [49]. Possibly, BVDV transmission by semen occurs in atypical cases of congenital persistent infection in pigs [49].

4. Final Consideration

The course of BVDV infection in pigs will depend on the virulence of the viral strain and the pig immune response [66] and may be limited [44]. Even so, the presence of the virus in the nasal secretions of infected animals demonstrated that pigs could act as a source of infection, thus facilitating the spread in the herd [26,27]. Although BVDV does not pose the same threat to pig herds as it poses to ruminants, it may lead to the development of a range of clinical signs and culminate in a serological cross-reaction with the CSFV, interfering negatively in classical swine fever monitoring and surveillance programs, and misleading diagnosis of the disease [10].

Author Contributions: All authors have made substantial contributions to this paper, including manuscript organization, writing, editing, and approving the final version. All authors have read and agreed to the published version of the manuscript.

Acknowledgments: The authors appreciate the support provided by Prof. Eduardo Furtado Flores Federal University of Santa Maria (UFSM) and Dra. Edviges Maristela Pituco (Biological Institute of São Paulo).

References

1. King, A.M.; Lefkowitz, E.; Adams, M.J.; Carstens, E.B. (Eds.) *Virus Taxonomy: Ninth Report of the International Committee on Taxonomy of Viruses*; Elsevier: Amsterdam, The Netherlands, 2011; Volume 9.
2. Houe, H. Economic impact of BVDV infection in dairies. *Biologicals* **2003**, *31*, 137–143. [CrossRef]
3. Moennig, V.; Becher, P. Pestivirus control programs: How far have we come and where are we going? *Anim. Health Res. Rev.* **2015**, *16*, 83–87. [CrossRef] [PubMed]
4. King, A.M.; Lefkowitz, E.J.; Mushegian, A.R.; Adams, M.J.; Dutilh, B.E.; Gorbalenya, A.E.; Kropinski, A.M. Changes to taxonomy and the International Code of Virus Classification and Nomenclature ratified by the International Committee on Taxonomy of Viruses (2018). *Arch. Virol.* **2018**, *163*, 2601–2631. [CrossRef]
5. Yeşilbağ, K.; Alpay, G.; Becher, P. Variability and global distribution of subgenotypes of bovine viral diarrhea virus. *Viruses* **2017**, *9*, 128. [CrossRef] [PubMed]
6. Ridpath, J.; Bauermann, F.V.; Flores, E.F. *Flaviviridae*. In *Virologia Veterinária*, 2nd ed.; Flores, E.F., Ed.; Editora UFSM: Santa Maria, Rio Grande do Sul, Brazil, 2007.
7. Kirklant, P.; Le Potier, M.F.; Vannier, P.; Sinlaison, D. *Pestiviruses*. In *Diseases of Swine*, 10th ed.; Zimmerman, J.J., Karriker, L., Ramirez, A., Schwartz, K.J., Stevenson, G.W., Eds.; Blackwell: Oxford, UK, 2012.
8. Ridpath, J.F. Bovine viral diarrhea virus: Global status. *Vet. Clin. N. Am. Food Anim. Pract.* **2010**, *26*, 105–121. [CrossRef] [PubMed]
9. Deng, Y.; Sun, C.Q.; Cao, S.J.; Lin, T.; Yuan, S.S.; Zhang, H.B.; Wen, X.T.; Tong, G.Z. High prevalence of bovine viral diarrhea virus 1 in Chinese swine herds. *Vet. Microbiol.* **2012**, *159*, 490–493. [CrossRef]
10. Loeffen, W.L.A.; Van Beuningen, A.; Quak, S.; Elbers, A.R.W. Seroprevalence and risk factors for the presence of ruminant pestiviruses in the Dutch swine population. *Vet. Microbiol.* **2009**, *136*, 240–245. [CrossRef]
11. Mosena, A.C.; Weber, M.N.; Cibulski, S.P.; Silva, M.S.; Paim, W.P.; Silva, G.S.; Silveira, S. Survey for pestiviruses in backyard pigs in southern Brazil. *J. Vet. Diag. Investig.* **2020**, *32*, 136–141. [CrossRef]

12. Almeida, H.M.S.; Gatto, I.R.H.; dos Santos, A.C.R.; Ferraudo, A.S.; Samara, S.I.; de Oliveira, L.G. A Cross-Sectional and Exploratory Geospatial Study of Bovine Viral Diarrhea Virus (BVDV) Infections in Swines in the São Paulo State, Brazil. *Pak. Vet. J.* **2017**, *37*, 470–474.
13. Gatto, I.R.H.; Linhares, D.C.L.; de Souza Almeida, H.M.; Mathias, L.A.; de Medeiros, A.S.R.; Poljak, Z.; de Oliveira, L.G. Description of risk factors associated with the detection of BVDV antibodies in Brazilian pig herds. *Trop. Anim. Health Prod.* **2018**, *50*, 773–778. [CrossRef]
14. Liess, B.; Moennig, V. Ruminant pestivirus infection in pigs. *Rev. Sci. Tech.* **1990**, *9*, 151–161. [CrossRef] [PubMed]
15. O'Connor, M.; Lenihan, P.; Dillon, P. Pestivirus antibodies in pigs in Ireland. *Vet. Rec.* **1991**, *129*, 269. [CrossRef] [PubMed]
16. Løken, T.; Krogsrud, J.; Larsen, I.L. Pestivirus infections in Norway. Serological investigations in cattle, sheep and pigs. *Acta. Vet. Scand.* **1991**, *32*, 27–34. [PubMed]
17. Graham, D.A.; Calvert, V.; German, A.; McCullough, S.J. Pestiviral infections in sheep and pigs in Northern Ireland. *Vet. Rec.* **2001**, *148*, 69–72. [CrossRef] [PubMed]
18. Jensen, M.H. Screening for neutralizing antibodies against hog cholera-and/or bovine viral diarrhea virus in Danish pigs. *Acta. Vet. Scand.* **1985**, *26*, 72–80.
19. Weber, M.N.; Pino, E.H.M.; Souza, C.K.; Mósena, A.C.S.; Sato, J.P.H.; de Barcellos, D.E.S.N.; Canal, C.W. First evidence of bovine viral diarrhea virus infection in wild boars. *Acta Sci. Vet.* **2016**, *44*, 1–5. [CrossRef]
20. Weber, M.N.; Silveira, S.; Machado, G.; Groff, F.H.; Mósena, A.C.; Budaszewski, R.F.; Dupont, P.M.; Corbellini, L.G.; Canal, C.W. High frequency of bovine viral diarrhea virus type 2 in Southern Brazil. *Virus Res.* **2014**, *19*, 117–124. [CrossRef]
21. Becher, P.; Ramirez, R.A.; Orlich, M.; Rosales, S.C.; König, M.; Schweizer, M.; Thiel, H.J. Genetic and antigenic characterization of novel pestivirus genotypes: Implications for classification. *Virology* **2003**, *311*, 96–104. [CrossRef]
22. Paton, D.J.; Done, S.H. Congenital infection of pigs with ruminant-type pestiviruses. *J. Comp. Pathol.* **1994**, *111*, 151–163. [CrossRef]
23. Terpstra, C.; Wensvoort, G. Natural infections of pigs with bovine viral diarrhea virus associated with signs resembling swine fever. *Res. Vet. Sci.* **1988**, *45*, 137–142. [CrossRef]
24. Paton, D.J.; Lowings, J.P.; Barrett, A.D.T. Epitope mapping of the gp53 envelope protein of bovine viral diarrhea virus. *Virology* **1992**, *190*, 763–772. [CrossRef]
25. Santos, A.C.R.; Nascimento, K.A.; Mechler, M.L.; Almeida, H.M.S.; Gatto, I.R.H.; Carnielli, L.G.F.; Pollo, A.S.; De Oliveira, L.G. Experimental infection and evaluation of airborne transmission and nose-to-nose contact of bovine viral diarrhea virus among weaned piglets. *AJBAS* **2017**, *11*, 12–19.
26. Nascimento, K.A.; Mechler, M.L.; Gatto, I.R.; Almeida, H.M.S.; Pollo, A.S.; Sant'Ana, F.J.; Oliveira, L.G.D. Evidence of bovine viral diarrhea virus transmission by back pond water in experimentally infected piglets. *Pesq. Vet. Bras.* **2018**, *38*, 1896–1901. [CrossRef]
27. Pereira, D.A.; Peron, J.B.; de Souza Almeida, H.M.; Baraldi, T.G.; Gatto, I.R.H.; Kasmanas, T.C.; de Oliveira, L.G. Experimental inoculation of gilts with bovine viral diarrhea virus 2 (BVDV-2) does not induce transplacental infection. *Vet. Microbiol.* **2018**, *225*, 25–30. [CrossRef]
28. Mechler, M.L.; dos Santos Gomes, F.; Nascimento, K.A.; de Souza-Pollo, A.; Pires, F.F.B.; Samara, S.I.; Pituco, M.E.; de Oliveira, L.G. Congenital tremor in piglets: Is bovine viral diarrhea virus an etiological cause? *Vet. Microbiol.* **2018**, *220*, 107–112. [CrossRef]
29. Gomes, F.S.; Mechler-Dreibi, M.L.; Gatto, I.R.H.; Storino, G.Y.; Pires, F.F.B.; Xavier, E.B.; Samara, S.I. Congenital persistent infection with bovine viral diarrhea virus not observed in piglets. *Can. Vet. J.* **2019**, *10*, 1220–1222.
30. Storino, G.Y.; Xavier, E.B.; Mechler-Dreibi, M.L.; Simonatto, A.; Gatto, I.R.H.; Oliveira, M.E.F.; de Oliveira, L.G. No effects of noncytopathic bovine viral diarrhea virus type 2 on the reproductive tract of experimentally inoculated boars. *Vet. Microbiol.* **2020**, *240*, 108512. [CrossRef]
31. Walz, P.H.; Baker, J.C.; Mullaney, T.P.; Kaneene, J.B.; Maes, R.K. Comparison of type I and type II bovine viral diarrhea virus infection in swine. *Can. J. Vet. Res.* **1999**, *63*, 119.
32. Walz, P.H.; Baker, J.C.; Mullaney, T.P.; Maes, R.K. Experimental inoculation of pregnant swine with type 1 bovine viral diarrhoea virus. *J. Vet. Med. Ser. B* **2004**, *51*, 191–193. [CrossRef]
33. Wieringa-Jelsma, T.; Quak, S.; Loeffen, W.L.A. Limited BVDV transmission and full protection against CSFV transmission in pigs experimentally infected with BVDV type 1b. *Vet. Microbiol.* **2006**, *118*, 26–36. [CrossRef]

34. Langohr, I.M.; Stevenson, G.W.; Nelson, E.A.; Lenz, S.D.; Wei, H.; Pogranichniy, R.M. Experimental co-infection of pigs with Bovine viral diarrhea virus 1 and Porcine circovirus-2. *J. Vet. Diag. Investig.* **2012**, *24*, 51–64. [CrossRef] [PubMed]
35. Chase, C.C. The impact of BVDV infection on adaptive immunity. *Biologicals* **2013**, *41*, 52–60. [CrossRef] [PubMed]
36. Iwasaki, A.; Medzhitov, R. Regulation of adaptive immunity by the innate immune system. *Science* **2010**, *327*, 291–295. [CrossRef] [PubMed]
37. Vilček, Š.; Nettleton, P.F. Pestiviruses in wild animals. *Vet. Microbiol.* **2006**, *116*, 1–12. [CrossRef]
38. Fan, X.Z.; Ning, Y.B.; Wang, Q.; Xu, L.; Shen, Q.C. Detection of bovine viral diarrhea virus as contaminant in classical swine fever virus live vaccine with RT-PCR. *Chin. J. Vet. Med.* **2010**, *46*, 8–10.
39. Houe, H.; Lindberg, A.; Moennig, V. Test strategies in bovine viral diarrhea virus control and eradication campaigns. *Eur. J. Vet. Diag. Investig.* **2006**, *18*, 427–436. [CrossRef]
40. Kliučinskas, R.; Lukauskas, K.; Milius, J.; Vyšniauskis, G.; Kliučinskas, D.; Šalomskas, A. Detection of bovine viral diarrhoea virus in saliva samples. *Bull. Vet. Inst. Pulawy* **2008**, *52*, 31–37.
41. Vilček, Š.; Strojny, L.; Ďurkovič, B.; Rossmanith, W.; Paton, D. Storage of bovine viral diarrhoea virus samples on filter paper and detection of viral RNA by a RT-PCR method. *J. Virol. Methods* **2001**, *92*, 19–22. [CrossRef]
42. Blank, W.A.; Henderson, K.S.; White, L.A. Virus PCR assay panels: An alternative to the mouse antibody production test. *Lab Anim.* **2004**, *33*, 26–32. [CrossRef]
43. Samara, S.I.; Dias, F.C.; Moreira, S.P.G. Ocorrência da diarréia viral bovina nas regiões sul do Estado de Minas Gerais e nordeste do Estado de São Paulo. *Braz. J. Vet. Res. Anim. Sci.* **2004**, *41*, 396–403. [CrossRef]
44. O'Sullivan, T.; Friendship, R.; Carman, S.; Pearl, D.L.; McEwen, B.; Dewey, C. Seroprevalence of bovine viral diarrhea virus neutralizing antibodies in finisher hogs in Ontario swine herds and targeted diagnostic testing of 2 suspect herds. *Can. Vet. J.* **2011**, *52*, 1342–1344. [PubMed]
45. Dahle, J.; Patzelt, T.; Schagemann, G.; Liess, B. Antibody prevalence of hog cholera, bovine viral diarrhoea and Aujeszky's disease virus in wild boars in northern Germany. *DTW* **1993**, *100*, 330–333.
46. Sedlak, K.; Bartova, E.; Machova, J. Antibodies to selected viral disease agents in wild boars from the Czech Republic. *J. Wildl. Dis.* **2008**, *44*, 777–780. [CrossRef] [PubMed]
47. Milićević, V.; Maksimović-Zorić, J.; Veljović, L.; Kureljušić, B.; Savić, B.; Cvetojević, Đ.; Radosavljević, V. Bovine viral diarrhea virus infection in wild boar. *Res. Vet. Sci.* **2018**, *119*, 76–78. [CrossRef]
48. Gatto, I.R.; Di Santo, L.G.; Storino, G.Y.; Sanfilippo, L.F.; Ribeiro, M.G.; Mathias, L.A.; De Oliveira, L.G. Serological survey of bovine viral diarrhea (BVDV-1), brucellosis, and leptospirosis in captive white-lipped peccaries (Tayassu pecari) from the Midwest region in Brazil. *Austral J. Vet. Sci.* **2020**, *52*, 37–42. [CrossRef]
49. Terpstra, C.; Wensvoort, G. A congenital persistent infection of bovine virus diarrhoea virus in pigs: Clinical, virological and immunological observations. *Vet. Q.* **1997**, *19*, 97–101. [CrossRef]
50. Thurmond, M.C. Virus Transmission. In *Bovine Viral Diarrhea Virus: Diagnosis, Management, and Control*; Goyal, S.M., Ridpath, J.F., Eds.; John Wiley & Sons: Hoboken, NJ, USA, 2008.
51. Ohmann, H.B. Experimental fetal infection with bovine viral diarrhea virus. II. Morphological reactions and distribution of viral antigen. *Can. J. Comp. Med.* **1982**, *46*, 363.
52. Scarratt, W.K. Cerebellar disease and disease characterized by dysmetria or tremors. *Vet. Clin. N. Am. Food Anim. Pract.* **2004**, *20*, 275–286. [CrossRef]
53. Grooms, D.L. Reproductive losses caused by bovine viral diarrhea virus and leptospirosis. *Theriogenology* **2006**, *66*, 624–628. [CrossRef]
54. Bachofen, C.; Vogt, H.R.; Stalder, H.; Mathys, T.; Zanoni, R.; Hilbe, M.; Peterhans, E. Persistent infections after natural transmission of bovine viral diarrhoea virus from cattle to goats and among goats. *Vet. Res.* **2013**, *44*, 32. [CrossRef]
55. Stewart, W.C.; Miller, L.D.; Kresse, J.I.; Snyder, M.L. Bovine viral diarrhea infection in pregnant swine. *Am. J. Vet. Res.* **1980**, *41*, 459–462. [PubMed]
56. Kulcsar, G.; Soos, P.; Kucsera, L.; Glavits, R.; Pálfi, V. Pathogenicity of a bovine viral diarrhoea virus strain in pregnant sows. *Acta. Vet. Hung.* **2001**, *49*, 117–120. [CrossRef] [PubMed]
57. Makoschey, B.; Liebler-Tenorio, E.M.; Biermann, Y.M.; Goovaerts, D.; Pohlenz, J.F. Leukopenia and thrombocytopenia in pigs after infection with bovine viral diarrhoea virus-2 (BVDV-2). *DTW* **2002**, *109*, 225–230.

58. Arruda, B.L.; Arruda, P.H.; Magstadt, D.R.; Schwartz, K.J.; Dohlman, T.; Schleining, J.A.; Victoria, J.G. Identification of a divergent lineage porcine pestivirus in nursing piglets with congenital tremors and reproduction of disease following experimental inoculation. *PLoS ONE* **2016**, *11*, e0150104. [CrossRef]
59. De Groof, A.; Deijs, M.; Guelen, L.; Van Grinsven, L.; Os-Galdos, V.; Vogels, W.; Suijskens, J. Atypical porcine pestivirus: A possible cause of congenital tremor type A-II in Newborn piglets. *Viruses* **2016**, *8*, 271. [CrossRef]
60. Schwarz, L.; Riedel, C.; Högler, S.; Sinn, L.J.; Voglmayr, T.; Wöchtl, B.; Rümenapf, T. Congenital infection with atypical porcine pestivirus (APPV) is associated with disease and viral persistence. *Vet. Res.* **2017**, *48*, 1. [CrossRef]
61. Gatto, I.R.H.; Harmon, K.; Bradner, L.; Silva, P.; Linhares, D.C.L.; Arruda, P.H.; Arruda, B.L. Detection of atypical porcine pestivirus in Brazil in the central nervous system of suckling piglets with congenital tremor. *Transbound. Emerg. Dis.* **2018**, *65*, 375–380. [CrossRef]
62. Maes, D.; Van Soom, A.; Appeltant, R.; Arsenakis, I.; Nauwynck, H. Porcine semen as a vector for transmission of viral pathogens. *Theriogenology* **2016**, *85*, 27–38. [CrossRef]
63. Choi, C.; Chae, C. Detection of classical swine fever virus in boar semen by reverse transcription–polymerase chain reaction. *J. Vet. Diag. Investig.* **2003**, *15*, 35–41. [CrossRef]
64. De Smit, A.J.; Bouma, A.; Terpstra, C.; Van Oirschot, J.T. Transmission of classical swine fever virus by artificial insemination. *Vet. Microbial.* **1999**, *67*, 239–249. [CrossRef]
65. Gatto, I.R.H.; Arruda, P.H.; Visek, C.A.; Victoria, J.G.; Patterson, A.R.; Krull, A.C.; Arruda, B.L. Detection of atypical porcine pestivirus in semen from commercial boar studs in the United States. *Transbound. Emerg. Dis.* **2018**, *65*, e339–e343. [CrossRef] [PubMed]
66. Penrith, M.L.; Vosloo, W.; Mather, C. Classical swine fever (hog cholera): Review of aspects relevant to control. *Transbound. Emerg. Dis.* **2011**, *58*, 187–196. [CrossRef] [PubMed]

6

Monitoring *Mycoplasma bovis* Diversity and Antimicrobial Susceptibility in Calf Feedlots Undergoing a Respiratory Disease Outbreak

Claire A.M. Becker [1,*], Chloé Ambroset [1], Anthéa Huleux [2,†], Angélique Vialatte [2,‡], Adélie Colin [2], Agnès Tricot [1], Marie-Anne Arcangioli [1] and Florence Tardy [2]

[1] UMR Mycoplasmoses des Ruminants, VetAgro Sup, Université de Lyon, 69280 Marcy-l'Etoile, France; chloe.ambroset@vetagro-sup.fr (C.A.); agnes.tricot@vetagro-sup.fr (A.T.); marie-anne.arcangioli@vetagro-sup.fr (M.-A.A.)

[2] UMR Mycoplasmoses des Ruminants, ANSES Laboratoire de Lyon, Université de Lyon, 69364 Lyon CEDEX 07, France; anthea.huleux@orange.fr (A.H.); angelique.vialatte@gmail.com (A.V.); adelie.colin@anses.fr (A.C.); florence.tardy@anses.fr (F.T.)

* Correspondence: claire.becker@vetagro-sup.fr

† Current Address: Cancer Research Centre of Lyon, 69008 Lyon, France.

‡ Current Address: Mylan Laboratories SAS, 01400 Châtillon-sur-Chalaronne, France.

Abstract: Bovine respiratory diseases (BRD) are widespread in veal calf feedlots. Several pathogens are implicated, both viruses and bacteria, one of which, *Mycoplasma bovis*, is under-researched. This worldwide-distributed bacterium has been shown to be highly resistant in vitro to the main antimicrobials used to treat BRD. Our objective was to monitor the relative prevalence of *M. bovis* during BRD episodes, its diversity, and its resistance phenotype in relation to antimicrobial use. For this purpose, a two-year longitudinal follow-up of 25 feedlots was organized and 537 nasal swabs were collected on 358 veal calves at their arrival in the lot, at the BRD peak and 4 weeks after collective antimicrobial treatments. The presence of *M. bovis* was assessed by real-time PCR and culture. The clones isolated were then subtyped (*polC* subtyping and PFGE analysis), and their susceptibility to five antimicrobials was determined. The course of the disease and the antimicrobials used had no influence on the genetic diversity of the *M. bovis* strains: The subtype distribution was the same throughout the BRD episode and similar to that already described in France, with a major narrowly-variable subtype circulating, st2. The same conclusion holds for antimicrobial resistance (AMR) phenotypes: All the clones were already multiresistant to the main antimicrobials used (except for fluoroquinolones) prior to any treatments. By contrast, changes of AMR phenotypes could be suspected for Pasteurellaceae in two cases in relation to the treatments registered.

Keywords: *Mycoplasma bovis*; antimicrobial resistance; Bovine Respiratory Disease; genetic diversity

---

1. Introduction

Bovine Respiratory Disease (BRD), also known as "shipping fever", is a very common and extremely costly disease impacting the beef cattle industry worldwide [1]. It is a complex viral and/or bacterial infection affecting the upper or lower respiratory tracts in cattle, with a particularly high prevalence in recently weaned calves within the first days or weeks of arrival at the feedlot [2]. Multiple stress factors (weaning, transportation, co-mingling in lots or in markets, changes in diet, weather changes, etc.) with additive effects are known to influence the susceptibility of calves to developing BRD [3]. The percentage of morbidity and mortality can reach 70% but varies with the management system in place, prevention programs and the kind of pathogens involved, bacteria being more often fatal than viruses alone [1]. The disease most often results from an overwhelming, dysregulated host immune response [4]. Classical clinical signs of bacterial BRD include fever over 40 °C, dyspnea, nasal discharge, coughing and depression with diminished or no appetite [2]. The most common viral agents associated with BRD include Bovine Herpes Virus type 1 (BHV-1), Parainfluenza-3 virus (PI3), Bovine Viral Diarrhea Virus (BVDV), Bovine Coronavirus (BCoV) and Bovine Respiratory Syncytial Virus (BRSV). The main bacteria are *Mannheimia haemolytica*, *Pasteurella multocida*, *Histophilus somni* and *Mycoplasma* (*M.*) *bovis* [5,6]. These agents are not all equivalent in terms of pathogenesis, duration of the clinical disease or shedding after exposure [5,6]. Viral agents are thought to be mainly initiators of the disease that then facilitate colonization by bacterial pathogens or aggravating factors during co-infection [7]. Among bacteria, *M. bovis* is still regarded as the least well-characterized BRD pathogen [6–8]. It has been reported to rapidly proliferate in the nasopharynx within the first 14 days of feedlot placement as a preliminary step in the development of BRD [3,9]. Asymptomatic carriage months or even years after an outbreak have been described but with a low prevalence and a role on transmission yet to be defined [10].

Prevention and control of BRD rely on metaphylaxis in high-risk herds (e.g., >1000 animals in the USA), bacterial vaccinations when available, but with controversial efficacies, and antimicrobial treatments of diseased animals [11,12]. Because feedlot management uses many antimicrobials, antimicrobial resistance (AMR) among the bacterial pathogens commonly associated with BRD has been increasingly reported worldwide [12,13]. *M. bovis* is no exception [14].

In France, previous studies have demonstrated the spread of an *M. bovis* clonal population with acquired resistance to most antimicrobial families except for fluoroquinolones [15–17]. However, these data capture a particular context of sampling that might not reflect the short-term evolution of isolates toward AMR. All these studies used strains collected in the framework of our network, Vigimyc, a "passive" surveillance network, the decision to test for mycoplasmas being solely on the initiative of the veterinarian [18]. Most often, a diagnosis for *Mycoplasma* is requested when all other analyses have proved negative or when a treatment failure is observed. Biased sampling might therefore result from using Vigimyc strains as they often originate from antimicrobials-treated animals. *Mycoplasma* species are known to evolve fast, and they develop AMR mainly through mutations in antimicrobial targets, which could be rapidly selected under antimicrobial pressure [19–22].

The present study was conducted to refine our understanding of relationships between antimicrobial use, AMR phenotype (as Minimum inhibitory concentration, MIC) and clonal diversity in *M. bovis* during BRD episodes. For that purpose, a longitudinal follow-up of 25 feedlots was conducted, with complete etiological exploration when BRD cases occurred, from the day of introduction to 4 weeks after the clinical peak. *M. bovis* isolate diversity per feedlot and per animal (by molecular subtyping and Pulsed-Field Gel Electrophoresis, PFGE) and AMR were analyzed before and after treatments. The relative persistence of *M. bovis* and Pasteurellaceae after antimicrobial treatment was also explored.

2. Results

2.1. M. bovis Was the Third Most Frequently Isolated Pathogen (in Association with Others) in Calf Feedlots at BRD Onset

During the 2016–2017 and 2017–2018 winters, 537 double nasal swabs (DNS) were sampled on 358 veal calves in 25 feedlots of Western France. Their characteristics are listed in Supplementary Table S1. Three sampling times were defined: introduction of the animals (T0), BRD peak (T1) and 4 weeks after collective antimicrobial treatment (T2) (Figure 1, Table 1). Four feedlots were excluded from the prevalence study as no BRD episode occurred.

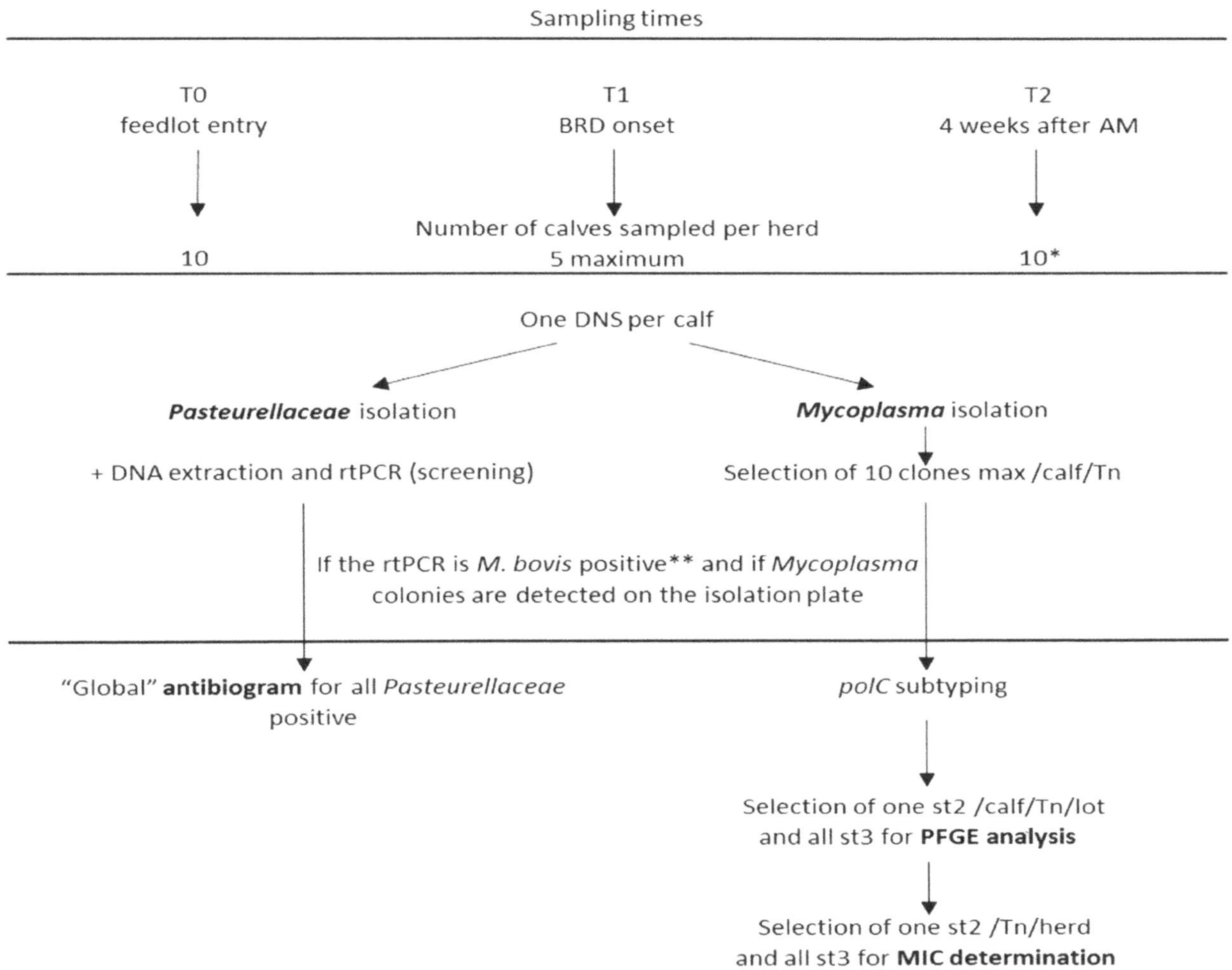

Figure 1. Workflow for sample collection and analyses. DNS, double nasal swab; AM, antimicrobial treatment. * If possible the same 10 calves were sampled at T0 and T2. ** Ct ≤ 37 in rtPCR.

Table 1. Number of double nasal swabs (DNS), calves harboring *M. bovis* (assessed with culture and real-time Polymerase Chain Reaction (rtPCR)) and clones isolated at each sampling time.

	T0	T1	T2	Total
DNS	271	115	151	537
Calves with *M. bovis* rtPCR	6 (2%)	59 (51%)	39/79 * (49%)	104
Calves with *M. bovis* culture	5 (2%)	60 (52%)	28 (19%)	93
Isolated clones	38	251	125	414

T0, feedlot entry; T1, BRD onset; T2, 4 weeks after antimicrobial treatment. * Not all T2 samples were tested by rtPCR (see Supplementary Table S1 for details).

At BRD onset (T1), the etiology was determined using a real-time Polymerase Chain Reaction (rtPCR) screening of seven pathogens (Figure 2). Out of the 21 feedlots where BRD occurred, 115 calves were tested, and *M. bovis* was detected in 51% of them (n = 59), with a mean Ct of 25.7 [20.4–35]. The positive calves (Ct ≤ 37) originated from 18 feedlots: Three feedlots had only calves negative for *M. bovis* (Supplementary Table S1). *M. bovis* ranked as the third most prevalent pathogen after *P. multocida* and the Coronavirus, this triple association being the most common coinfection, calves being frequently infected by more than one pathogen. The proportion of calves found positive at T1 by a culture approach was very similar to that from rtPCR (52%, n = 60) (Table 1). We note that for some calves in different lots (e.g., ME, Supplementary Table S1), cultures were initially positive for *M. bovis*, but no clones could be successfully retrieved from plates, mainly due to coinfections with *M. bovirhinis*.

By contrast, *M. bovis* was seldom detected at feedlot entry (T0). Detection rate was 2%: 5/271 calves by culture and 6/271 by rtPCR, with a mean Ct of 36.7 [25.4–36.8], this difference being compatible with a weak infectious load in the positive calves. Four weeks after the antimicrobial treatment (T2), the presence of *M. bovis* remained high as determined by rtPCR (49%, 39/79, 12/13 feedlots being positive (Supplementary Table S1) with a mean Ct of 30.4 [23.6–36.7]. These Ct values suggest that at this stage of clinical recovery, the viable *Mycoplasma* load was rather low, as the proportion of calves positive by culture was only 17% (25/151 calves, 13/24 lots being considered positive, see Supplementary Table S1).

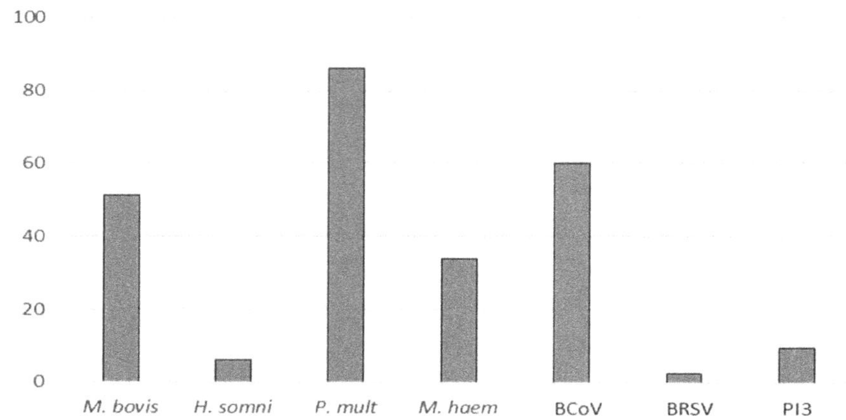

Figure 2. Proportions of calves harboring the different pathogens as assessed by rtPCR at BRD onset (T1, n = 115 calves tested).

The different pathogens tested, indicated on x-axis, are *Mycoplasma bovis* (*M. bovis*), *Histophilus somni* (*H. somni*), *Pasteurella multocida* (*P. mult*), *Mannheimia haemolytica* (*M. haem*), Bovine Coronavirus (BCoV), Bovine Respiratory Syncytial Virus (BRSV) and Parainfluenza 3 virus (PI3). Y-axis, percentage of calves infected with each pathogen.

2.2. The Diversity of Clones Does Not Differ at Different Sampling Times and Is Similar to the Reference Population of Vigimyc Isolates

The number of isolated clones per feedlot (with a maximum of 10 per calf) selected from agar plates, with their characteristics, is given in Supplementary Table S1. Out of the 414 clones retrieved from the 93 calves sampled at different times in the 25 feedlots, 400 were subtyped using the *polC* subtyping scheme as proposed earlier [15]. Most (313/400, 78%) st2 was recovered, but st3 was also present (86/400, 21%). Both subtypes could be found in the same feedlot at the same sampling time, but no calf was shown to harbor both subtypes at one sampling time. For this reason, we further analyzed the proportion of subtypes per calf at each sampling time, which we considered thereafter as our epidemiological unit. This proportion was of 81% calves having a st2 *M. bovis* (Figure 3A), while 18% had a st3 *M. bovis*. Surprisingly, a new st was defined in the French scheme for one calf (T2-RO-1647, black on Figure 3) showing 15 SNPs with respect to the reference sequence of PG45^{TS} (11 out of 15 SNPs in common with the st3 sequence). The subtype determined using the MLST scheme of Register was ST45 (legacy scheme, ST124) [23,24].

The st proportions were identical between different sampling times (Figure 3B). No clear evolution of subtypes proportions was observed along the study, whatever the antimicrobials used in the herds

(Supplementary Table S2). Some calves harbored the same st in T1 and T2 (e.g., HA-8680 with st2 or NE-6423 with st3), whereas others had a different st at the two sampling times (e.g., NE-8907 st2 then st3 or CA-8149 st3 then st2), suggesting a potential contamination by another strain in the course of the fattening period.

The overall proportions of the st in the study (calculated on calf numbers) was compared to the diversity retrieved among the strains of the Vigimyc network over the past six years (Figure 3A). The same epidemiological tendency was observed between the study strains and the Vigimyc strains: The st2 *polC* subtype was the most prevalent, while the proportion of st3 was similar at each sampling date in this study (19%).

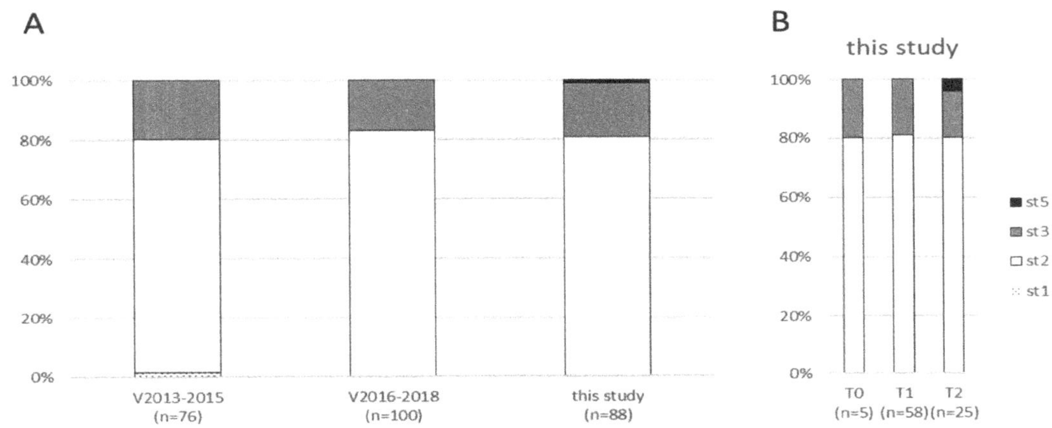

Figure 3. Subtype proportions of French strains of the Vigimyc network over the past 6 years and the clones of this study determined by *polC* subtyping. (**A**) Global comparison between Vigimyc strains and those from the present study and (**B**) detailed proportions of st according to sampling times (T0, T1, T2) in this study. X-axis, category of strains (Vigimyc, V, with different sampling year or this study); y-axis, proportion of each subtype. Numbers in brackets under each lane indicate the number of strains tested.

A restricted panel of clones was then analyzed by PFGE to further evaluate their relatedness. We first evaluated intra-st2 diversity by analyzing all the clones from two feedlots. All the st2 clones retrieved from eight sampled calves showed a unique, identical PFGE pattern, with no difference between calves or feedlots (data not shown). Consequently, in further analyses, for st2, only one clone per calf and per sampling time was selected. Because an increased diversity was expected from st3 clones [15] and as these were less numerous, they were all tested by PFGE. The PFGE patterns were homogeneous for all the st2 clones (Branch A in Figure 4) while the st3 clones showed more diversity (Branches B to I, in Figure 4, see also Supplementary Table S2). This within-st3 diversity was observed at different levels, i.e., different feedlots, different calves, or even different clones isolated from the same calf (e.g., T1-FO-0494-c3 or c11 * in Figure 4). However, no correlation was established between the PFGE profiles and the treatment history or sampling date. The st5 clone was found in a specific, different branch (J in Figure 4), showing a more distant profile.

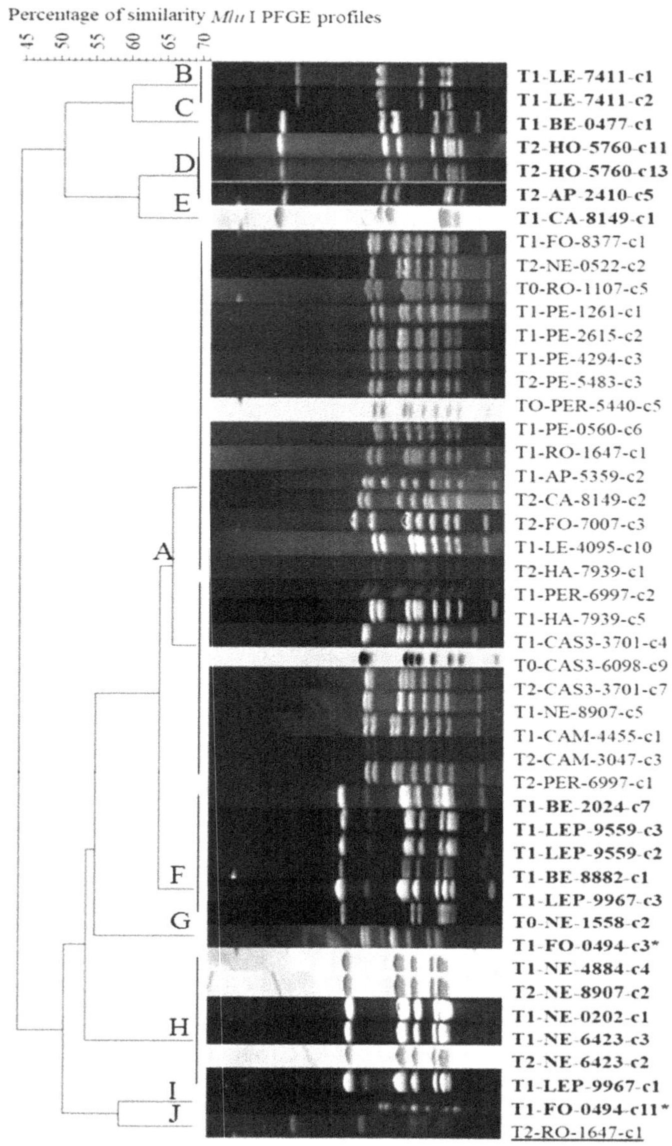

Figure 4. Cluster analysis of 46 *M. bovis* clones based on their Pulse Field Gel Electrophoresis (PFGE)-*MluI* profiles using the Dice coefficient and UPGMA method. The resulting degree of similarity is indicated on the scale on the top left corner (similarity cut-off value set at 70%). *M. bovis* clones are characterized by the sampling time, feedlot name, calf number and clone number. (**A**) cluster of st2 strains; (**B–I**) clusters of st3 strains (bold); J, branch for the clone of new st5 (underlined); the asterisk indicates 2 clones coming from the same calf with different PFGE profiles.

2.3. *M. bovis Field Isolates Are Already Multiresistant to Antimicrobials before Any Treatment in the Lot*

Antimicrobial susceptibility was tested on 39 clones representative of the various genetic subtypes or macrorestriction profiles and the different sampling times, i.e., one representative clone of st2 per feedlot and per sampling time and one representative clone per PFGE cluster per calf and per sampling time for st3 (see Supplementary Table S2). As no breakpoints are available for *M. bovis*, clinical breakpoints for Pasteurellaceae were used for interpretation of the results [25] and the MIC90 for the French *M. bovis* population (as calculated from Gautier Bouchardon et al., 2014 for recent isolates, collected between 2010 and 2012 [16]) are also indicated (blue double arrows in Figure 5). Whatever the sampling time, all the clones were resistant to oxytetracycline, tilmicosin and florfenicol (Figure 5A,B,D), except for one susceptible and three intermediary strains for florfenicol (Figure 5D).

By contrast, most of the clones showed a low MIC of enrofloxacin (≤0.25 μg/mL, Figure 5C), except for three clones with a slight increase in MIC (0.5–1 μg/mL). These three clones were isolated from three different feedlots (see Supplementary Table S1): in one of these, oxolinic acid was used once to treat some calves before T1. No relationship was observed between MIC and sampling time, or with subtype.

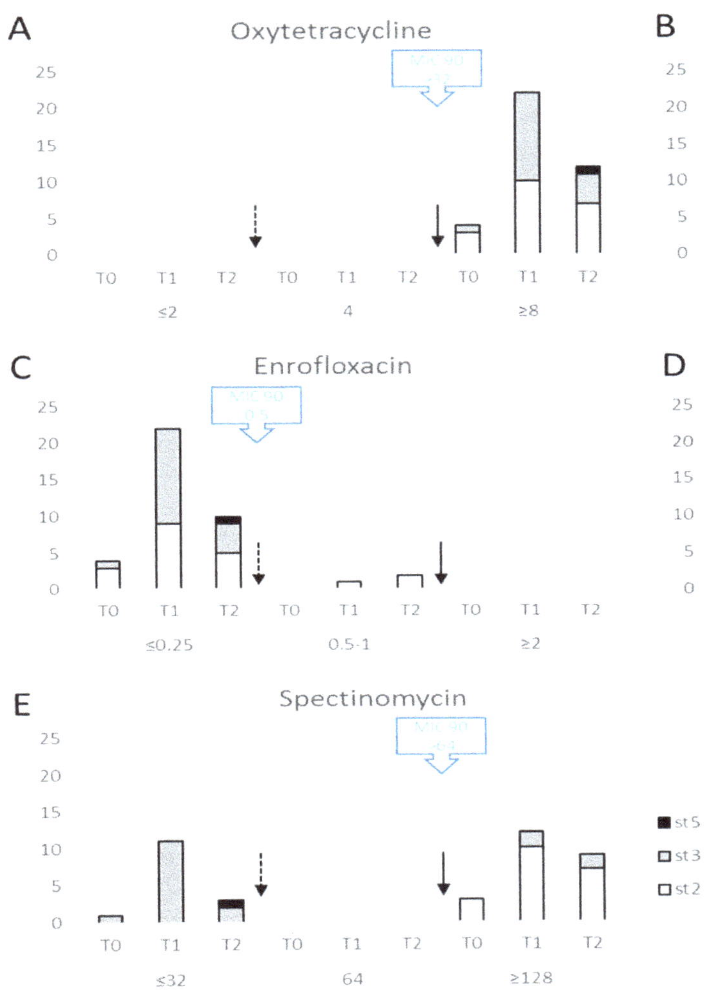

Figure 5. Minimum Inhibitory Concentrations (MICs) for 5 antimicrobial molecules for 39 clones according to their genetic st (*polC* subtyping) and sampling date. (**A**) Oxytetracycline, (**B**) Tilmicosin, (**C**) Enrofloxacin, (**D**) Florfenicol, (**E**) Spectinomycin. X-axis, MIC classes detailed with sampling times; y-axis, number of isolates. Arrows indicate the threshold for Pasteurellaceae when available; dotted arrow, susceptible to intermediate MIC; plain arrow, intermediate to resistant MIC. Blue rectangles with arrow indicate the MIC90 for the French *M. bovis* strains collected between 2010–2012 [16] (oxytetracycline > 32, tilmicosin > 128, enrofloxacin 0.5, florfenicol 16, spectinomycin > 64).

For spectinomycin, 15/39 strains showed surprisingly low MICs (Figure 5E) that classify them as susceptible according to CLSI [25]. They were from T0, T1 or T2 but showed the common characteristic of being of st3 (in one case st5). This contrasted with previous data obtained on French strains (MIC90 > 64 μg/mL for strains collected in 2010–2012 [16]). To further analyze this discrepancy, 33 strains isolated between 2011 and 2018 (mainly st3 and a few st2 as control, see Supplementary Table S1) through the Vigimyc network were selected and their MICs for spectinomycin analyzed (Figure 6). A third of the strains (33.3%) were susceptible to spectinomycin, irrespective of subtype.

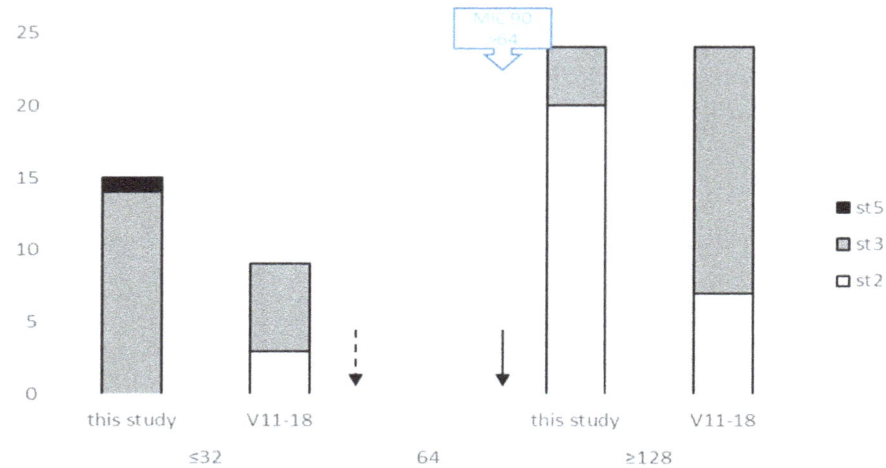

Figure 6. Distribution of *M. bovis* strains MICs for spectinomycin as a function of their origin and genetic subtype (*polC* subtyping). X-axis, spectinomycin MICs for sets of strains (either from Vigimyc and isolated between 2011 to 2018, V11-18, or from this study); y-axis, number of isolates. Arrows indicate the threshold for Pasteurellaceae when available; dotted arrow, susceptible to intermediate MIC; plain arrow, intermediate to resistant MIC. Blue rectangle with arrow indicates the MIC90 for the French *M. bovis* strains collected between 2010–2012 [16] (spectinomycin > 64).

No correlation could be found between antimicrobial treatments used in the feedlots (Supplementary Table S1) and either MIC or genetic subtype, whatever the substance used. No selection was observed as a result of the various treatments used in the feedlots.

2.4. *Antimicrobial Resistance Profile of Pasteurellaceae Is Different from That of M. bovis*

M. bovis and Pasteurellaceae were co-isolated in 13 occurrences (five different feedlots, different sampling times) (see Supplementary Table S2 and Figure S1). In these 13 occurrences of co-isolation, the antimicrobial susceptibility profiles of Pasteurellaceae were examined by the disk method. *P. multocida* strains were mainly sensitive to amoxicillin, tulathromycin, tylosin, spectinomycin, florfenicol, enrofloxacin and marbofloxacin but resistant to tetracycline. In one feedlot (CAM) we detected strains resistant to tulathromycin. The sole strain of *M. haemolytica* that was isolated in the study (T1, herd NE) was resistant to amoxicillin, intermediate for enrofloxacin and tulathromycin and susceptible for the other antimicrobials.

In two feedlots (CAS5 and NE), collective antimicrobial treatments could have helped to select resistant strains. In CAS5 where doxycycline was used as metaphylaxis at the BRD peak, isolates were resistant to tetracycline at T1 and T2 but not at T0 (Supplementary Figure S1A,D). In NE, where spectinomycin was used individually, though not for the sampled calves, isolates were resistant to spectinomycin at T1 and T2 but not at T0 (Supplementary Figure S1E).

Pasteurellaceae remained globally largely more susceptible to antimicrobials than *M. bovis*. Although it is hard to conclude on a small number of strains, it seems that treatment influenced Pasteurellaceae antimicrobial susceptibility patterns, as the selection of resistant isolates was observed in two situations.

3. Discussion

In the present study, out of 25 monitored feedlots, 21 experienced a BRD episode, of which 18 were positive for *M. bovis*, among other pathogens, at the disease peak (T1). This high prevalence confirms the major contribution of *M. bovis* in BRD in this context of feedlots where animals of several origins are comingled [26]. *M. bovis* was most often associated with other pathogens, such as *P. multocida* and the Coronavirus (Figure 2), also frequently reported in BRD episodes [3,27]. Nevertheless, these prevalence results may be related to our sampling choice, i.e., nasal swabs. The Bovine Coronavirus was indeed shown to be detected in higher proportions in superficial samplings than in the lower respiratory tract samples, such as bronchoalveolar lavages [28]. The overall mycoplasmal load per calf was high at the disease peak, with a mean Ct of 25.7. Nonetheless, in 2/4 feedlots with no BRD episode, we were able to detect *M. bovis*-positive calves at T2, suggesting a potential asymptomatic circulation of the pathogen in the absence of any clinical disease as already suggested [8]. The weak prevalence observed at T0 (2% of positive calves) seems a true picture of the actual circulation of *M. bovis* in dairy herds in France [29], calves reared in feedlots mainly coming from dairy herds.

Four weeks after antimicrobial treatment (T2), when acute clinical signs of BRD were over, 49% of the calves remained rtPCR-positive for *M. bovis* against 51% at T1, indicating failed microbial clearance by treatments. However, the increase in the mean Ct to 30.4 and the low proportion of calves tested positive by culture (19%) suggest that at this stage of clinical recovery, the viable *Mycoplasma* load was significantly reduced. At T2, the proportion of *M. bovis*-positive animals estimated by culture was comparable to that recorded by our epidemiosurveillance network Vigimyc (15%, [18]). This suggests that most often, in day to day diagnosis, mycoplasmas are searched for only after antimicrobial treatment, remaining an etiology explored in case of failure of clinical improvement after chemotherapy.

We further showed that the overall genetic diversity of strains, assessed by *polC* subtyping [15] and PFGE analysis [30], was unmodified either by the ongoing BRD episode or by the associated antimicrobial treatments. The proportion of the two main *polC* subtypes currently circulating in France was comparable at each sampling time (feedlot entry, BRD peak and 4 weeks after the peak), i.e., 80% st2 and 20% st3. This proportion was also comparable to that of diagnosis strains collected in the framework of the Vigimyc surveillance network [15]. This confirms that our network, in its current operating procedures [18], is able to collect strains representative of those circulating in France and so is a real resource for monitoring genetic diversity and AMR.

PFGE patterns confirmed that st3 strains were more variable than st2 strains [15], but once again, this diversity was not related to any particular evolution of BRD or antimicrobial treatments. Both subtypes could be found circulating in the same herd, although no calf was detected harboring both subtypes at any one time. Considering the marked polymorphisms between st2 and st3, it is unlikely that the switch of subtypes observed on some calves over time (from T1 to T2, st2→st3 or st3→st2) could result from genetic evolution of the strains in such a short interval. The most likely scenario is co-circulation within a lot or a calf of the two subtypes, a possibility not observed here but previously reported and one becoming more prevalent at the time of sampling. Interestingly, a different subtype, never detected before in France, namely st5, was found in the RO feedlot. It had already been described in North America (ST124, in the legacy MLST scheme or ST45 in the revised scheme of Register [31,32]). Further genomic and phylogenetic characterization of this strain is ongoing, especially to establish phylogenetic relationships between the three subtypes.

As expected from studies around the world, our MIC data confirmed the overall multiresistance of *M. bovis* strains. For all the antimicrobials, resistance levels were the same as reported recently elsewhere [12,33–41]: *M. bovis* strains were resistant to tetracyclines, macrolides and florfenicol (with a few intermediate strains). However, we were further able to demonstrate that strains were already resistant before any antimicrobial treatment and that their MIC patterns were not changed in the course of the BRD episode and the associated chemotherapy. These results show that resistant clones are not selected during the disease episode but that clones circulating in France are already multiresistant. Fluoroquinolones remain the only antimicrobials with low MICs, which might be due to their restricted use in veterinary medicine owing to their classification as critically important antimicrobials. For this family, although we could fear an MIC increase for st3 due to a greater ability to fix mutations in vitro under subinhibitory concentrations of enrofloxacin [19], we observed the same susceptibility profiles for both subtypes. The few strains showing a slight increase in MIC of enrofloxacin to an intermediate level were st2, most strains of both subtypes being susceptible. The hypothesis of the spread since the year 2000 of a dominant multiresistant clone is thus confirmed [15] and we further rule out the possibility of the co-existence of susceptible clones.

The situation was different for Pasteurellaceae, for which we were partly able to correlate antimicrobial treatments and change in susceptibility profiles. We managed to gather data on antimicrobial use, although stockbreeders did not always continuously record treatments, which resulted in some incomplete data [40] (Supplementary Table S2). However, potential acquisition of AMR was recorded in two feedlots (CAS5 and NE), where the targeted antimicrobials had been used. This underlines the fact that acquisition of AMR may not have the same dynamics for *M. bovis* and for Pasteurellaceae. For the latter, AMR may arise during the BRD course under the influence of chemotherapy as already demonstrated by the apparition or spreading of new clones [42]. We were able to illustrate this fact only in two herds, because of the difficulty to retrieve Pasteurellaceae from nasal swabs that are often polymicrobial [43].

One unexpected finding in this study was the diversity of susceptibility profiles for spectinomycin, contrasting with previous observations that classified *M. bovis* as 100% resistant to this drug in France [16]. The decrease in spectinomycin MICs in France could signal a reappearance of more susceptible profiles, which are observed elsewhere in the world [33,34]. This mixed situation, with the coexistence of highly and poorly spectinomycin-resistant strains is very similar to what has been described in Hungary [38]. It would be of interest to investigate whether it is associated with a true reversion of antimicrobial resistance genotypes, with notably mutations (and reversions) in the *rrs* genes at position 1192 as previously reported [22,34].

4. Materials and Methods

4.1. Sampling Campaigns

A total of 537 veal calves were sampled in 25 fattening units located in Western France from November to April 2016–2017 and November to April 2017–2018. The size of each feedlot, ranging from 22 to 519 heads, and the antimicrobial treatments used during the observation periods were recorded (for more details see Supplementary Tables S1 and S2). Figure 1 summarizes the sampling and analysis workflow. In each herd, 10 randomly chosen calves were sampled using double nasal swabs (DNS) when introduced in the feedlot (T0). When a BRD episode occurred in the feedlot and before any collective antimicrobial treatment (T1), DNS were taken from five diseased calves. Four weeks after the end of the collective antimicrobial treatment (T2), the ten calves sampled at T0 were re-sampled, if possible. All DNS (T0, T1, T2) were sent, dry, at 4 °C, within at most two days after sampling, to the Anses laboratory. One swab was used for Pasteurellaceae isolation on Columbia agar plate containing 5% sheep blood (Biomérieux) and then for nucleic acid extraction (see hereafter). Another swab was used for *Mycoplasma* isolation (see below).

4.2. Nucleic Acid Extraction from Swabs and rtPCR Amplifications

Nucleic acids were extracted from swabs using the simplified protocol described previously [44]. Briefly, swabs were squeezed and sterilely cut in a tube containing a lysis buffer (TRIS 0.1 M, Tween 20 0.05% and proteinase K 0.24 mg/mL). They were heated for 1 h at 60 °C and then for 15 min at 95 °C to inactivate the proteinase. Real-time PCR (rtPCR) was performed on these bulk extracts using LSI VetMAX Screening pack Ruminant Respiratory Pathogens (ThermoFisher) to detect the various pathogens responsible for BRD (*M. bovis*, *Histophilus somni*, *Pasteurella multocida*, *Mannheimia haemolytica*, Coronavirus, Respiratory Syncytial Virus and Parainfluenza 3) (at T1), or with VetMAX™ *M. bovis* Kit (ThermoFisher) to only assess *M. bovis* presence (at T0 and T2), according to the manufacturer's recommendations. The Ct cut-off for *M. bovis*-positiveness was set at $\leq$ 37 according to the recommendation of Wisselink et al. [45].

4.3. Isolation and Identification of M. bovis Isolates

Swabs were seeded on plates containing a PPLO agar medium modified as previously described [46], with addition of 0.1% of Tween 80 for specific inhibition of *M. bovirhinis* potential contamination [47]. Plates were incubated for 4 days at 37 °C in 5% CO_2. A maximum of 10 clones per calf and per sampling point were randomly selected with a wooden toothpick, further cultured in 2 mL PPLO broth and identified using membrane filtration dot-immunobinding tests (MF-Dot) as previously described [48]. As the number of picked clones per calf varied with the quality of the isolation, each calf at one sampling time (T0, T1 or T2) was considered as a single epidemiological unit.

A set of *M. bovis* isolates from a collection kept at Anses, Lyon Laboratory and mostly derived from the French national surveillance network for mycoplasmosis in ruminants (Vigimyc) [18] were included in the study as a "reference" population for both subtyping and antimicrobial resistance.

4.4. Strain Subtyping by Sequence Analysis of the Housekeeping Gene polC and Pulse Field Gel Electrophoresis (PFGE)

Genomic DNA was extracted from 200 µL of each clone culture using QIAamp® DNA Minikit (Qiagen), and the *M. bovis* clones were all subtyped using *polC* sequence analysis as previously described [15] (Figure 1).

One isolate yielded a new *polC* subtype and was further analyzed to determine its subtype according to the MLST scheme of Register et al. ([24]; https://pulmlst.org/bovis/), by a whole genome resequencing approach. Briefly, a DNA sample was sequenced using an Illumina MiSeq technology generating 2 × 300-bp pair-end reads (MiSeq 600 cycles V3 kit, Biofidal, Vaux-en-Velin, France). A total of 1,443,759 reads were generated for each R*, resulting in an average coverage of 860 X. Trimmed reads (using Trimmomatic-0.36) were aligned to two reference genomes, namely PG45 (refseq NC_014760.1) and JF4278 (a corrected version provided by Bern University).

After quality control of the alignments, the variants were identified and annotated using GATK4 v4.0.10.0 (https://software.broadinstitute.org/gatk). The filtered output vcf files were then used to retrieve the different Register loci sequences [24].

A sub-panel of clones was selected (one st2 per calf at each sampling time and per lot and all st3, Figure 1 and Supplementary Table S1) to be further subtyped by Pulse-Field Gel Electrophoresis (PFGE) with the *MluI* enzyme as previously described [30]. Briefly, mycoplasma cells from overnight cultures were embedded in low melt agarose plugs and lysed by proteinase K before DNA overnight restriction using endonucleases. The macrorestriction fragments were separated by electrophoresis on a CHEF-DR III system (Bio-Rad) in 1% agarose gel, in TBE 0.5% at 14 °C, for 24h, with an included angle of 120°. Images were analyzed with the software Bionumerics GelCompar II v6.6 (Applied Maths NV, Sint-Martens-Latem, Belgium). The similarity analysis was carried out using the Dice coefficient (position tolerance 1.5%) and a dendrogram was constructed using the UPGMA method.

4.5. Antimicrobial Susceptibility Testing of M. bovis and Pasteurellaceae

The susceptibility of the selected *M. bovis* clones was tested using Minimum inhibitory concentration (MICs) assays as previously described [17] for the five antimicrobial classes mostly used to treat BRD in the field and known to be potentially active against *Mycoplasma* spp: quinolones (enrofloxacin), tetracyclines (oxytetracycline), phenicols (florfenicol), aminoglycosides (spectinomycin) and macrolides (tilmicosin). Briefly, clones were plated on PPLO agar plates containing twofold increasing antimicrobial concentrations, either as a full range of antimicrobial dilutions or only for a few concentrations corresponding to the CLSI clinical breakpoints for Pasteurellaceae, a family known to colonize the same body niche [25]. At least two experiments were conducted, and the modes of the different results were retained as the final MIC values. For some strains, the different experiments did not allow us to conclude on a single MIC value: an MIC interval was defined (Supplementary Table S2) but was not represented in Figure 5.

Antibiograms for Pasteurellaceae were outsourced at the Laboratoire Vétérinaire Départemental du Rhône. For each sample positive for both *M. bovis* and Pasteurellaceae, a mix of Pasteurellaceae-like colonies with similar phenotype was collected from the Columbia agar plate, identified with an API 20E gallery and tested for resistance with the standardized diffusion method in agar (norm NF U47-107) for the same five antimicrobial classes tested for *M. bovis* (depending on the available disks): quinolones (enrofloxacin and marbofloxacin), tetracyclines (tetracycline), phenicols (florfenicol), aminoglycosides (spectinomycin) and macrolides (tylosin and tulathromycin). The β-lactam amoxicillin known to be active against Pasteurellaceae was also tested. Zone diameters were interpreted according to the CLSI standards [25].

5. Conclusions

This study demonstrates that *M. bovis* is an important player in feedlot BRD. Its prevalence is weak at entry but rapidly increases to reach a peak at the disease onset. It can circulate in the absence of clinical episodes and remain present even after antimicrobial treatments, which can result in clinical recovery without mycoplasmal clearance. The disease course and the associated chemotherapy did not affect the genetic diversity or AMR patterns of strains circulating in a lot. The strains observed in this longitudinal study reflected the general population circulating in France, with one major clone multiresistant to the main antimicrobials used in BRD, also retrieved by our surveillance network.

Author Contributions: F.T., M.-A.A., C.B. designed the study. M.-A.A. and F.T. supervised the sampling campaign. A.C., A.H., A.T., A.V., C.A. and C.A.M.B. did the experiments. C.A., C.A.M.B. and F.T. analyzed the results and drafted the manuscript. C.A.M.B. and F.T. reviewed and edited the manuscript. All the authors reviewed the manuscript. All authors have read and agreed to the published version of the manuscript.

Acknowledgments: The authors are grateful to the veterinarians who sampled the calves and gave access to antimicrobial treatment data. Special thanks go to François Poumarat and Maryne Jaÿ, respectively former and current manager of Vigimyc, who made surveillance data available.

References

1. Urban-Chmiel, R.; Grooms, D.L. Prevention and Control of Bovine Respiratory Disease. *J. Livest. Sci.* **2012**, *3*, 27–36.
2. Snowder, G.D.; Van Vleck, L.D.; Cundiff, L.V.; Bennett, G.L. Bovine respiratory disease in feedlot cattle: Environmental, genetic, and economic factors. *J. Anim. Sci.* **2006**, *84*, 1999–2008. [CrossRef]
3. Cirone, F.; Padalino, B.; Tullio, D.; Capozza, P.; Losurdo, M.; Lanave, G.; Pratelli, A. Prevalence of Pathogens Related to Bovine Respiratory Disease Before and After Transportation in Beef Steers: Preliminary Results. *Animals* **2019**, *9*, 1093. [CrossRef] [PubMed]
4. McGill, J.L.; Sacco, R.E. The Immunology of Bovine Respiratory Disease: Recent Advancements. *Vet. Clin. N. Am. Food Anim. Pract.* **2020**, in press. [CrossRef]
5. Grissett, G.P.; White, B.J.; Larson, R.L. Structured Literature Review of Responses of Cattle to Viral and Bacterial Pathogens Causing Bovine Respiratory Disease Complex. *J. Vet. Intern. Med.* **2015**, *29*, 770–780. [CrossRef] [PubMed]
6. Amat, S.; Holman, D.B.; Timsit, E.; Schwinghamer, T.; Alexander, T.W. Evaluation of the Nasopharyngeal Microbiota in Beef Cattle Transported to a Feedlot, With a Focus on Lactic Acid-Producing Bacteria. *Front. Microbiol.* **2019**, *10*, 1988. [CrossRef] [PubMed]
7. Taylor, J.D.; Fulton, R.W.; Lehenbauer, T.W.; Step, D.L.; Confer, A.W. The epidemiology of bovine respiratory disease: What is the evidence for predisposing factors? *Can. Vet. J.* **2010**, *51*, 1095–1102. [PubMed]
8. Maunsell, F.P.; Woolums, A.R.; Francoz, D.; Rosenbusch, R.F.; Step, D.L.; Wilson, D.J.; Janzen, E.D. *Mycoplasma bovis* infections in cattle. *J. Vet. Intern. Med.* **2011**, *25*, 772–783. [CrossRef]
9. Holman, D.B.; Timsit, E.; Amat, S.; Abbott, D.W.; Buret, A.G.; Alexander, T.W. The nasopharyngeal microbiota of beef cattle before and after transport to a feedlot. *BMC Microbiol.* **2017**, *17*, 70. [CrossRef]

10. Calcutt, M.J.; Lysnyansky, I.; Sachse, K.; Fox, L.K.; Nicholas, R.A.J.; Ayling, R.D. Gap analysis of *Mycoplasma bovis* disease, diagnosis and control: An aid to identify future development requirements. *Transbound. Emerg. Dis.* **2018**, *65*, 91–109. [CrossRef]
11. Amat, S.; Timsit, E.; Baines, D.; Yanke, J.; Alexander, T.W. Development of Bacterial Therapeutics against the Bovine Respiratory Pathogen *Mannheimia haemolytica*. *Appl. Environ. Microbiol.* **2019**, *85*, e01359-19. [CrossRef] [PubMed]
12. Stanford, K.; Zaheer, R.; Klima, C.; McAllister, T.; Peters, D.; Niu, Y.D.; Ralston, B. Antimicrobial Resistance in Members of the Bacterial Bovine Respiratory Disease Complex Isolated from Lung Tissue of Cattle Mortalities Managed with or without the Use of Antimicrobials. *Microorganisms* **2020**, *8*, 288. [CrossRef] [PubMed]
13. De Donder, K.D.; Apley, M.D. A Review of the Expected Effects of Antimicrobials in Bovine Respiratory Disease Treatment and Control Using Outcomes from Published Randomized Clinical Trials with Negative Controls. *Vet. Clin. N. Am. Food Anim. Pract.* **2015**, *31*, 97–111. [CrossRef]
14. Gautier-Bouchardon, A.V. Antimicrobial Resistance in *Mycoplasma* spp. *Microbiol. Spectr.* **2018**, 6. [CrossRef]
15. Becker, C.A.M.; Thibault, F.M.; Arcangioli, M.-A.; Tardy, F. Genotypic evolution of *Mycoplasma bovis* isolates collected in France over the last 35 years. In Proceedings of the Progress in Human and Animal Mycoplasmology, Istanbul, Turkey, 3–5 June 2015; p. 60.
16. Gautier-Bouchardon, A.V.; Ferre, S.; Le Grand, D.; Paoli, A.; Gay, E.; Poumarat, F. Overall Decrease in the Susceptibility of *Mycoplasma bovis* to Antimicrobials over the Past 30 Years in France. *PLoS ONE* **2014**, *9*, e87672. [CrossRef]
17. Khalil, D.; Becker, C.A.M.; Tardy, F. Monitoring the decrease in susceptibility to ribosomal RNAs targeting antimicrobials and its molecular basis in clinical *Mycoplasma bovis* isolates over time. *Microb. Drug Resist.* **2017**, *23*, 799–811. [CrossRef]
18. Poumarat, F.; Jarrige, N.; Tardy, F. Principe et bilan du réseau Vigimyc consacré à l'épidémiosurveillance des mycoplasmoses des ruminants en France. *Euroref. Cah. Réf.* **2014**, *12*, 24–29.
19. Khalil, D.; Becker, C.A.M.; Tardy, F. Alterations in the Quinolone Resistance-Determining Regions and Fluoroquinolone Resistance in Clinical Isolates and Laboratory-Derived Mutants of *Mycoplasma bovis*: Not All Genotypes May Be Equal. *Appl. Environ. Microbiol.* **2016**, *82*, 1060–1068. [CrossRef]
20. Sato, T.; Higuchi, H.; Yokota, S.-i.; Tamura, Y. *Mycoplasma bovis* isolates from dairy calves in Japan have less susceptibility than a reference strain to all approved macrolides associated with a point mutation (G748A) combined with multiple species-specific nucleotide alterations in 23S rRNA. *Microbiol. Immunol.* **2017**, *61*, 215–224. [CrossRef]
21. Sato, T.; Okubo, T.; Usui, M.; Higuchi, H.; Tamura, Y. Amino Acid Substitutions in GyrA and ParC Are Associated with Fluoroquinolone Resistance in *Mycoplasma bovis* Isolates from Japanese Dairy Calves. *J. Vet. Med. Sci.* **2013**, *75*, 1063–1065. [CrossRef]
22. Sulyok, K.M.; Kreizinger, Z.; Wehmann, E.; Lysnyansky, I.; Bányai, K.; Marton, S.; Jerzsele, Á.; Rónai, Z.; Turcsányi, I.; Makrai, L.; et al. Mutations Associated with Decreased Susceptibility to Seven Antimicrobial Families in Field and Laboratory-Derived *Mycoplasma bovis* Strains. *Antimicrob. Agents Chemother.* **2017**, 61. [CrossRef] [PubMed]
23. Register, K.B.; Lysnyansky, I.; Jelinski, M.D.; Boatwright, W.D.; Waldner, M.; Bayles, D.O.; Pilo, P.; Alt, D.P. Comparison of Two Multilocus Sequence Typing Schemes for *Mycoplasma bovis* and Revision of the PubMLST Reference Method. *J. Clin. Microbiol.* **2020**, in press. [CrossRef]
24. Register, K.B.; Thole, L.; Rosenbush, R.F.; Minion, F.C. Multilocus sequence typing of *Mycoplasma bovis* reveals host-specific genotypes in cattle versus bison. *Vet. Microbiol.* **2015**, *175*, 92–98. [CrossRef] [PubMed]
25. Clinical and laboratory standards institute. *Performance Standards for Antimicrobial Disk and Dilution Susceptibility Tests for Bacteria Isolated From Animals*, 3rd ed.; Clinical and Laboratory Standards Institute: Wayne, PA, USA, 2015.
26. Caswell, J.L.; Bateman, K.G.; Cai, H.Y.; Castillo-Alcala, F. *Mycoplasma bovis* in respiratory disease of feedlot cattle. *Vet. Clin. N. Am. Food Anim. Pract.* **2010**, *26*, 365–379. [CrossRef] [PubMed]
27. Decaro, N.; Campolo, M.; Desario, C.; Cirone, F.; D'abramo, M.; Lorusso, E.; Greco, G.; Mari, V.; Colaianni, M.L.; Elia, G.; et al. Respiratory Disease Associated with Bovine Coronavirus Infection in Cattle Herds in Southern Italy. *J. Vet. Diagn. Investig.* **2008**, *20*, 28–32. [CrossRef] [PubMed]
28. Doyle, D.; Credille, B.; Lehenbauer, T.W.; Berghaus, R.; Aly, S.S.; Champagne, J.; Blanchard, P.; Crossley, B.; Berghaus, L.; Cochran, S.; et al. Agreement Among 4 Sampling Methods to Identify Respiratory Pathogens

in Dairy Calves with Acute Bovine Respiratory Disease. *J. Vet. Intern. Med.* **2017** *31*, 954–959. [CrossRef]

29. Arcangioli, M.; Chazel, M.; Sellal, E.; Botrel, M.; Bezille, P.; Poumarat, F.; Calavas, D.; Le Grand, D. Prevalence of *Mycoplasma bovis* udder infection in dairy cattle: Preliminary field investigation in southeast France. *N. Z. Vet. J.* **2011**, *59*, 75–78. [CrossRef]
30. Arcangioli, M.A.; Aslan, H.; Tardy, F.; Poumarat, F.; Le Grand, D. The use of pulsed-field gel electrophoresis to investigate the epidemiology of *Mycoplasma bovis* in French calf feedlots. *Vet. J.* **2012**, *192*, 96–100. [CrossRef]
31. Register, K.B.; Jelinski, M.D.; Waldner, M.; Boatwright, W.D.; Anderson, T.K.; Hunter, D.L.; Hamilton, R.G.; Burrage, P.; Shury, T.; Bildfell, R.; et al. Comparison of multilocus sequence types found among North American isolates of *Mycoplasma bovis* from cattle, bison, and deer, 2007–2017. *J. Vet. Diagn. Investig.* **2019**, *31*, 899–904. [CrossRef]
32. Yair, Y.; Borovok, I.; Mikula, I.; Falk, R.; Fox, L.K.; Gophna, U.; Lysnyansky, I. Genomics-based epidemiology of bovine *Mycoplasma bovis* strains in Israel. *BMC Genom.* **2020**, *21*, 70. [CrossRef]
33. Cai, H.Y.; McDowall, R.; Parker, L.; Kaufman, E.I.; Caswell, J.L. Changes in antimicrobial susceptibility profiles of *Mycoplasma bovis* over time. *Can. J. Vet. Res.* **2019**, *83*, 34–41. [PubMed]
34. Hata, E.; Harada, T.; Itoh, M. Relationship between Antimicrobial Susceptibility and Multilocus Sequence Type of *Mycoplasma bovis* Isolates and Development of a Method for Rapid Detection of Point Mutations Involved in Decreased Susceptibility to Macrolides, Lincosamides, Tetracyclines, and Spectinomycin. *Appl. Environ. Microbiol.* **2019**, *85*, e00575-19. [CrossRef] [PubMed]
35. Heuvelink, A.; Reugebrink, C.; Mars, J. Antimicrobial susceptibility of *Mycoplasma bovis* isolates from veal calves and dairy cattle in the Netherlands. *Vet. Microbiol.* **2016**, *189*, 1–7. [CrossRef] [PubMed]
36. Klein, U.; de Jong, A.; Youala, M.; El Garch, F.; Stevenin, C.; Moyaert, H.; Rose, M.; Catania, S.; Gyuranecz, M.; Pridmore, A.; et al. New antimicrobial susceptibility data from monitoring of *Mycoplasma bovis* isolated in Europe. *Vet. Microbiol.* **2019**, *238*, 108432. [CrossRef]
37. Lysnyansky, I.; Ayling, R.D. *Mycoplasma bovis*: Mechanisms of resistance and trends in antimicrobial susceptibility. *Front. Microbiol.* **2016**, *7*. [CrossRef]
38. Sulyok, K.M.; Kreizinger, Z.; Fekete, L.; Hrivnak, V.; Magyar, T.; Janosi, S.; Schweitzer, N.; Turcsanyi, I.; Makrai, L.; Erdelyi, K.; et al. Antibiotic susceptibility profiles of *Mycoplasma bovis* strains isolated from cattle in Hungary, Central Europe. *BMC Vet. Res.* **2014**, *10*, 256. [CrossRef]
39. Jelinski, M.; Kinnear, A.; Gesy, K.; Andrés-Lasheras, S.; Zaheer, R.; Weese, S.; McAllister, A.T. Antimicrobial Sensitivity Testing of *Mycoplasma bovis* Isolates Derived from Western Canadian Feedlot Cattle. *Microorganisms* **2020**, *8*, 124. [CrossRef]
40. Anholt, R.M.; Klima, C.; Allan, N.; Matheson-Bird, H.; Schatz, C.; Ajitkumar, P.; Otto, S.J.; Peters, D.; Schmid, K.; Olson, M.; et al. Antimicrobial Susceptibility of Bacteria That Cause Bovine Respiratory Disease Complex in Alberta, Canada. *Front. Vet. Sci.* **2017**, 4. [CrossRef]
41. Klein, U.; de Jong, A.; Moyaert, H.; El Garch, F.; Leon, R.; Richard-Mazet, A.; Rose, M.; Maes, D.; Pridmore, A.; Thomson, J.R.; et al. Antimicrobial susceptibility monitoring of *Mycoplasma hyopneumoniae* and *Mycoplasma bovis* isolated in Europe. *Vet. Microbiol.* **2017**, *204*, 188–193. [CrossRef]
42. Woolums, A.R.; Karisch, B.B.; Frye, J.G.; Epperson, W.; Smith, D.R.; Blanton, J.; Austin, F.; Kaplan, R.; Hiott, L.; Woodley, T.; et al. Multidrug resistant *Mannheimia haemolytica* isolated from high-risk beef stocker cattle after antimicrobial metaphylaxis and treatment for bovine respiratory disease. *Vet. Microbiol.* **2018**, *221*, 143–152. [CrossRef]
43. Van Driessche, L.; Valgaeren, B.R.; Gille, L.; Boyen, F.; Ducatelle, R.; Haesebrouck, F.; Deprez, P.; Pardon, B. A Deep Nasopharyngeal Swab Versus Nonendoscopic Bronchoalveolar Lavage for Isolation of Bacterial Pathogens from Preweaned Calves With Respiratory Disease. *J. Vet. Intern. Med.* **2017**, *31*, 946–953. [CrossRef] [PubMed]
44. Vilei, E.M.; Bonvin-Klotz, L.; Zimmermann, L.; Ryser-Degiorgis, M.P.; Giacometti, M.; Frey, J. Validation and diagnostic efficacy of a TaqMan real-time PCR for the detection of *Mycoplasma conjunctivae* in the eyes of infected Caprinae. *J. Microbiol. Methods* **2007**, *70*, 384–386. [CrossRef] [PubMed]
45. Wisselink, H.J.; Smid, B.; Plater, J.; Ridley, A.; Andersson, A.M.; Aspan, A.; Pohjanvirta, T.; Vahanikkila, N.; Larsen, H.; Hogberg, J.; et al. A European interlaboratory trial to evaluate the performance of different PCR methods for *Mycoplasma bovis* diagnosis. *BMC Vet. Res.* **2019**, *15*, 12. [CrossRef] [PubMed]

46. Poumarat, F.; Longchambon, D.; Martel, J.L. Application of dot immunobinding on membrane filtration (MF dot) to the study of relationships within "*M. mycoides* cluster" and within "glucose and arginine-negative cluster" of ruminant mycoplasmas. *Vet. Microbiol.* **1992**, *32*, 375–390. [CrossRef]
47. Shimizu, T. Selective medium for the isolation of *Mycoplasma bovis* from nasal discharges of pneumonic calves. *Res. Vet. Sci.* **1983**, *34*, 371–373. [CrossRef]
48. Poumarat, F.; Perrin, B.; Longchambon, D. Identification of ruminant mycoplasmas by dot immunobinding on membrane filtration (MF dot). *Vet. Microbiol.* **1991**, *29*, 329–338. [CrossRef]

7

Prevalence and Genetic Diversity of Atypical Porcine Pestivirus (APPV) Detected in South Korean Wild Boars

SeEun Choe [1], Gyu-Nam Park [1], Ra Mi Cha [1], Bang-Hun Hyun [1], Bong-Kyun Park [1,2] and Dong-Jun An [1,*]

1 Virus Disease Division, Animal and Plant Quarantine Agency, Gimchen, Gyeongbuk-do 39660, Korea; ivvi59@korea.kr (S.C.); changep0418@gmail.com (G.-N.P.); rami.cha01@korea.kr (R.M.C.); hyunbh@korea.kr (B.-H.H.); parkx026@korea.kr (B.-K.P.)

2 College of Veterinary Medicine, Seoul University, Gwanak-ro, Gwanak-gu, Seoul 08826, Korea

* Correspondence: andj67@korea.kr.

Abstract: Atypical porcine pestivirus (APPV), currently classified as *pestivirus K*, causes congenital tremor (CT) type A-II in piglets. Eighteen APPV strains were identified from 2297 South Korean wild boars captured in 2019. Phylogenetic analysis of the structural protein E2 and nonstructural proteins NS3 and Npro classified the APPV viruses, including reference strains, into Clades I, II and III. Clade I was divided into four subclades; however, the strains belonging to the four subclades differed slightly, depending on the tree analysis, the NS3, E2, and Npro genes. The maximum-likelihood method was assigned to South Korean wild boar APPV strains to various subclades within the three trees: subclades I.1 and I.2 in the E2 tree, subclade I.1 in the Npro tree, and subclades I.1 and I.4 in the NS3 ML tree. In conclusion, APPV among South Korean wild boars belonging to Clade I may be circulating at a higher level than among the South Korean domestic pig populations.

Keywords: APPV; wild boar; ML tree; Clade; pestivirus

---

1. Introduction

Pestiviruses are highly variable single-stranded RNA genome viruses belonging to the family *Flaviviridae*. The genus *Pestivirus* includes animal pathogens that are of worldwide socioeconomic significance—these include bovine viral diarrhea virus (BVDV, *pestivirus A–B*), classical swine fever virus (CSFV, *pestivirus C*), and border disease virus (BDV, *pestivirus D*) [1]. Other *Pestiviruses* include *Pestivirus E* (pronghorn pestivirus), *Pestivirus F* (Bungowannah virus), *Pestivirus G* (giraffe pestivirus), *Pestivirus H* (Hobi-like pestivirus), *Pestivirus I* (Aydin-like pestivirus), and *Pestivirus J* (rat pestivirus) [1].

A novel genetically distinct strain of *pestivirus K*, named atypical porcine pestivirus (APPV), was first identified in the USA in 2015 [2]. It was also identified in Germany, the Netherlands, Austria, Spain, China, Hungary, Brazil, and Sweden in 2016–18 [3–8]. In South Korea, the first case of APPV, which causes congenital tremor (CT) type A-II in suckling piglets, was identified in 2017 [9]. Although APPV has been found in animals with no clinical signs, there is clear evidence that it is associated with CT type A-II in newborns [10]. The presence of APPV in domestic pigs was confirmed repeatedly in several countries in Europe, North and South America, and Asia [2,11], and in wild boars from countries in Europe [10,12,13]. Clinically, healthy pigs and wild boars may have an epidemiological role as vehicles for APPV.

Pestivirus genomes can be classified into genogroups and sub-genogroups [14,15]. Phylogenetic analysis of the E2 and Npro proteins divided APPV into at least four (A–D) [5,16] or five (A–E) different genogroups [17].

In this study, we describe the detection and genetic characterization of APPV in wild boars from South Korea.

2. Material and Methods

2.1. Wild Boars

To satisfy the OIE requirements for the surveillance of wild boars and feral pigs in Classical Swine Fever-free countries, wild boars have been hunted (in co-operation with the Korean Pork Producers Association and the South Korea government) since 2010. Immediately after hunting, blood samples were collected from wild boars captured in nine provinces of South Korea and transported to the APQA. Blood samples from 2297 wild boars (1126 males, 1045 females, and 126 unknown), captured in 2019, were screened for APPV.

2.2. Reverse Transcription-Polymerase Chain Reaction (RT-PCR) of APPV

RT-PCR was performed to detect APPV [12,16]. Briefly, total RNA was extracted from 100 μL of whole blood using the QIAamp viral RNA mini kit (Qiagen, Cat. No. 52904. Hilden, Germany). Extracted RNA was reverse-transcribed using SuperScript III (Invitrogen, Cat. No. 18080093. Carlsbad, CA, USA). For APPV screening and sequencing, PCR was performed using primers designed to target areas of the conserved NS3-encoding region, as described previously [12]. Primers targeting the E2 and Npro genes were used to amplify the complete nucleotide sequences, as described previously [16]. The amplification products were purified using the QIAquick Gel Extraction Kit (Qiagen, Cat. No. 28704. Hilden, Germany) and used directly for sequencing (Cosmogentech Co., Seoul, Korea). PCR and serum neutralization tests were used to detect viral antigens and antibodies specific for CSFV and BVDV in APPV-positive samples, as described previously [18].

2.3. Phylogenetic Analysis of APPV

Multiple nucleotide sequence alignment was carried out by the Clustal X alignment program [19] using APPV sequences available in GenBank as references, and BLAST software (NCBI, Bethesda, Rockville, MD, USA). Outgroup strains comprised *pestiviruses A–H*. The partial sequences of NS3, derived from 18 APPVs detected in South Korean wild boars, were compared with 86 reference sequences (including eight outgroup strains) from Asia, North America, and Europe. The complete E2 sequence of four APPVs and the complete Npro sequence data of five APPVs detected in South Korean wild boars were compared with 70 (including ten outgroup strains) and 69 reference sequences (including ten outgroup strains), respectively. Nucleotide sequences of the NS3, E2, and Npro regions were analyzed phylogenetically using the maximum-likelihood (ML) method, with the Tamura–Nei model and bootstrap analysis (n = 1000) within MEGA 7.0 software (State College, PA, USA) with default parameters [20]. The ML tree was based on rates among sites (Gamma distributed with invariant sites (G+I)) and the ML heuristic method (Nearest-neighbor-interchange (NNI)). The partial NS3 sequences of 18 APPV strains (accession numbers: MT501737–MT501754), the complete E2 sequences of four APPV strains (accession numbers: MT501733–MT501736), and the complete Npro sequences of five APPV strains (accession numbers: MT501555–MT501759) detected in South Korean wild boars were deposited in GenBank.

2.4. Ethical Approval

The authors confirm that the work complies with the ethical policies of the journal. The work was approved by the Institutional Animal Care and Use Committee of the Animal and Plant Quarantine Agency (APQA) (Approval Number: 2019-448).

3. Results

3.1. Geographic Prevalence of APPV

Eighteen APPV strains were identified in 2297 blood samples collected from wild boars in 2019, suggesting that the prevalence of APPV is 0.78%. Of the APPV-positive wild boars, 15 were male (15/18, 83.3%), two were female (2/18, 11.1%), and one was of unknown sex (1/18, 5.6%). APPV strains were detected in wild boars from six provinces and of various weights (seven <30 kg; seven 30–60 kg; four >60 kg). Among the 18 APPVs detected in South Korean wild boars, five were detected in Gyeongnam (GN, 5/292; 1.71%), four in Gangwon (GW, 4/609; 0.66%), three each in Gyeonggi (GG, 3/452; 0.66%) and Chungnam (CN, 3/288; 0.35%), two in Chungbuk (CB, 2/204; 0.98%), and one in Gyeongkuk (GB, 1/275; 0.36%), as shown in Figure 1. All APPV-positive samples were negative for anti-CSFV and BVDV antibodies and antigens.

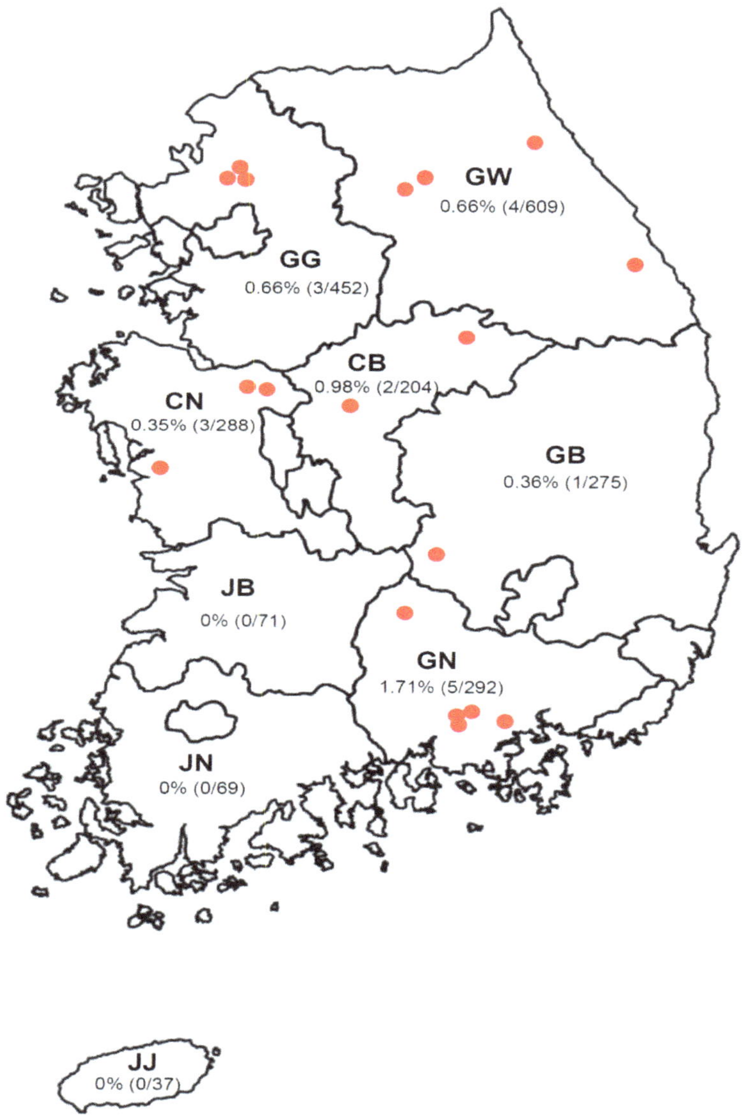

Figure 1. Locations in which APPV-positive wild boars were captured. Locations in which wild boars were captured are marked by a red dot. GW: Gangwon; GG: Gyeonggi; GN: Gyeongnam; GB, Gyeongbuk; JN: Jennam; JB: Jenbuk; CN: Chungnam; CB: Chungbuk; JJ: Jeju.

3.2. ML Trees Based on NS3 Sequences

The NS3 sequences (767 nucleotides (nt)) of the 18 APPVs detected from wild boars were 87.7–99.9% identical at the nt level and 96.5–100% identical at the amino acid (aa) level. ML tree analysis of NS3, E2, and Npro sequences revealed that *Pestivirus* strains were clearly divided into two groups: *Pestivirus K* (APPVs) and Other *Pestiviruses* (*A–H*), as shown in Figures 2–4). All APPVs were classified into three large Clades (I, II, and III) and four smaller subclades (I.1, I.2, I.3, and I.4), as shown in Figures 2–4). ML analysis of the NS3 sequences of the 18 APPVs from South Korean wild boars were included in Clade I (16 in subclade I.1 and two in subclade I.4), as shown in Figure 2. The nt sequence identity between the South Korean APPVs in subclades I.1 and I.4 was 86.8–88.7%; however, identity at the aa sequence level was 95.7–97.6%.

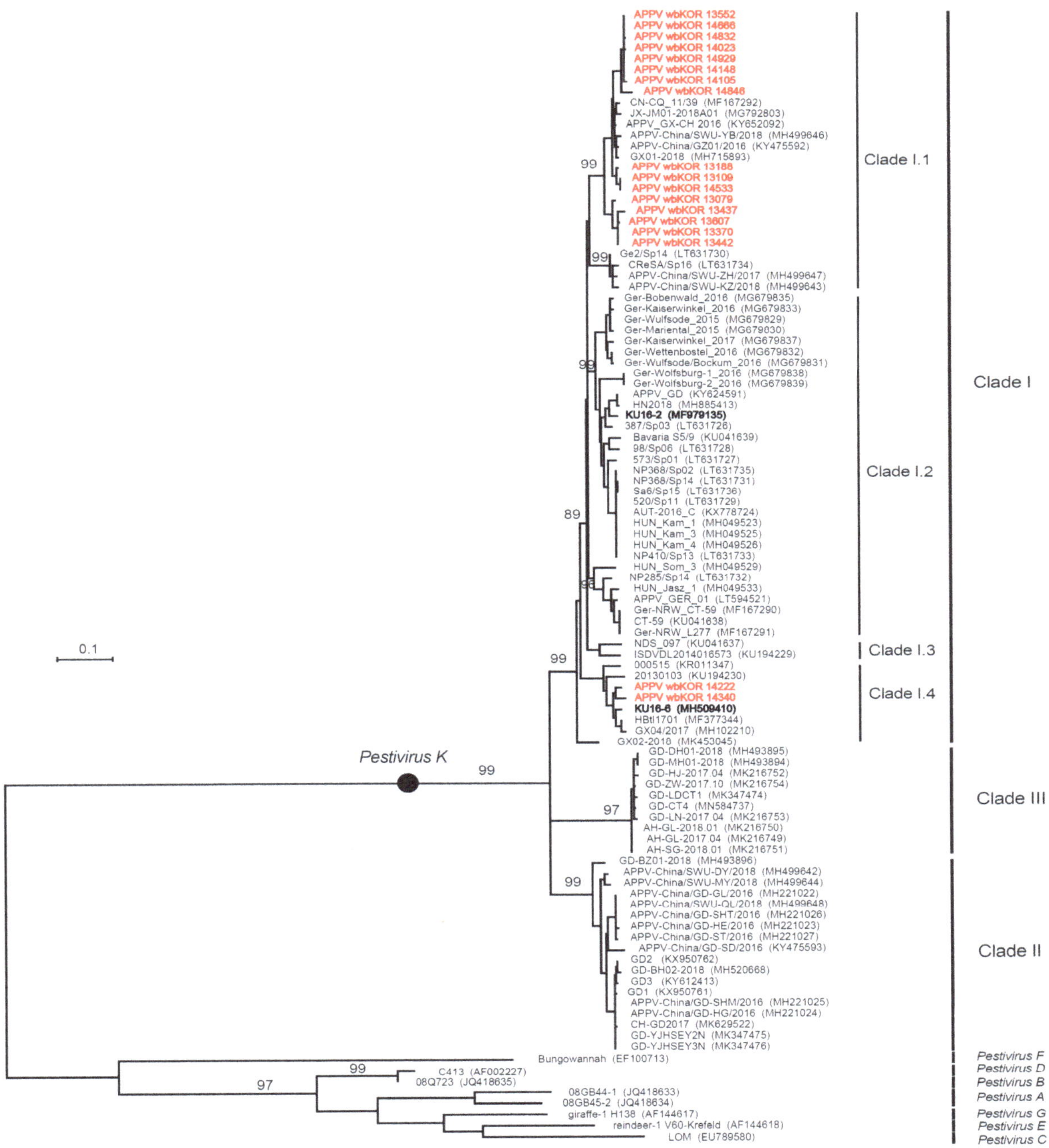

Figure 2. Phylogenetic tree of South Korean wild boar APPVs, based on NS3 sequences. The phylogenetic tree was constructed using the ML method (based on the Tamura–Nei model), with bootstrap analysis

($n = 1000$), in MEGA 7.0 software. The 767 nt NS3 sequences of 18 APPVs from South Korean wild boars were compared with 86 reference sequences (including eight outgroup strains: *pestiviruses A–G*) from Asia, North America, and Europe. The Log likelihood (Log L) is −10,191.77, and only bootstrap values ≥70 are indicated on the nodes. South Korean wild boar APPV strains and South Korean domestic pig APPV strains are denoted by red bold and black bold letters. The scale bar indicates the number of nucleotide substitutions per site.

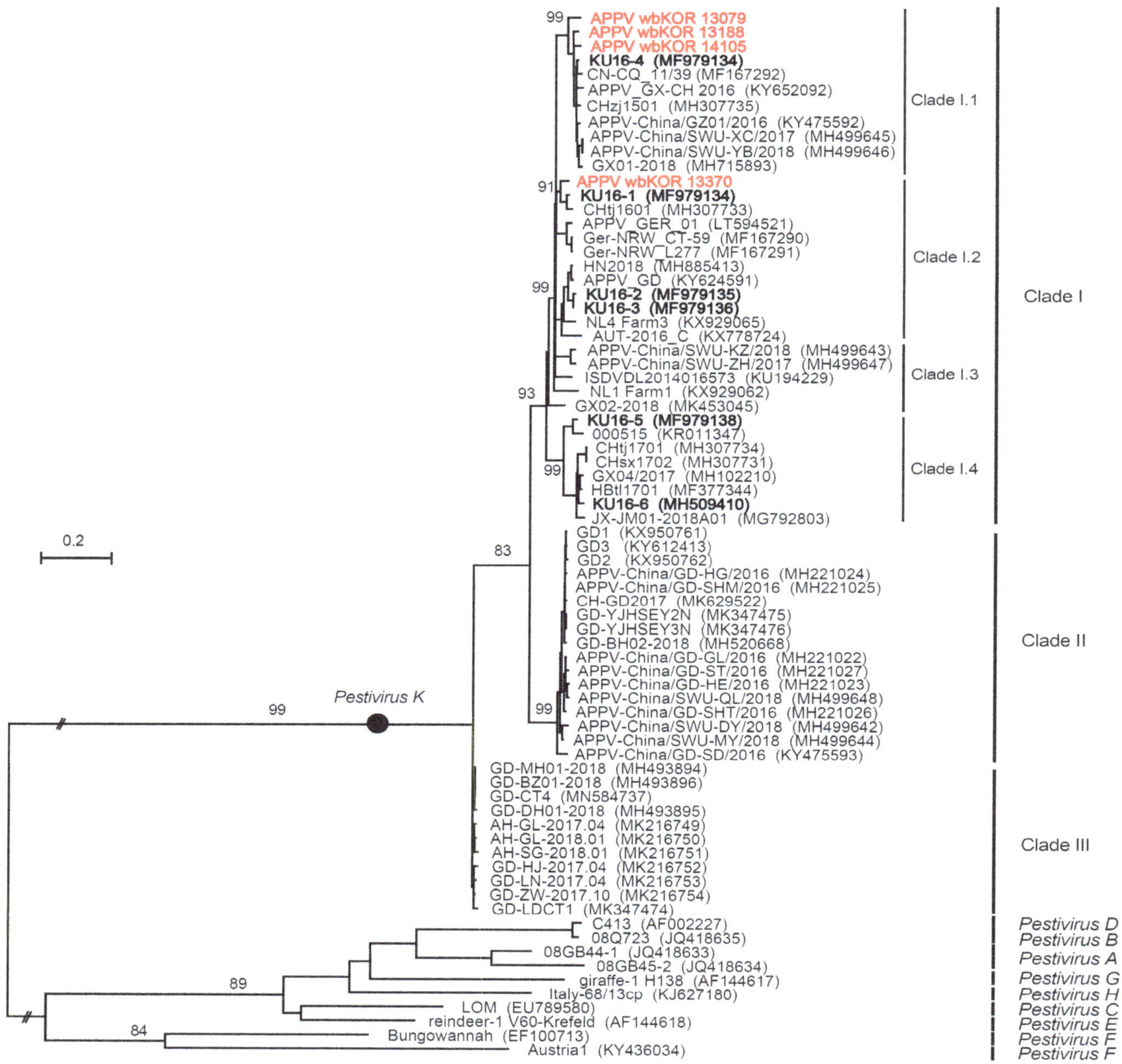

Figure 3. ML tree of South Korean wild boar APPVs, based on E2 sequences. The phylogenetic tree (Log L, −11,438.12) was constructed using the ML method (based on the Tamura–Nei model), with bootstrap analysis ($n = 1000$). The complete E2 sequences of four APPVs detected in South Korean wild boars were compared with 70 reference sequences (including ten outgroup strains: *pestiviruses A–H*).

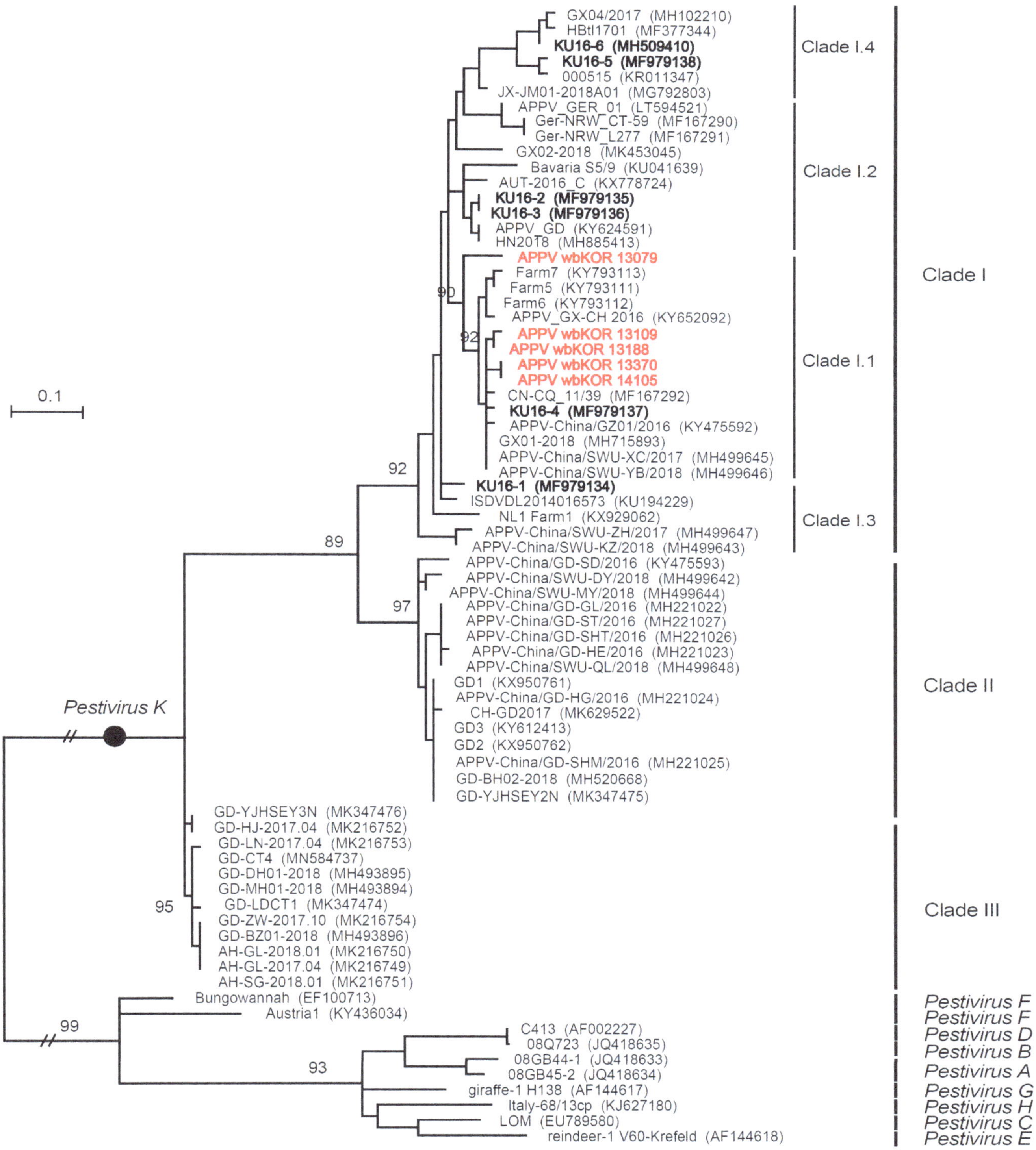

Figure 4. ML tree of South Korean wild boar APPV, based on Npro sequences. The phylogenetic tree (Log L: −5113.82) was constructed using the ML method (based on the Tamura–Nei model), with bootstrap analysis ($n = 1000$). The complete Npro sequences of five APPV detected in South Korean wild boars were compared with 69 reference sequences (including ten outgroup strains: *pestiviruses A–H*).

The 767-nt NS3 sequences of the 16 South Korean wild boar APPVs (Subclade I.1) and 8 APPVs isolated from German wild boars (Subclade I.2), as shown in Figure 2, were 90.9–92.0% identical at the nt level and 97.6–99.2% identical at the aa level. Moreover, NS3 sequences from the two South Korean wild boar APPVs (subclade I.4) and of the eight German wild boar APPVs (subclade I.2) were 88.1–88.9% identical at the nt level and 96.1–97.3% identical at the aa level.

3.3. ML Trees for the E2 Sequences

The E2 sequences (723 nt) from four South Korean wild boar APPVs (wbKOR 13079, -13188, -14105, and -13370) were 91.3–94.3% identical at the nt level and 95.4–97.1% identical at the aa level. ML analysis of the E2 sequences categorized them as Clade I (three in subclade I.1 and one in subclade I.2), as shown in Figure 3. By contrast, six APPVs from South Korean domestic pigs belonged to three subclades (one to subclade I.1, three to subclade I.2, and two to subclade I.4), as shown in Figure 3. The four South Korean wild boar APPVs and six South Korean domestic pig APPVs were 87.4–94.3% identical at the nt level and 94.2–98.8% identical at the aa level. The E2 sequences from the four South Korean wild boar APPVs and the 17 other APPVs in Clade II were 84.4–85.1% identical at the nt level and 94.2–96.3% identical at the aa level, whereas the four South Korean wild boar APPVs and 11 other APPVs in Clade III were 81.5–82.7% identical at the nt level and 90.0–92.5% identical at the aa level.

3.4. ML Trees for the Npro Sequences

The Npro sequences (540 nt) of five APPVs from South Korean wild boars (wbKOR 13079, -13109, -13188, -14105, and -13370) were 92.6–98.7% identical at the nt level and 93.9–99.4% identical at the aa level. ML analysis of the Npro sequences categorized them as Clade I (all five belonged to subclade I.1), as shown in Figure 4. The six APPVs from South Korean domestic pigs were distributed among all subclades (one in subclade I.1, two in subclade I.2, one in subclade I.3, and one in subclade I.4), as shown in Figure 4. The nt sequence identity between the five South Korean wild boar APPVs and the six South Korean domestic pig APPVs was 85.0–95.4%, whereas the aa sequences were 89.4–95.0% identical. The Npro sequences of the five South Korean wild boar APPVs and the 16 APPVs in Clade II were 79.3–80.5% identical at the nt level and 80.6–83.9% identical at the aa level, whereas the sequences from the five South Korean wild boar APPVs and the 12 APPVs in Clade III were 77.0–80.4% identical at the nt level and 80.6–81.1% identical at the aa level.

4. Discussion

Some retrospective studies suggest that APPVs were circulating widely for decades before the recent reports describing their detection [21,22]. An early study identified an APPV strain from samples obtained from piglets with CT; qRT-PCR of samples from a pig herd in the USA revealed an APPV prevalence of 6% [2]. Another study reported APPVs in CT-affected piglets from many countries, which further supports the potential relationship between APPV and CT type A-II [3]. In South Korea, APPV sequences from the domestic pig samples collected in 2016 had been submitted to GenBank (accession numbers: MF979135, MH509410), and the first identification of APPV was reported in suckling piglets with CT in 2017 [9]. Moreover, an APPV detection rate of 2.4–22% was reported in apparently healthy pigs in the USA and Germany [6,12,23]. A recent study of serum samples from apparently healthy pigs revealed that the prevalence of APPV in Europe was 2.3–17.5%, and that in China it was 5–11% [11]. All of these results demonstrate that APPV is highly prevalent in both apparently healthy pigs and CT-affected pigs, suggesting that the virus may have spread worldwide.

Wild boars are susceptible to APPV infection, although the role of this species in the epidemiology of the virus is unknown [13]. A very recent finding is that the prevalence of APPV in serum samples from wild boars in Europe is 0.23–19%, suggesting that wild boars may be a reservoir for APPV [10,12,13]. All wild boars sampled in this study, including APPV-positive wild boars, were considered healthy (based on their behavior) before hunting. The prevalence of APPV among South Korean wild boars is low, as in Spain (0.23%) and Italy (0.69%) [10,13]; however, this is in contrast to the high prevalence detected in northern Germany (19%) [12]. Furthermore, serological investigations in wild boars revealed an antibody detection rate of 52% in northern Germany, where APPV seems to be endemic among wild boars in many areas [12].

Phylogenetic analysis revealed that APPV sequences (complete or partial polyprotein) exhibit high genetic diversity between strains detected in different countries and species (domestic pigs or wild boars), and that they form independent clusters according to geographic location [24].

Recently, phylogenetic analysis in China revealed a high level of genetic variation among APPVs: three Clades (I–III), with four subgroups (1–4) in Clade I [25]. Sequence analysis of the APPV NS3, E2, and Npro genes, followed by the construction of ML trees, classified them into three Clades—APPVs isolated from China were assigned to all Clades, whereas APPVs isolated from Asia, North America, and European countries belonged only to Clade I [25,26]. APPV strains isolated from South Korean wild boars and South Korean domestic pigs belonged to Clade I, without a preference for any particular subclade. This means that APPVs may have high the potential for spreading between wild boars and domestic pigs. In the three ML trees (NS3, E2, and Npro) constructed for this study, Clade I contained four subclades; however, the APPV strains contained within these subclades were not clearly distinguished by the three ML trees. A previous study suggests that recombination events occur between Clades (Clades II and III) or within a Clade (Clade I) [25]. Therefore, further research is needed to determine whether the difference in subclade of South Korean APPV strains in three ML trees are because of the recombination events within Clade I.

5. Conclusions

Here, we present the first report of APPV detected in South Korean wild boars. We found that the overall prevalence of APPV in South Korean wild boars was low (0.78%). South Korean wild boars harbor genetically diverse APPV strains belonging to Clade I. Wild boars may be an important virus reservoir for APPV. More epidemiological information will help to establish effective control measures and to eradicate the virus from affected pig herds in the future.

Author Contributions: Conceptualization, S.C. and B.-K.P.; methodology, G.-N.P. and R.M.C.; writing—review and editing, B.-H.H. and D.-J.A. All authors have read and agreed to the published version of the manuscript.

References

1. Smith, D.B.; Meyers, G.; Bukj, J.; Gould, E.A.; Monath, T.; Scott Muerhoff, A.; Pletnev, A.; Rico-Hesse, R.; Stapleton, J.T.; Simmonds, P.; et al. Proposed revision to the taxonomy of the genus Pestivirus, family Flaviviridae. *J. Gen. Virol.* **2017**, *98*, 2016–2112. [CrossRef]
2. Hause, B.; Collin, E.A.; Peddireddi, L.; Yuan, F.; Chen, Z.; Hesse, R.A.; Anderson, G. Discovery of a novel putative atypical porcine pestivirus in pigs in the United States. *J. Gen. Virol.* **2015**, *96*, 2994–2998. [CrossRef] [PubMed]
3. Yuan, J.; Han, A.; Li, J.; Huang, Y.; Yang, J.; Ding, H.; Zhang, J.; Zhu, M.; Zhang, Y.; Liao, J.; et al. Atypical porcine pestivirus as a novel type of pestivirus in pigs in China. *Front. Microbiol.* **2017**, *8*, 862. [CrossRef] [PubMed]
4. Beer, M.; Wernlike, K.; Drager, D.; Hoper, D.; Pohlmann, A.; Bergermann, C.; Hoffmann, B. High prevalence of highly variable atypical porcine pestiviruses found in Germany. *Transboud. Emerg. Dis.* **2016**, *64*, e22–e26. [CrossRef]
5. De Groof, A.; Deijs, M.; Guelen, K.; van Grinsven, L.; van Os-Galdos, L.; Vogels, W.; van der Hoek, L. Atypical porcine pestivirus: A possible cause of congenital tremor type A-II in newborn piglets. *Viruses* **2016**, *8*, 271. [CrossRef]
6. Postel, A.; Hansmann, F.; Baechlein, C.; Fischer, N.; Alawi, M.; Grundhoff, A.; Becher, P. Presence of atypical porcine pestivirus (APPV) genome in newborn piglets correlates with congenital tremor. *Sci. Rep.* **2016**, *6*, 27735. [CrossRef] [PubMed]
7. Schwarz, L.; Riedel, C.; Hogler, S.; Sinn, L.J.; Voglmayr, T.; Wochtl, B.; Lamp, B. Congenital infection with atypical porcine pestivirus (APPV) is associated with disease and viral persistence. *Vet. Res.* **2017**, *48*, 1–14. [CrossRef]

8. Gatto, I.R.H.; Harmon, K.; Bradner, L.; Silva, P.; Kinhares, D.C.L.; Arruda, P.H.; de Oliverira, L.G.; Arruda, B.L. Detection of atypical porcine pestivirus in Brazil in the central nervous system of suckling piglets with congenital tremor. *Transboud Emerg. Dis.* **2018**, *65*, 375–380. [CrossRef]
9. Kim, S.; Jeong, C.; Yoon, S.; Lee, K.; Yang, M.; Kim, B.; Lee, S.Y.; Kang, S.J.; Kim, W.I. Detection of atypical porcine pestivirus (APPV) from a case of congenital tremor in Korea. *Korean. J. Vet. Sev.* **2017**, *40*, 209–213.
10. Enrica, S.; Saloni, C.; Lelli, D.; Barbieri, I.; Moreno, A.; Loris, G.; Lavazza, A. Molecular Survey and Phylogenetic Analysis of Atypical Porcine Pestivirus (APPV) Identification in Swine and Wild Boar from Northern Italy. *Viruses.* **2019**, *11*, 1142.
11. Postel, A.; Meyer, D.; Cagatay, G.N.; Feliziani, F.; De Mia, G.M.; Fischer, N.; Grundho_, A.; Mili´cevi´c, V.; Deng, M.C.; Chang, C.Y.; et al. High Abundance and Genetic Variability of Atypical Porcine Pestivirus in Pigs from Europe and Asia. *Emerg. Infect. Dis.* **2017**, *23*, 2104–2107. [CrossRef] [PubMed]
12. Cagatay, G.N.; Antos, A.; Meyer, D.; Maistrelli, C.; Keuling, O.; Becher, P.; Postel, A. Frequent infection of wild boar with atypical porcine pestivirus (APPV). *Transboud Emerg. Dis.* **2018**, *65*, 1087–1093. [CrossRef] [PubMed]
13. Colom-Cadena, A.; Ganges, L.A.; Munoz-Gonsalez, S.; Castillo-Contreras, R.; Alejandro Bochorquez, J.; Rosell, R.; Seglaes, J.; Marco, I.; Cabezon, O. Atypical porcine pestivirus in wild boar (Sus Scrofa), Spain. *Vet. Rec.* **2018**, *183*, 569. [CrossRef] [PubMed]
14. Weber, M.N.; Streck, A.F.; Silveira, S.; Mosena, A.C.S.; da Silva, M.S.; Canal, C.W. Homomolgours recombination in pestiviruses: Identification of three putative novel events between different subtypes/ genogroups. *Infect. Genet. Evol.* **2015**, *30*, 2109–2224. [CrossRef] [PubMed]
15. Greiser-Wilke, I.; Depner, K.; Fritzemeier, J.; Haas, L.; Moenning, V. Application of a computer program for genetic typing of classical swine fever virus isolates from Germany. *J. Virol. Methods.* **1998**, *75*, 141–150. [CrossRef]
16. Zhang, H.; Wen, W.; Hao, G.; Hu, Y.; Chen, H.; Qian, P.; Li, X. Phylogenetic and genomic characterization of a novel atypical porcine pestivirus in China. *Transboud Emerg. Dis.* **2018**, *65*, e202–e204. [CrossRef] [PubMed]
17. Zhou, K.; Yue, H.; Tang, C.; Ruan, W.; Zhou, Q.; Zhang, B. Prevalence and genome characteristics of atypical porcine pestivirus in Southwest China. *J. Gen. Virol.* **2019**, *100*, 84–88. [CrossRef] [PubMed]
18. Choe, S.; Kim, J.H.; Kim, K.S.; Song, S.; Kang, W.C.; Kim, H.J.; Park, G.N.; Cha, R.M.; Cho, I.S.; Hyun, B.H.; et al. Impact of a live attenuated classical swine fever virus introduced onto Jeju Island, a CSF-free area. *Pathogens.* **2019**, *8*, 251. [CrossRef]
19. Thompson, J.D.; Gibson, T.J.; Plewniak, F.; Jeanmougin, F.; Higgins, D.G. The CLUSTAL_X windows interface: Flexible strategies for multiple sequence alignment aided by quality analysis tools. *Nucleic Acids Res.* **1997**, *25*, 4876–4882. [CrossRef]
20. Kumar, S.; Stecher, G.; Tamura, K. MEGA7: Molecular Evolutionary Genetics Analysis Version 7.0 for Bigger Datasets. *Mol. Biol. Evol.* **2016**, *33*, 1870–1874. [CrossRef]
21. Muñoz-González, S.; Canturri, A.; Pérez-Simó, M.; Bohórquez, J.A.; Rosell, R.; Cabezón, O.; Segalés, J.; Domingo, M.; Ganges, L. First report of the novel atypical porcine pestivirus in Spain and a retrospective study. *Transbound Emerg. Dis.* **2017**, *64*, 1645–1649. [CrossRef] [PubMed]
22. Kaufmann, C.; Stalder, H.; Sidler, X.; Renzullo, S.; Gurtner, C.; Grahofer, A.; Schweizer, M. Long-Term Circulation of Atypical Porcine Pestivirus (APPV) within Switzerland. *Viruses.* **2019**, *11*, 653. [CrossRef] [PubMed]
23. Saitou, N.; Nei, M. The neighbor-joining method: A new method for reconstructing phylogenetic trees. *Mol. Biol. Evol.* **1987**, *4*, 406–426. [PubMed]
24. Gatto, I.; Sonalio, K.; Oliveira, L. Atypical porcine pestivirus (APPV) as a New Species of Pestivirus in Pig Production. *Front. Vet. Sci.* **2019**, *6*, 35. [CrossRef] [PubMed]
25. Guo, Z.; Wang, L.; Qaio, S.; Deng, R.; Zhang, G. Genetic characterization and recombination analysis of atypical porcine pestivirus. *Infect. Genet. Evol.* **2020**, *81*, 104259. [CrossRef] [PubMed]
26. Yan, X.L.; Li, Y.Y.; He, L.L.; Wu, J.L.; Tang, X.Y.; Chen, G.H.; Mai, K.J.; Wu, R.T.; Li, Q.N.; Chen, Y.H.; et al. 12 novel atypical porcine pestivirus genomes from neonatal piglets with congenital tremors: A newly emerging branch and high prevalence in China. *Virology.* **2019**, *533*, 50–58. [CrossRef]

8

Fetal Lymphoid Organ Immune Responses to Transient and Persistent Infection with Bovine Viral Diarrhea Virus

Katie J. Knapek [1,2,†,‡], Hanah M. Georges [1,†], Hana Van Campen [1,2], Jeanette V. Bishop [1], Helle Bielefeldt-Ohmann [3], Natalia P. Smirnova [1,§] and Thomas R. Hansen [1,*]

[1] Department of Biomedical Sciences, Colorado State University, Fort Collins, CO 80523, USA; kjknapek@central.uh.edu (K.J.K.); h.georges@colostate.edu (H.M.G.); hana.van_campen@colostate.edu (H.V.C.); jeanette.bishop@colostate.edu (J.V.B.); natalia.smirnova@sidelinesoft.com (N.P.S.)

[2] Department of Microbiology, Immunology and Pathology, Colorado State University, Fort Collins, CO 80523, USA

[3] Australian Infectious Diseases Research Centre and School of Veterinary Science, The University of Queensland, St. Lucia, QLD 4072, Australia; h.bielefeldtohmann1@uq.edu.au

[*] Correspondence: thomas.hansen@colostate.edu.

[†] These authors contributed equally to this work.

[‡] Current Address: Department of Animal Care Operations, University of Houston, Houston, TX 77004, USA.

[§] Current Address: Beckman Coulter Life Sciences, Loveland, CO 80538, USA.

Abstract: Bovine Viral Diarrhea Virus (BVDV) fetal infections occur in two forms; persistent infection (PI) or transient infection (TI), depending on what stage of gestation the fetus is infected. Examination of lymphoid organs from both PI and TI fetuses reveals drastically different fetal responses, dependent upon the developmental stage of the fetal immune system. Total RNA was extracted from the thymuses and spleens of uninfected control, PI, and TI fetuses collected on day 190 of gestation to test the hypothesis that BVDV infection impairs the innate and adaptive immune response in the fetal thymus and spleen of both infection types. Transcripts of genes representing the innate immune response and adaptive immune response genes were assayed by Reverse Transcription quatitative PCR (RT-qPCR) ($2^{-\Delta\Delta Cq}$; fold change). Genes of the innate immune response, interferon (IFN) inducible genes, antigen presentation to lymphocytes, and activation of B cells were downregulated in day 190 fetal PI thymuses compared to controls. In contrast, innate immune response genes were upregulated in TI fetal thymuses compared to controls and tended to be upregulated in TI fetal spleens. Genes associated with the innate immune system were not different in PI fetal spleens; however, adaptive immune system genes were downregulated, indicating that PI fetal BVDV infection has profound inhibitory effects on the expression of genes involved in the innate and adaptive immune response. The downregulation of these genes in lymphocytes and antigen-presenting cells in the developing thymus and spleen may explain the incomplete clearance of BVDV and the persistence of the virus in PI animals while the upregulation of the TI innate immune response indicates a more mature immune system, able to clear the virus.

Keywords: bovine viral diarrhea virus; fetus; thymus; immune response

---

1. Introduction

Bovine viral diarrhea viruses (BVDV) cause significant economic losses in all sectors of cattle production worldwide [1–4]. BVDVs are small single-stranded RNA viruses belonging to the Pestivirus genus in the family Flaviviridae [5]. Isolates of BVDV are classified into two genotypes, type 1 and type 2, with several subtypes and two biotypes: cytopathic (cp) and noncytopathic (ncp) [6]. Acute BVDV infection of immunocompetent cattle results in diverse clinical presentations, including subclinical infection, fever, nasal and/or ocular discharge, pneumonia, severe systemic disease, hemorrhage, and peracute death [7]. Importantly, BVDV infection of pregnant cattle results in fetal infection and reproductive losses, including early embryonic death, abortion, and stillbirth [8–11]. If maternal infection with ncp BVDV occurs prior to 125 days of gestation, the fetus becomes persistently infected (PI) with the virus and is born without BVDV-specific antibodies [12,13]. PI animals will shed BVDV throughout life, serving as the main source of infection for other cattle. BVDV infection of pregnant cows after 150 days of gestation results in a transient infection (TI) of the fetus. These TI calves are born with BVDV-specific antibodies indicative of a functional adaptive immune response and clearance of the virus [9,14,15]. Virus-specific immune responses in the bovine fetus develops between days 125 and 150; therefore, BVDV infection during this time may result in either a PI or TI, depending on the individual fetuses [16]. The differences in the outcomes of PI and TI fetal infections have been attributed to the maturation and function of the fetal immune system at the time of infection [17].

At least two explanations have been tendered to explain the persistence of BVDV in PI cattle. First, ncp BVDV has been shown to inhibit type I interferon (IFN) induction in vitro through the actions of virally encoded RNase (E^{rns}) and the N-terminal protease (N^{pro}) (reviewed in [18–21]). The latter N^{pro} degrades *interferon regulatory factor 3* (IRF3), thus inhibiting the transcription of IFNB and its antiviral activity in adjacent cells [22–24]. E^{rns} binds to and degrades double-stranded RNA (dsRNA), preventing its binding to cells and induction of IFNs [25]. Inhibition of the IFN response by N^{pro} and E^{rns} allows BVDV to persist and replicate in cells. Conversely, in an in vivo model, mutations of these two viral genes affecting their functions negate persistent infection [26]. In another in vivo model using BVDV strain Pe515nc, fetuses were inoculated in utero (amniotic fluid) and collected on days 3, 5, and 7 post-inoculation [27]. BVDV was confirmed in fetal tissues; however, an innate immune response was not seen, suggesting an inhibition of the fetal innate immune response to BVDV [27]. A second explanation of BVDV persistence in fetal infections might be that BVDV does not inhibit the IFN response, but instead, another unknown mechanism is responsible for persistence. Previously, we observed that bovine fetuses whose dams were inoculated with ncp BVDV 96B2222 on day 75 of gestation had a peak in BVDV RNA in fetal blood on day 97 of gestation, 21 days post-maternal inoculation (dpmi), followed by a 10-fold decrease in viral RNA on days 192 and 245 of gestation, suggesting partial viral clearance by an active immune response in the PI fetus, or possibly a decrease in infected cell types/numbers [28–30]. Interferon stimulated genes (ISG), such as *ISG15*, *protein kinase RNA-activated* (*PKR*), as well as the RNA helicases: *DEAD Box Protein 58* (*DDX58*), also known as *retinoic acid-inducible gene* (*RIGI*), *melanoma differentiation-associated protein 5* (*MDA5*); and *DExH-box helicase 58* (*DHX58*) were also shown to be chronically upregulated in the PI animal postnatally [31]. These results indicate that PI fetuses and placenta respond to BVDV with an innate immune response, albeit somewhat reduced compared to TI fetuses [28,29,31]. These findings indicate that the fetus responds to ncp BVDV infection with an innate immune response, much like the innate response to ncp BVDV infection in postnatal calves shown by Palomares et al. (2013); hence, inhibition of the innate immune response by viral proteins does not entirely explain viral persistence in vivo [32]. Another in vivo postnatal model used BVDV strain 11,249, which was previously shown to inhibit the IFN response in vitro [33]. The study revealed that in vivo, this BVDV strain does induce IFN responses [33]. The stimulation of an IFN response to BVDV has been exhibited in in vitro studies, in vivo fetal infection studies, and in vivo postnatal infections. Differences in these theories could be explained by differences in BVDV strains used and/or differences in experimental models. It is important to examine these differences and theories when considering the results of the present study.

An additional explanation for viral persistence is that the presence of BVDV during the development of the T cell repertoire permits its antigens to be accepted as "self" antigens, resulting in a state referred to as immunotolerance in which elements of the adaptive immune system do not respond to viral antigens and do not clear the virus from fetal tissues [34]. We hypothesize that ncp BVDV fetal infection early in gestation (<125 days) interferes with T cell development in the bovine fetal thymus during a critical period in which T cells are selected based on their recognition of self-antigens, affecting T cell response to BVDV in the spleen, resulting in immunotolerance to the virus and persistent infection in the calf. BVDV fetal infection later in gestation (>150 days) results in an active innate immune response, which clears the virus infection and causes a delay in antigen-specific T and B cell responses. To examine the effect of ncp BVDV infection on the bovine fetal thymus and spleen, transcripts of genes representative of the innate and adaptive immune response pathways were compared with control fetuses collected on day 190 of gestation.

2. Materials and Methods

2.1. Animals

Animal experiments were performed as previously described [28,34]. All animal experiments were approved by the Institutional Animal Care and Use Committees at the University of Wyoming, approval 05-265A-02 (19/10/2005) and 08-16A-01 (11/01/09). BVDV antigen negative and seronegative yearling Hereford heifers were synchronized for estrus (ovulation) and artificially inseminated with BVDV-free semen. Pregnancy was confirmed by ultrasound examination on days 35 to 40 and on day 70 of gestation.

2.2. Experimental Design: BVDV Inoculation and Fetal Collections

A power analysis was performed, and a group of 6 animals per treatment group (control, TI, and PI) was determined to be appropriate for a power of 1. Therefore, 18 unvaccinated pregnant heifers were randomly placed into treatment groups and inoculated intranasally with 2 mL culture media to generate sham-treated controls ($n = 6$) or with media containing 4.4 $\log_{10}$ $TCID_{50}/_{mL}$ of ncp BVDV2 strain 96B2222 on day 75 of gestation to generate PI ($n = 6$) fetuses and on day 175 to generate TI ($n = 6$) fetuses [34]. Treatment groups were kept in widely separated pens and fed at the end of feeding rounds to minimize viral transmission. To capture the fetal immune response during maternal seroconversion (in the PI group), day 190 of gestation was chosen for fetal collections. Eighteen fetuses were collected by Cesarean section and necropsied on day 190 of gestation. Samples of fetal thymuses and spleens were frozen in liquid nitrogen and stored at −80 °C.

2.3. RNA Extraction and RT-qPCR

Total RNA from 70 mg of frozen thymus and 50 mg of frozen spleen was isolated using TRIzol reagent according to the manufacturer's instructions (Invitrogen ThermoFisher, Rockford, IL, USA). The isolated RNA was treated with DNase I (Qiagen, Germantown, MD, USA) and purified using the RNeasy MiniElute Cleanup Kit (Qiagen, Germantown, MD, USA). RNA concentration and 260/280 and 260/230 ratios were measured using the NanoDrop 1000 Spectrophotometer (ThermoScientific, Rockford, IL, USA). The primer sequences and gene accession numbers are listed in Table 1. One μg of RNA was reverse transcribed to synthesize cDNA using iScript™ Reverse Transcription Supermix (Bio-Rad, Hercules, CA, USA). Reverse transcription quantitative polymerase chain reaction (RT-qPCR) was performed with iQ™ SYBR® Green Supermix (Bio-Rad, Hercules, CA, USA). Each cDNA reaction was diluted (1:5 for thymus and 1:10 for spleen) with RNase-free water. Primers were used at 3 μM concentration. Each sample was assayed in duplicate wells on a 384-well plate. Four biological replicates of RT-qPCR plates were performed at one cycle of 95 °C for 3 min, 40 cycles of 95 °C for 30 s, 58 °C for 30 s, and 72 °C for 15 s with a final 5 min elongation in a LightCycler-480 Instrument (Roche, Basel, Switzerland). Upon completion of RT-qPCR, melting curve analysis was performed to assess the quality of amplification.

Table 1. Primers utilized for RT-qPCR.

Gene	Sequence	Accession	Efficiency
18S	FW: GAACGAGACTCTGGCATGC REV: CTGAACGCCACTTGTCCCTC	NR_036642	102%
DDX58	FW: GAGCACTGGTGGATGCCTTA REV: GCTGTCTCTGTTGGTTCGGA	XM_024996055.1	157%
IRF7	FW: GCCTCCTGGAAAACCAACTT REV: CCTTATGAGGGTCGGTAGGGG	NM_001105040.1	127%
NFKB	FW: CGAGGTTCGGTTCTACGAGG REV: TGCAGGAACACGGGTTACAGG	NM_001102101.1	134%
IFNB	FW: TCCAGCACATCTTCGGCATT REV: TTCCCTAGGTGGGGAACGAT	NM_174350.1	104%
ISG15	FW: GGTATCCGAGCTGAAGCAGTT REV: ACCTCCCTGCTGTCAAGGT	NM_174366	115%
STAT4	FW: TTCTTCCCATGTCGCCAAGT REV: AACCAGATGTGATTGTTGGCA	NM_001083692.2	104%
IFI30	FW: GCATGCAGCTCTTGCACATC REV: GGCCCCAAGAGTTCTTACCC	NM_001101251.2	131%
PSMB9	FW: ATCTACCTGGCCACCATCAC REV: AGGAGAGTCCGAGGAAGGAG	NM_001034388	115%
PSMB8	FW: ACTGGAAGGCAGCACAGAGT REV: ATTGTGCTTAGTGGGGCATC	NM_001040480	124%
B2M	FW: AFTAAGCCGCAGTGGAGGT Rev: CGCAAAACACCCTGAAGACT	AC_000167.1	123%
CXCL10	FW: ACACCGAGGCACTACGTTCT Rev: TAAGCCCAGAGCTGGAAAGA	CB533091	121%
CXCL16	FW: CTTGTGAGGGCAGATTGTGA Rev:GGTCAATAGCTGGTTAGTTGTGAA	CK770974	105%
CD4	FW: GGGCAGAACGGATGTCTCAA REV: ATAGGTCTTCTGGAGCCGGT	NM_001103225.1	110%
CD8a	FW: TACATCTGGGCTCCCTTGGT REV: CCACAGGCCTGGGACATTTG	NM_174015.1	130%
CD8b	FW: AGCTGAGTGTGTTGATGTTCT REV: TTCTGAGTCACCTGGGTTGG	NM_001105344.2	93%
CD79b	FW: TGATTCCCGGGCTCAACAAC REV: CTGCCAGATCCGGGAACAAG	XM_002696068.6	160%

DDX58: DExD/H-Box Helicase 58; *IRF7*: Interferon Regulatory Factor 7; *NFKB*: Nuclear Factor Kappa-Light-Chain -Enhancer of Activated B Cells; *IFNB*: Interferon Beta; *ISG15*: Interferon Stimulated Gene 15; *STAT4*: Signal Transducer and Activator of Transcription 4; *IFI30*: IFI30 Lysosomal Thiol Reductase; *PSMB9*: Proteasome 20S Subunit Beta 9; *PSMB8*: Proteasome 20S Subunit Beta 8; *B2M*: Beta-2-Microglobulin; *CXCL10*: C-X-C Motif Chemokine Ligand 10; *CXCL*: C-X-C Motif Chemokine Ligand 16. FW: Forward primer; REV: Reverse Primer.

2.4. RT-qPCR Targets and Validation

RT-qPCR targets for each tissue were chosen based on current knowledge and available tissue. Targets shared between the thymus and spleen were chosen to understand basic changes in both the innate and adaptive branches of the immune system. For the innate immune branch, targets chosen were *DDX58, NFKB, IRF7, IFNB*, and *ISG15*. For the adaptive branch, targets chosen were *PSMB9, IFI30, CD4, CD8A, CD8B*, and *CD79B*. Thymic tissue samples were more abundant than the spleen, allowing for additional targets to be studied in the thymus; *STAT1, IFI6, CXCL10, CXCL16, CXCR6, TAP1, B2M, CIITA*, and *CD46*. These results can be found in Table A1. A previous study which used a microarray to study BVDV-infected spleens indicated *STAT4* and *PSMB8* as targets of interest specific for splenic samples [35]. Therefore, both *STAT4* and *PSMB8* were additional targets for splenic samples in this study. BVDV viral RNA was also targeted to confirm tissue infection in TI and PI fetuses. These results can also be found in Table A1. Standard RT-qPCR primers were validated and evaluated based on MIQE guidelines [36].

2.5. Morphogenesis of Thymus during Bovine Fetal Development and Effect of In Utero BVDV Infection

Fetal thymus and spleen samples were fixed for 48 h in 10% neutral-buffered formalin, transferred into 70% ethanol, and paraffin-embedded. Four to 5 μm sections were cut and stained with eosin and hematoxylin (H&E). Microscopic assessment was performed with special attention to the components of the reticulo-endothelial network, myeloid, and lymphoid cells, including where the latter two cell types appear in the organ primordium. The relative cortical-to-medulla ratio was assessed, including full encirclement of the medulla by cortical thymocytes. Additionally, attention was paid to myoid cells and Hassall's corpuscles in terms of appearance, frequency, and size.

2.6. Statistical Analysis

RT-qPCR data are presented according to MIQE guidelines and statistically analyzed using the $2^{-\Delta\Delta Cq}$ method [37]. Briefly, the Δ quantification cycle (C_q; also known as C_t) was calculated by subtracting the mean C_q of the reference gene (18S rRNA), within the treatment group, from the C_q of the target gene (same treatment group as the reference). The average of the Δ C_q for controls for the target gene were then subtracted from each infection treatment Δ C_q, for the same target gene as controls, to calculate the fold change ($2^{-\Delta\Delta Cq}$). Statistical analysis of data obtained by RT-qPCR ($2^{-\Delta\Delta Cq}$) was performed in GraphPad Prism 8 (GraphPad Software, San Diego, CA, USA). The data were checked for normality using Shapiro-Wilks test; normally distributed data were analyzed with a one-way ANOVA and Dunnett's multiple comparisons test, while non-normally distributed data were analyzed with a Kruskal-Wallis test and Dunn's multiple comparisons test. Significant differences were at $p < 0.05$ and tendencies/trends were at $p < 0.10$. Data are presented as the mean ± SEM. Graphical data represents $2^{-\Delta\Delta Cq}$ of which statistical analysis was run. In the text, fold change is presented for ease of understanding up- and down-regulation. For $2^{-\Delta\Delta Cq}$ values > 1, fold changes were reported as averaged $2^{-\Delta\Delta Cq}$ values. For $2^{-\Delta\Delta Cq}$ values between 0 and 1 (down regulation), the negative inverse ($-1/(2^{-\Delta\Delta Cq})$) was calculated and reported as fold change.

3. Results

3.1. Detection of BVDV RNA Expression in Thymus and Spleen and BVDV Receptor CD46 in Fetal Thymuses

BVDV RNA was not detected in any of the control fetal thymus RNA samples and was present in 6 of 6 PI and 5 of 6 TI fetal thymic RNA samples with PI thymuses having 9.7- to 68.8-fold higher BVDV RNA concentrations compared to TI thymuses (Figure 1A). PI fetal spleens had a significantly increased amount of BVDV RNA ($p < 0.001$, $2^{-\Delta\Delta Cq} = 3037$-fold greater) compared to controls ($2^{-\Delta\Delta Cq} = 1.0$) and very low amounts of BVDV RNA in TI fetal spleens (Figure 1B). The concentration of BVDV receptor *CD46* mRNA in PI fetal thymuses was decreased 6.2-fold ($p < 0.001$) and increased in TI fetal thymuses ($p < 0.05$) compared to controls on day 190 (Figure 1C).

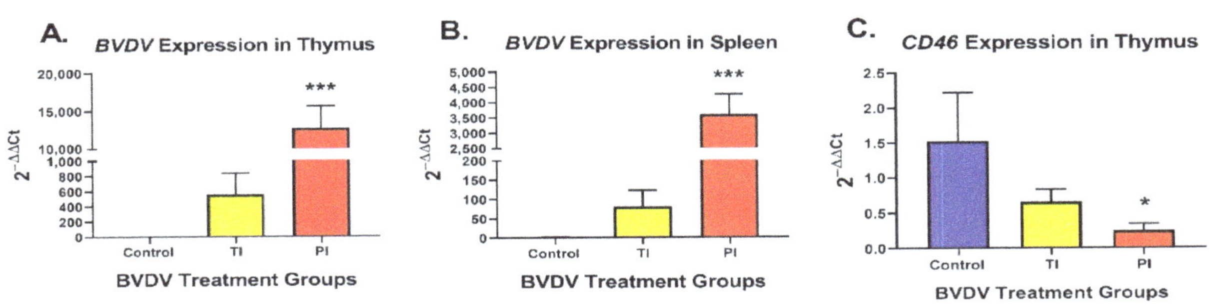

Figure 1. Bovine Viral Diarrhea Virus (BVDV) expression in (**A**) thymus and (**B**) spleen samples (Control, TI, and PI). Expression of BVDV was significantly upregulated in PIs compared to controls in both thymic and splenic samples. Expression of BVDV in TIs was higher than controls, but not significant due to individual variation. (**C**) BVDV receptor CD46 expression in thymus (Control, TI, and PI). *CD46* expression was significantly down-regulated in PI thymuses. Control: Uninfected, blue; TI: Transiently Infected, yellow; PI: Persistently Infected, red. * $p < 0.05$, *** $p < 0.001$.

3.2. Thymic Responses

3.2.1. Innate Immune Responses in TI and PI Fetal Thymuses

In TI fetal thymuses, mRNA concentrations were significantly increased ($p < 0.01$) for the innate immune response genes *NFKB* (1.5-fold) and *IRF7* (4.5-fold) compared to controls on day 190 (15 dpmi). Neither *DDX58*, *IFNB*, nor *ISG15* were significantly different than the controls (Figure 2).

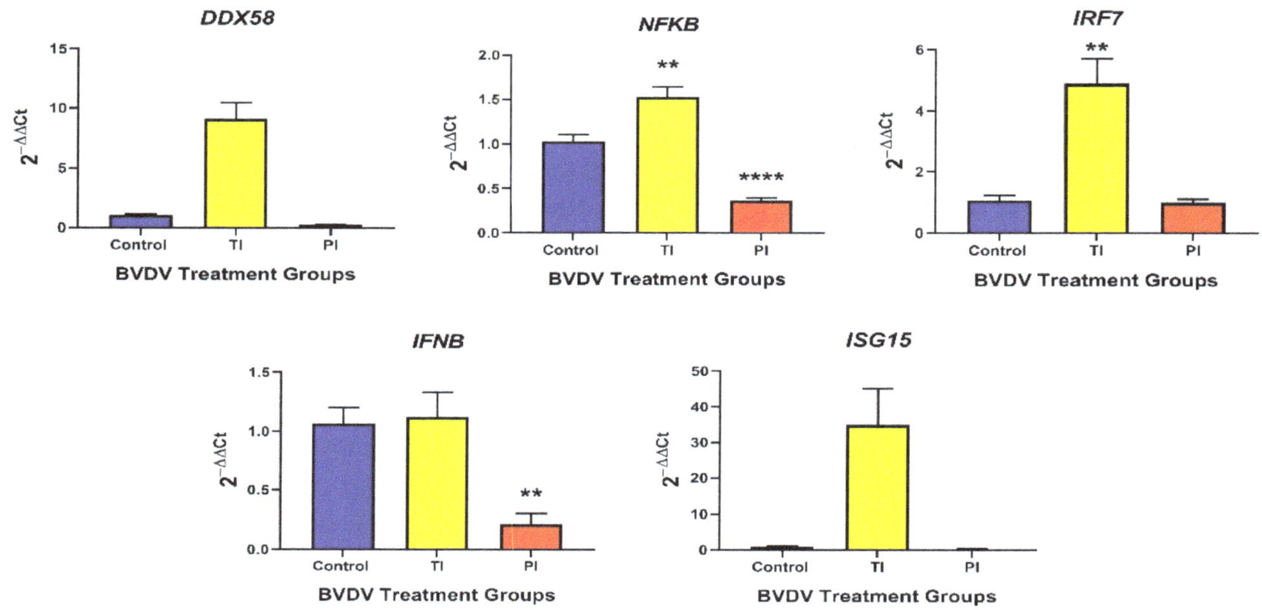

Figure 2. Control, TI, and PI thymus transcripts associated with the innate immune response. Interferon transcriptional regulators *NFKB* and *IRF7* were significantly upregulated in TI fetuses compared to controls. In PI fetal thymuses, only IFN transcriptional regulator *NFKB* and *IFNB* were down-regulated compared to control fetuses. TI: Transiently Infected, PI: Persistently Infected, ** $p < 0.01$, **** $p < 0.0001$.

In the PI fetal thymuses, the mRNAs of the innate response genes *NFKB* (−2.8-fold) and *IFNB* (6.0-fold) were significantly downregulated in PI thymuses compared to controls on day 190 ($p < 0.01$) (Figure 2); whereas *DDX58*, *IRF7*, and *ISG15* concentrations remained at control levels and were not significantly different between control and PI thymuses. A trending decrease in the type I IFN stimulated transcripts *STAT1* (−22.7-fold; Table A1) was found in PI fetal thymuses compared to controls ($p < 0.10$), which was consistent with the observed downregulation of *IFNB*. Type II IFN stimulated transcripts, transitional responses from the innate to adaptive immune response, *IFI16* (−11.3-fold, trend $p < 0.10$) and *CXCL16* (−22.4-fold, $p < 0.05$) were similarly down-regulated (Table A1). *CXCR6* mRNA concentration was not different between control and PI fetal thymuses (Table A1).

3.2.2. Adaptive Immune Responses in TI and PI Fetal Thymuses

In TI fetal thymuses, the expression of *MHC I* mRNA *PSMB9* (Figure 3), *TAP1* (Table A1), and *B2M* (Table A1) were not significantly different from controls. T cell markers *CD8A*, *CD8B*, and *CD4* and activated B cell marker *CD79B* mRNAs were not significantly different in TI fetal thymuses compared to controls.

The relative expression of MHC I antigen presentation pathway genes *PSMB9* (−5.2-fold), *TAP1* (−5.5-fold), and *B2M* (−27.9-fold) transcripts were significantly decreased in PI fetal thymuses relative to controls on day 190 of gestation ($p < 0.05$) (Figure 3, Table A1 respectively). CTL co-receptors *CD8A* (−16.2-fold) and *CD8B* (−9.6-fold) mRNA concentrations were significantly decreased in PI fetal thymuses compared to the controls on day 190 of gestation ($p < 0.05$) (Figure 3). *CIITA* (−3.4-fold, trend $p < 0.10$) and *CD4* (−8.1-fold, $p < 0.0001$) mRNA associated with MHC II antigen presentation were significantly decreased in PI fetal thymuses on day 190 (Table A1 and Figure 3, respectively). Activated B cell marker, *CD79B*, mRNA concentration was significantly decreased (−3.8-fold) in PI fetal thymuses compared to control ($p < 0.001$) thymuses at day 190 of gestation (Figure 3).

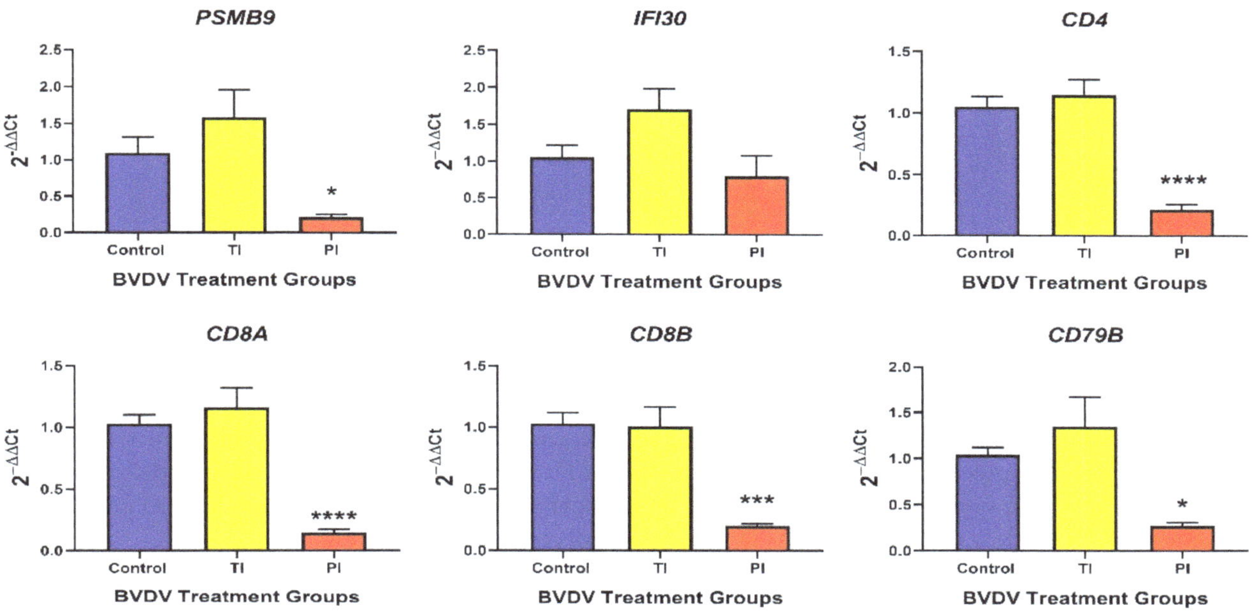

Figure 3. Thymic (Control, TI, and PI) transcript expression associated with the adaptive immune response. No significant differences were found in TI fetal thymuses compared to controls. However, all adaptive genes, with the exception of *IFI30*, were significantly down-regulated in PI fetal thymuses compared to controls. TI: Transiently Infected, PI: Persistently Infected. * $p < 0.05$, *** $p < 0.001$, **** $p < 0.0001$.

3.2.3. Morphogenesis and Histology of the Thymus during Bovine Fetal Development and the Effect of in Utero BVDV Infection

There were no discernible differences between the control or PI fetuses with regard to the thymus morphology at day 190. The morphology of the fetal thymus had attained almost a neonatal appearance, with the cortex having expanded to completely surround the medulla, and the cortico-medullary ratio being ≥2. The medulla contained large, often complex Hassall's corpuscles, large numbers of myoid cells, and eosinophilic granulocytes. The latter could be seen throughout the medulla, but appeared in highest frequency in the cortico-medullary border zone. The myoid cells were large, round cells with a deeply eosinophilic cytoplasm, either homogenous or with finely fibrillar patterning. The almost euchromatic nucleus was round and centrally located, or more oval and acentric. A small amount of chromatin clumping along the nuclear membrane and occasionally a small nucleolus was present. These cells may, in some cases, be considered "single-cell" Hassall's corpuscles.

3.3. Splenic Responses

3.3.1. Innate Immune Responses in TI and PI Fetal Spleens

DDX58 (25-fold; $p < 0.05$), IRF7 (22-fold; $p < 0.05$), and ISG15 (160-fold; $p < 0.05$) mRNA were upregulated in TI fetal spleens compared to controls, whereas *NFKB* and *IFNB* mRNA concentrations remained at basal levels and were not significantly different (Figure 4). The innate immune response in PI fetal spleens was similar to controls with only *NFKB* being significantly downregulated in PI fetal spleens compared to controls (0.1532-fold, $p < 0.05$, Figure 4).

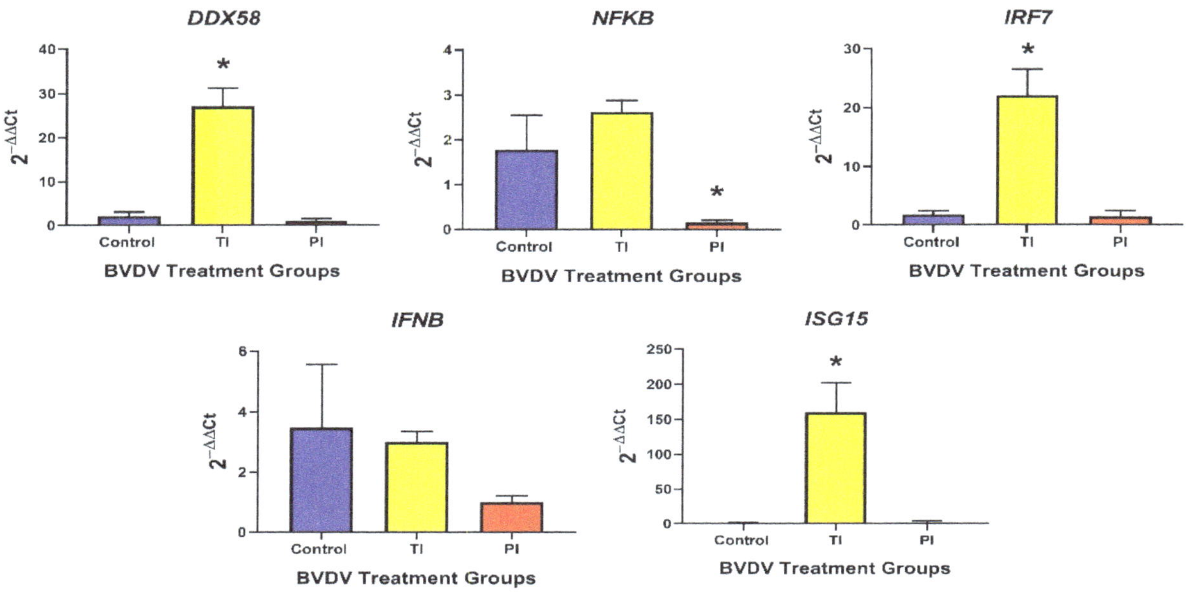

Figure 4. Spleen (Control, TI, and PI) expression of transcripts associated with the innate immune response. TI fetal spleens exhibited an upregulation of *DDX58*, *IRF7*, and *ISG15* compared to controls, indicating an active type I IFN response. In PI fetal spleens, only *NFKB* was downregulated compared to controls. TI: Transiently Infected, PI: Persistently Infected. * $p < 0.05$.

3.3.2. Adaptive Immune Responses in TI and PI Fetal Spleens

Adaptive immune response genes, such as *STAT4* (Figure 5), *PSMB9* (MHC class I, Table A1), and *IFI30* (MHC class II; Figure 5) were significantly upregulated in TI spleens compared to controls (5.54-fold, $p < 0.01$; 12.9-fold, $p < 0.05$ respectively); however, *PSMB8* (MHC class I) was not significantly different between the two groups (Figure 5). T and B lymphocyte markers, *CD4, CD8A, CD8B*, and *CD79B*, were not different in TI compared to the control spleen (Figure 5).

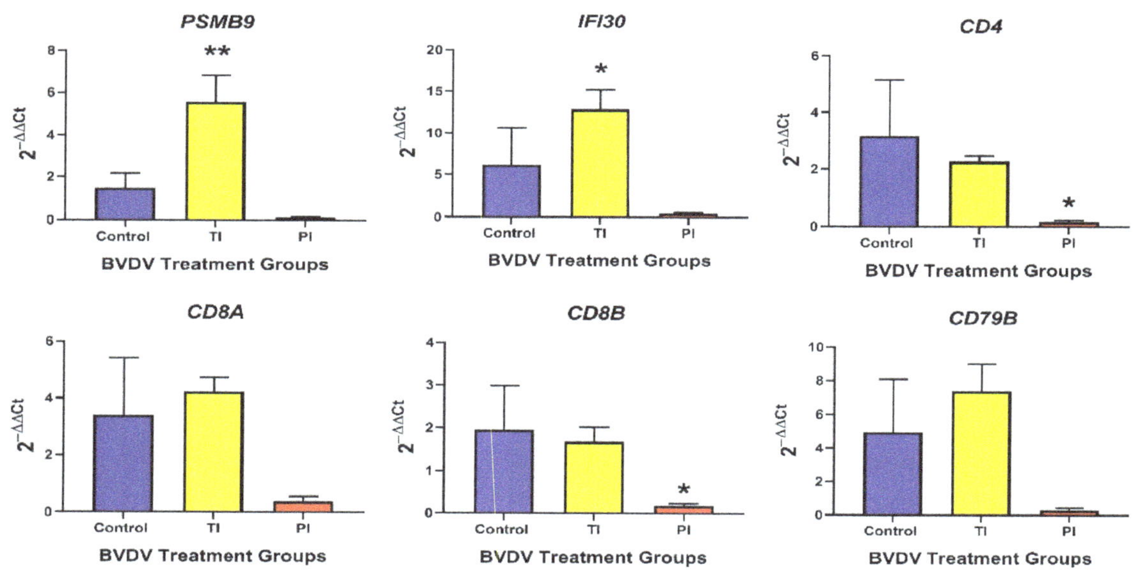

Figure 5. Splenic (Control, TI, and PI) expression of transcripts associated with the adaptive immune response. In TI fetal spleens, only *PSMB9* and *IFI30*, associated with antigen presentation, were significantly different to the controls. In PI fetal spleens, T cell markers *CD4* and *CD8A* were significantly downregulated compared to controls. TI: Transiently Infected, PI: Persistently Infected. * $p < 0.05$, ** $p < 0.01$.

In PI fetal spleens, *STAT4* (Table A1), *PSMB8/9* (Table A1 and Figure 5, respectively), and *IFI30* (Figure 5) were not differentially expressed compared to control fetal spleens. PI fetal spleens exhibited a downregulation of T lymphocyte markers mRNA (*CD4*, and *CD8B*) compared to controls (0.1465-fold, $p < 0.5$; 0.4005-fold, $p < 0.05$, respectively) (Figure 5) but T lymphocyte marker *CD8A* and B lymphocyte marker *CD79B* were not significantly different between the two groups.

4. Discussion

4.1. Transient Infection on Day 175 of Gestation Elicits an Immunocompetent Response in the Bovine Fetal Thymus and Spleen on Day 190

BVDV takes approximately 7–14 days to cross the placenta and infect the fetus following intranasal inoculation of the dam [38]. The TI fetal spleens and thymuses collected at day 190 of gestation, 15 days post-maternal infection were positive for BVDV RNA, indicating that the fetuses were infected for 1–7 days, which is sufficient time to have elicited an innate immune response in all TI fetuses and initial adaptive responses in some TI fetuses.

The rudimentary thymus is first detected around day 27 of gestation in ruminants with colonization and lymphoid development occurring at day 42 of gestation. Day 42 progenitor cells come from the fetal liver until the bone marrow develops and matures enough (around day 70) to take over as the primary source of thymocytes [39]. The bovine fetal thymus contains a discernable cortico-medullary delineation by day 42, Hassall's corpuscles by day 65, and IgM positive cells by day 70 to 100 [40]. In addition to T lymphocytes and prothymocytes of T cell lineage, the postnatal thymus contains thymic epithelial cells, myoid cells, fibroblasts, dendritic cells, macrophages and miscellaneous neutrophils, eosinophils and B cells [41,42]. These cell types would be present in the thymus at the time of maternal inoculation with BVDV (75 dpmi and 175 dpmi) and subsequent fetal infection in this experimental model. In utero BVDV infections have been shown to result in thymic hypoplasia in bovine fetuses characterized by marked lymphocyte depletion in the cortex, accompanied by hypertrophy of the epithelial stroma and infiltration by monocytes and mature macrophages with BVDV antigens primarily localized to macrophages [43–45].

The innate immune gene transcripts, *NFKB*, and *IRF7* were significantly upregulated in TI fetal thymuses indicative of a robust activation of the innate immune response to BVDV, which agrees with previous findings [34,35,38]. Significant changes were not observed in adaptive response genes, including the T cell marker transcripts, *CD8A*, *CD8B*, *CD4*, or B cell activation marker *CD79B* compared to controls, as expected due to the short course between fetal infection and tissue collection. In addition, the thymus is a primary lymphoid organ responsible for the selection and maturation of T cells but with limited antigen-specific immune responses. The decreased BVDV RNA concentrations in TI thymuses compared to PI thymuses, however, is supportive evidence that TI fetuses were able to mount an effective immune reaction against the virus. Despite the ability of TI fetuses to clear the virus, BVDV fetal infection during day 175–190 of gestation occurs during a critical stage of thymus and spleen development, as well as T cell selection and maturation in the thymus. BVDV fetal infection during this stage of fetal development may alter the animal's ability to fight other infections postnatally.

The spleen is a secondary lymphoid organ responsible for rapid immune responses to bloodborne pathogens like BVDV. During embryonic development, mesenchymal progenitor cells differentiate into marginal reticular cells, fibroblastic reticular cells, and follicular dendritic cells (reviewed in [46]). These cells will contribute to the spleen stroma and begin to form the white pulp, a lymphocyte-rich area which is the site of antigen-specific immune responses to blood-borne pathogens [46]. White pulp establishment occurs at approximately 15 weeks of gestation in humans, assumed to be a similar time point for cattle [40,46]. At this early time point, few B cells cluster around splenic arterioles, and 3 weeks later, are joined by T cells [46]. The T cells form the periarteriolar sheath (PALS), while the B cells form a follicle around the PALS [46]. Lymphocyte infiltration is believed to occur well after persistent infection with BVDV. However, TI fetuses were infected following the establishment of the white pulp and lymphocyte infiltration of the spleen. This may play a large role in the transient and persistent infection of BVDV in fetuses, as discussed later.

In TI fetal spleens, the cytoplasmic sensor mRNA *DDX58*, transcriptional factor *IRF7*, and interferon-stimulated gene *ISG15* were upregulated indicating the detection of BVDV RNA by the immune system of TI fetuses and activation of the innate immune response. Transcripts for genes associated with antigen presentation, *PSMB9* and *IFI30*, were upregulated in the TI fetal spleen, suggesting that the antigen processing mechanisms of cells had been stimulated. However, transcripts for T and B cell markers were not increased as viral peptide presentation in the context of MHC I and MHC II would not have stimulated the proliferation of T and B cells in the short time period between fetal infection and tissue collection. In addition, T and B cell activation may also have been delayed in the TI fetuses. BVDV is known to inhibit lymphocyte activation, resulting in delayed T and B cell responses during acute infections of postnatal animals [47,48]. The low amounts of BVDV RNA detected in the TI fetal spleen compared to PI fetal spleens suggest the innate immune mechanisms effectively inhibited viral replication prior to the elaboration of an adaptive immune response. Additionally, the fetal spleen is assumed to have both T and B cells on day 105 of gestation. It can be assumed these lymphocytes in the spleen, once activated, contribute to the clearance of the virus, seen in TI postnatal animals [9,15].

4.2. PI Thymus and Spleen Exhibit Diminished or Inhibited Immune Responses at Day 190 of Gestation

The mechanism of BVDV PI is controversial. Some of the first in vitro studies on BVDV infection concluded that BVDV infection blocked the host's interferon response contributing to the persistence of BVDV in fetuses infected before day 120 of gestation [21,23,24]. In a paper published in 2001, the authors infected fetuses in utero (through amniotic fluid) on day 60 of gestation and collected fetuses 3, 5, and 7 days post-maternal inoculation [27]. It was concluded that ncp BVDV inhibits the fetal IFN response [27]. Subsequently, using a model of maternal infection, the fetal IFN response was stimulated by BVDV 22 days post-maternal infection [28,31,34,35,38]. However, it is important to note the differences in BVDV strains used and the differences in experimental models. This current study follows several others with similar experimental models and the same BVDV strain that have demonstrated an active innate immune response in PI fetuses soon after the establishment of fetal infection. The discussion below highlights these previous findings [28,31,34,35,38].

Previously, it was established that the early gestation bovine fetus (day 75) could respond to ncp BVDV infection with an innate immune response indicated by the upregulation of cytosolic dsRNA sensors in fetal blood and spleen, type I IFNs in cotyledons, and ISGs in fetal tissues, including the liver and spleen [28,31,38]. Moreover, the IFNG protein, an important bridge between the innate and the adaptive immune response, was detected in the amniotic fluid and fetal blood, and *IFNG* mRNA was upregulated in liver, spleen, and thymus of PI fetuses 14–22 dpmi (89–97 days of gestation) [34]. The activation of these genes corresponded with a reduction in BVDV titer in PI fetal blood at day 190 and 245, suggesting partial clearance of the virus by an active innate immune response; however, BVDV continued to be present in fetal tissues, albeit at a reduced level (reviewed in [14,28,34]). We hypothesized that the persistence of ncp BVDV was due to exhaustion of the initial innate immune response, and impaired steps in the adaptive immune response leading to incomplete viral clearance in the PI fetus. In support of this hypothesis, two innate immune response mRNAs, *NFKB* and *IFNB*, the bridging mRNA *CXCL16*, and the adaptive immune response mRNAs, *PSMB9*, *TAP1*, *B2M*, *CD8A*, *CD8B*, *CD4*, and *CD79B*, were found to be significantly decreased on day 190 in PI fetal thymuses compared to controls, and T cell marker mRNAs (*CD4* and *CD8B*) were significantly downregulated in the PI spleen. However, as discussed below, it is believed attenuation of the immune system may be caused by Treg development, instead of our original hypothesis of immune system exhaustion [35,49–51].

DDX58 binds to and recognizes viral RNA in the innate immune system pathway. A reduction in *DDX58* concentrations could negatively impact the ability of fetal cells to respond to BVDV RNA and subsequently impair the induction of IFN antiviral activities. Persistent inhibition of NFKB has been associated with inappropriate immune cell development or delayed cell growth. For example, mice null for NFKB signaling molecules have impaired thymic medullary epithelial cell formation and autoimmune disease [52]. The transcription factor NFKB is both induced by type 1 IFNs and is a transcriptional regulator of cytokine expression, including IFNB and IFNG [53]. The decreased *IFNB* mRNA observed in the PI fetal thymus on day 190 coincided with the decreased expression of *NFKB* and the IFNI-inducible gene mRNAs, *ISG15* and *CXCL16*. Reduced *IFNB* mRNA may be explained by a paucity of dendritic cells in the PI fetal thymus at this stage of development; however, differences in the dendritic cell population between PI and control thymuses collected on day 190 were not observed histologically. IFI16 is a cytosolic sensor for viral RNA/DNA, which transcriptionally regulates the expression of type I IFNs in a positive manner [54]. The trended downregulation of *IFI16* observed in the PI thymus could explain the decreased expression of *IFNB*.

The PI fetal thymus exhibited differences in the innate immune response genes at day 190 compared to those previously observed in the fetal spleen and blood. *DDX58, MDA5,* and *ISG15* were previously observed to be increased in PI fetal blood from day 97 to day 192, and *ISG15* was increased in the PI fetal spleen, bone marrow, caruncle, and cotyledon, reflecting an active innate response in these tissues [28,31]. In contrast, *NFKB* and *IFNB* were significantly downregulated in PI fetal thymuses on day 190, but only *NFKB* was downregulated in spleens. A previous study by our group indicated a significant down-regulation of *IFNB* in day 190 PI fetal spleens, but no significant change in *NFKB* [35]. These studies were independent, and although results differ slightly, they both indicate an inhibition of the innate immune response 115 days post-maternal infection. Regulatory T cells (Tregs) originate in the thymus during fetal development and create tolerance of self in the developing fetus to prevent autoimmune disorders [49,50]. Due to the fetal BVDV infection occurring early in fetal development, prior to lymphocyte infiltration in the spleen, it is possible the Treg cells are creating tolerance to the BVDV viral antigen, allowing the virus to continue replication without an immune response from the host [49,50]. The development of Tregs in the thymus could be contributing to the difference in immune gene expression between the thymus and spleen [49,50]. On day 190 of gestation in PI animals, Tregs may be inhibiting an immune response in the thymus first before the Treg cells migrate to the periphery and reach the spleen.

Thymic concentrations of adaptive immune response transcripts, such as MHC I antigen presentation (*PSMB9, TAP1,* and *B2M*), CTL co-receptors *CD8A* and *CD8B*, and T cell marker CD4 were also decreased in PI fetal thymuses compared to controls consistent with an impaired adaptive immune response. The reduction in antigen presentation gene transcripts in PI fetal thymuses were associated with reduced *CD79B*, a component of antigen recognition and activation in B cells. In this study, *PSMB9* expression in PI thymuses was decreased at day 190 of gestation, suggesting a reduction in the normal function of the immunoproteasome [55]. Following proteolysis of viral proteins by the immunoproteasome, TAP1 transports peptides to the endoplasmic reticulum (ER) where peptides bind to MHC class I molecules for presentation on the cell membrane. Decreased *TAP1* concentrations could negatively impact antigen presentation to immune cells. In addition, *B2M* mRNA in PI thymuses was significantly decreased at day 190 compared to controls. The B2M protein assembles with the MHC I molecule in the ER to form a stable MHC I complex necessary for antigen binding. When B2M is not present, MHC I remains in the ER, and the MHC I complex is not expressed on the cell surface [56]. Decreased expression of *B2M* would result in additional dysfunction of the endogenous viral antigen presentation mechanism. In PI fetal spleens, *PSMB9* and *IFI30* were not significantly different compared to controls. This contradicts a previous study in which PSMB9 and IFI30 were significantly downregulated in day 190 PI spleens compared to controls [35]. This difference between the studies reflect increased individual variability between controls in the present study or possibly due to slight variation in infection/fetal collection times. The difference in the expression of antigen presentation mRNAs between the spleen and thymus may be indicative of APC and lymphocyte migration from the primary lymphoid organ, that is, the thymus, to secondary lymphoid organs, such as the spleen. In secondary lymphoid organs, such as the spleen, APCs reside and actively survey the blood and lymph for antigens; thus, the secondary lymphoid organs will have higher gene expression of mature APCs and lymphocyte markers [57].

Cytotoxic T cells recognize peptides presented in the context of the MHC I and B2M complex on target cells by the T cell receptor (TCR) and co-receptor, CD8. Antigen recognition by the CD8-TCR complex triggers the release of perforin, granzymes and cytokines from the lytic granules of CTL. *CD8A* and *CD8B* mRNA concentrations in PI fetal thymuses and *CD8B* in spleens were significantly decreased at day 190, suggesting either a reduced number of CTLs or decreased CD8A/B expressed per cell. Similarly, *CD4*, the co-receptor of the T cell receptor on T helper cells, mRNA was decreased in PI fetal thymuses and spleens at day 190 compared to controls and may reflect a decrease in T helper cells or the number of co-receptors per T helper cell. Supporting the results in a previous study, a reduction in BVDV-specific CTLs, T helper cells, or in antigen recognition would negatively impact the clearance of BVDV-infected cells in the thymus, spleen, and other fetal tissues, thus contributing to viral persistence [35].

The B-cell antigen receptor complex-associated protein Beta chain, *CD79B*, is part of the B lymphocyte antigen receptor complex and is required for T cell-dependent activation of B cells. In cooperation with CD79A, CD79B activates B cells through the interaction with CD4 T cells. After this interaction, B cells then have the capability to proliferate, secrete antibodies, cytokines, and chemokines, and initiate memory cell formation [58]. CD79B gene expression was decreased in PI thymuses on day 190 compared to controls, but were not downregulated in PI fetal spleens. However, a previous study by our group did find a decrease in CD79B expression in PI fetal spleens [35]. This difference may be due to individual variation of animals in the current study or slight differences in infection/collection timing. A sustained decrease in CD79B expression could result in the depletion of B cells later in gestation or postnatally, contributing to the overall deficit in adaptive immunity, failed viral clearance, and BVDV persistence. The outcome would be apparent immunotolerance to BVDV and the inability of PI animals to combat secondary viral and bacterial infections, such as bovine respiratory disease in postnatal life.

CD46 has been shown to be a receptor for BVDV entry [59,60]. CD46 is a regulator of complement activation through its interaction with plasma serine protease factor I, which cleaves complement factors C3b and C4b to prevent cell injury from complement attack. The concentration of *CD46* was significantly decreased in PI fetal thymuses compared to controls at day 190. The reduced concentration of *CD46* in the PI thymuses may reflect a general diminishment of constitutively expressed cellular mRNAs due to viral mechanisms that usurp cellular transcriptional machinery in favor of the production of viral proteins [61]. Alternatively, expression of the BVDV receptor might be inhibited in response to the binding of BVDV to its receptor and the presence of high viral titers during persistent infection. The downregulation of *CD46* in PI thymuses might also reduce the regulatory activity of CD46 on the complement system and increase the vulnerability of host cells to complement-mediated injury. A soluble form of CD46 which neutralizes BVDV in vitro is present in adult bovine plasma and may play a role in viral clearance in postnatal acute infections. However, soluble CD46 is not found in fetal or neonatal serum, and is therefore unlikely to impact PI fetal BVDV infections [62].

The comparison of TI and PI fetal immune responses in developing lymphoid organs has not been previously examined in experimental settings. Unfortunately, bovine-specific antibodies for the genes of interest are unavailable, and limited this study to RNA expression only. The inability to obtain protein data does limit interpretation. However, the results of this transcriptome study exhibit a drastic difference in immune response competence and maturity between PI and TI fetuses. The upregulation of the innate immune response of TI lymphoid organs, along with the inability of BVDV levels to be significantly different than controls indicate that the TI fetus is effectively fighting the virus, unlike the PI fetus. The timepoint of TI fetal collections may have been too early to capture the activation of the adaptive immune response, or the virus is possibly able to temporarily inhibit the adaptive immune response. It is further hypothesized that although the TI fetuses are able to respond appropriately to the virus, this viral insult during fetal development epigenetically alters the TI animals' DNA and causes further immune-related issues postnatally. This will require further studies postnatally.

5. Conclusions

Although animals infected with BVDV in utero may be born morphologically normal, ncp BVDV fetal infection has significant effects on the expression of innate and adaptive immune responses. In TI animals infected late in gestation, the immune system is developed enough to fight and clear the virus prior to or following parturition. We interpret these RT-qPCR data to reflect an active and upregulated innate immune response in TI thymuses and spleens, seen as an increase in type I IFN transcriptional regulators (Figure 6). In the case of PI fetuses, the virus infects the fetus prior to complete immune system development, ultimately causing drastic attenuation of the immune system, possibly due to the fetus identifying the virus as "self" (Figure 6). Specifically, the downregulation of genes, including type I IFN transcriptional regulators, antigen presentation, and T cell markers in PI fetal tissues was found. These trends in TI and PI fetuses were seen in both the thymic and splenic tissues, suggesting that these changes occur simultaneously in tissues critical for immune system education and development (Figure 6). These types of changes are believed to affect the infected animals postnatally, possibly through epigenetic changes.

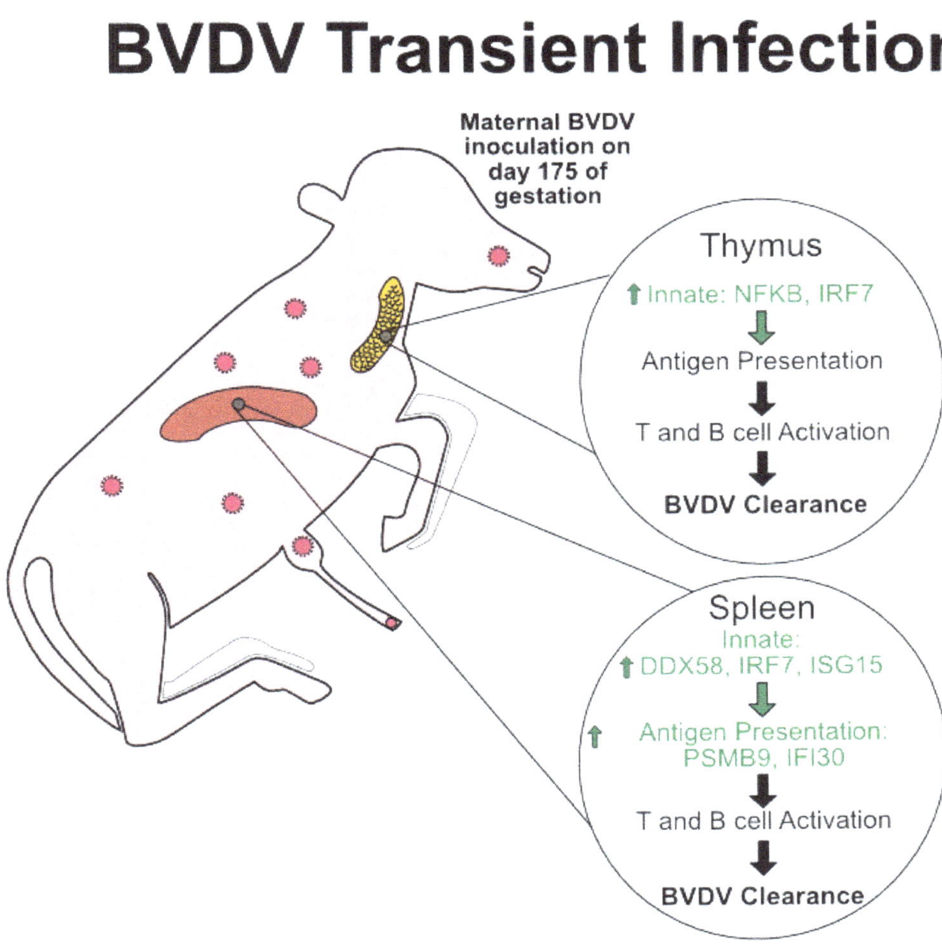

Figure 6. *Cont.*

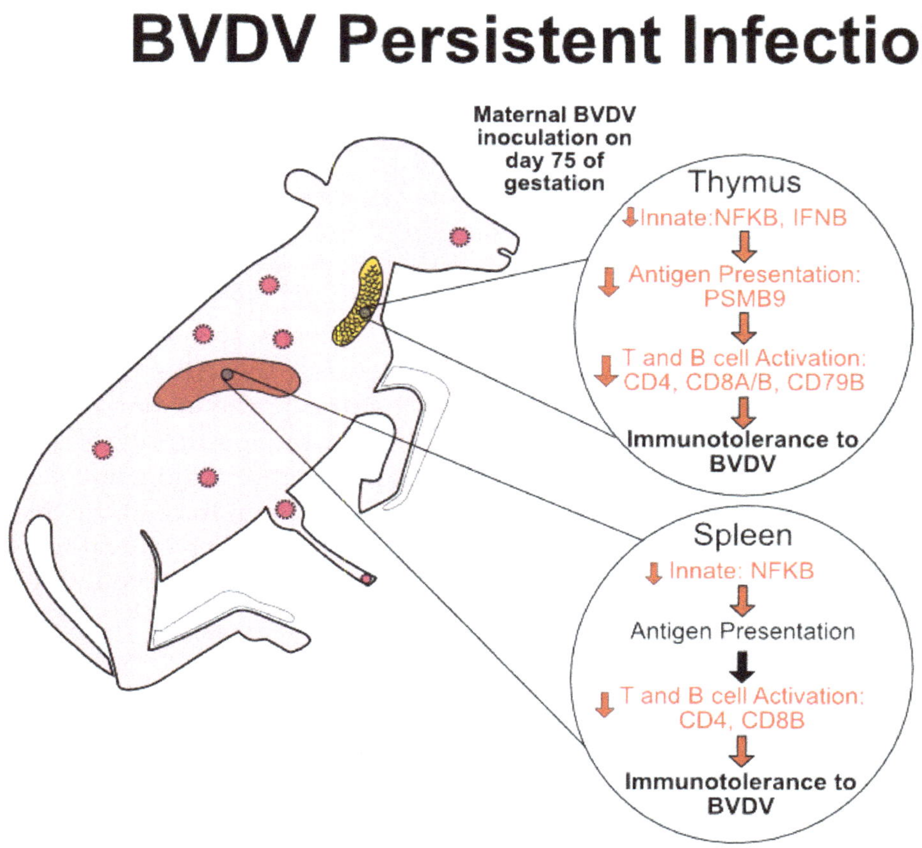

Figure 6. Graphic summarizing significant changes in fetal immune responses based on type of infection and tissue, as interpreted by RT-qPCR analysis. BVDV transient infection represents a fetal infection after gestational day 160 in which the fetus is able to clear the virus. Trends include an upregulation in genes associated with the innate immune response. Day 190 of collections may have been too early to capture an adaptive immune response in TI fetuses. However, we hypothesize that these pathways contribute to BVDV clearance in TI animals. BVDV-persistent infection represents a fetal infection before gestational day 120 in which the fetus is unable to clear the virus. Trends include a drastic down-regulation of the innate and adaptive branches of the immune system, and may lead to immunotolerance of the fetus to BVDV. In future studies, TI BVDV clearance and PI immunotolerance will be studied further with protein targets and flow cytometry. Green text, up arrow left of text, and listed genes represent pathways and genes which were significantly upregulated, as determined by RT-qPCR. Red text, down arrow left of text, and listed genes represent pathways and genes which were significantly downregulated as determined by RT-qPCR.

Author Contributions: Conceptualization, K.J.K. and T.R.H.; methodology, N.P.S., K.J.K.; validation, K.J.K., H.M.G., N.P.S.; formal analysis K.J.K., H.M.G., H.V.C.; investigation, K.J.K., H.M.G., H.V.C., H.B.-O.; resources, J.V.B.; writing—original draft preparation, K.J.K., H.M.G.; writing—review and editing, H.V.C., H.B.-O., T.R.H.; visualization, K.J.K., H.M.G.; supervision, J.V.B., H.B.-O.; project administration, T.R.H.; funding acquisition, T.R.H., H.M.G. All authors have read and agreed to the published version of the manuscript.

Acknowledgments: The authors would like to thank Ann Hess for her assistance with statistical analysis.

Appendix A

Table A1. Table of genes and their expression in respective tissues. These genes were not measured in both tissues, only one tissue.

Tissue	Target	Control Mean	Control SEM	TI Mean	TI SEM	PI Mean	PI SEM	TI v. C *p* value	PI v. C *p* value
Thymus	*STAT1*	1.32	0.48	2.29	0.21	0.04	0.01	0.58	0.07
Thymus	*IFI6*	1.10	0.20	2.09	0.49	0.10	0.02	0.09	0.09
Thymus	*CXCL10*	1.24	0.35	3.10	1.20	0.27	0.12	0.99	0.11
Thymus	*CXCL16*	1.22	0.34	1.21	0.27	0.05	0.01	0.99	0.01
Thymus	*CXCR6*	1.40	0.57	1.64	0.41	0.48	0.15	0.99	0.53
Thymus	*TAP1*	1.09	0.20	1.07	0.21	0.20	0.06	0.99	0.01
Thymus	*B2M*	1.17	0.31	1.33	0.24	0.04	0.01	0.89	0.01
Thymus	*CIITA*	1.19	0.27	1.35	0.35	0.35	0.08	0.99	0.08
Spleen	*STAT4*	1.62	0.83	2.25	0.51	0.32	0.04	0.43	0.08
Spleen	*PSMB8*	1.66	0.79	6.09	1.40	0.06	0.02	0.21	0.07

SEM: Standard Error Mean; TI: Transient Infection; PI: Persistent Infection; C: Control; STAT1: Signal Transducer and Activator of Transcription 1; IFI6: Interferon Alpha Inducible Protein 6; CXCL10: C-X-C Motif Chemokine Ligand 10, CXCL16: C-X-C Motif Chemokine Ligand 16; TAP1: Transporter 1 ATP Binding Cassette Subfamily B Member; B2M: Beta-2-Microglobulin; CIITA: Class II Major Histocompatibility Complex Transactivator; STAT4: Signal Transducer and Activator of Transcription 4; PSMB8: Proteasome 20S Subunit Beta 8.

References

1. Moennig, V.; Houe, H.; Lindberg, A. BVD control in Europe: Current status and perspectives. *Anim. Health Res. Rev.* **2005**, *6*, 63–74. [CrossRef] [PubMed]
2. Larson, R.; Pierce, V.; Grotelueschen, D.; Wittum, T. Economic evaluation of beef cowherd screening for cattle persistently-infected with bovine viral diarrhea virus. *Bov. Pract.* **2002**, *36*, 106–112.
3. Pinior, B.; Firth, C.L.; Richter, V.; Bakran-Lebl, K.; Trauffler, M.; Dzieciol, M.; Hutter, S.E.; Burgstaller, J.; Obritzhauser, W.; Winter, P.; et al. A systematic review of financial and economic assessments of bovine viral diarrhea virus (BVDV) prevention and mitigation activities worldwide. *Prev. Vet. Med.* **2017**, *137*, 77–92. [CrossRef]
4. Richter, V.; Bakran-Lebl, K.; Baumgartner, W.; Obritzhauser, W.; Käsbohrer, A.; Pinior, B. A systematic worldwide review of the direct monetary losses in cattle due to bovine viral diarrhoea virus infection. *Vet. J.* **2017**, *220*, 80–87. [CrossRef]
5. Simmonds, P.; Becher, P.; Bukh, J.; Gould, E.A.; Meyers, G.; Monath, T.; Muerhoff, S.; Pletnev, A.; Rico-Hesse, R.; Smith, D.B.; et al. ICTV Virus Taxonomy Profile: Flaviviridae. *J. Gen. Virol.* **2017**, *98*, 2–3. [CrossRef]
6. Tautz, N.; Tews, B.A.; Meyers, G. The Molecular Biology of Pestiviruses. *Nat. Eng. Resist. Plant Viruses Part II* **2015**, *93*, 47–160. [CrossRef]
7. Bielefeldt-Ohmann, H. The Pathologies of Bovine Viral Diarrhea Virus Infection. *Vet. Clin. N. Am. Food Anim. Pract.* **1995**, *11*, 447–476. [CrossRef]
8. Brownlie, J.; Clarke, M.C.; Howard, C.J.; Pocock, D.H. Pathogenesis and epidemiology of bovine virus diarrhoea virus infection of cattle. *Ann. Rech. Vet. Ann. Vet. Res.* **1987**, *18*, 157–166.
9. Kendrick, J.W. Bovine viral diarrhea-mucosal disease virus infection in pregnant cows. *Am. J. Vet. Res.* **1971**, *32*, 533–544.
10. Lanyon, S.; Hill, F.I.; Reichel, M.P.; Brownlie, J. Bovine viral diarrhoea: Pathogenesis and diagnosis. *Vet. J.* **2014**, *199*, 201–209. [CrossRef] [PubMed]
11. Olafson, P.; Maccallum, A.D.; Fox, F.H. An apparently new transmissible disease of cattle. *Cornell Vet.* **1946**, *36*, 205–213.
12. Coria, M.F.; McClurkin, A.W. Duration of active and colostrum-derived passive antibodies to bovine viral diarrhea virus in calves. *Can. J. Comp. Med. Rev. Can. Med. Comp.* **1978**, *42*, 239–243.
13. McClurkin, A.W.; Littledike, E.T.; Cutlip, R.C.; Frank, G.H.; Coria, M.F.; Bolin, S.R. Production of cattle immunotolerant to bovine viral diarrhea virus. *Can. J. Comp. Med. Rev. Can. Med. Comp.* **1984**, *48*, 156–161.
14. Hansen, T.R.; Smirnova, N.P.; Webb, B.T.; Bielefeldt-Ohmann, H.; Sacco, R.E.; Van Campen, H. Innate and adaptive immune responses to in utero infection with bovine viral diarrhea virus. *Anim. Health Res. Rev.* **2015**, *16*, 15–26. [CrossRef] [PubMed]
15. Brownlie, J.; Clarke, M.; Howard, C. Experimental production of fatal mucosal disease in cattle. *Vet. Rec.* **1984**, *114*, 535–536. [CrossRef]

16. Van Campen, H. Bovine Viral Diarrhea. In Proceedings of the Range Beef Cow Symposium, Rapid City, SD, USA, 9–11 December 1997; University of Nebraska-Lincoln Commons: Rapid City, SD, USA, 1997.
17. Potgieter, L.N. Immunology of Bovine Viral Diarrhea Virus. *Vet. Clin. N. Am. Food Anim. Pract.* **1995**, *11*, 501–520. [CrossRef]
18. Schweizer, M.; Peterhans, E. Pestiviruses. *Annu. Rev. Anim. Biosci.* **2014**, *2*, 141–163. [CrossRef]
19. Peterhans, E.; Schweizer, M. BVDV: A pestivirus inducing tolerance of the innate immune response. *Biology* **2013**, *41*, 39–51. [CrossRef]
20. Baigent, S.J.; Goodbourn, S.; McCauley, J.W. Differential activation of interferon regulatory factors-3 and -7 by non-cytopathogenic and cytopathogenic bovine viral diarrhoea virus. *Vet. Immunol. Immunopathol.* **2004**, *100*, 135–144. [CrossRef]
21. Baigent, S.J.; Zhang, G.; Fray, M.D.; Flick-Smith, H.; Goodbourn, S.; McCauley, J.W. Inhibition of Beta Interferon Transcription by Noncytopathogenic Bovine Viral Diarrhea Virus Is through an Interferon Regulatory Factor 3-Dependent Mechanism. *J. Virol.* **2002**, *76*, 8979–8988. [CrossRef]
22. Chen, Z.; Rijnbrand, R.; Jangra, R.K.; Devaraj, S.G.; Qu, L.; Ma, Y.; Lemon, S.M.; Li, K. Ubiquitination and proteasomal degradation of interferon regulatory factor-3 induced by Npro from a cytopathic bovine viral diarrhea virus. *Virology* **2007**, *366*, 277–292. [CrossRef] [PubMed]
23. Gil, L.H.; Ansari, I.H.; Vassilev, V.; Liang, D.; Lai, V.C.; Zhong, W.; Hong, Z.; Dubovi, E.J.; Donis, R.O. The amino-terminal domain of bovine viral diarrhea virus Npro protein is necessary for alpha/beta interferon antagonism. *J. Virol.* **2006**, *80*, 900–911. [CrossRef] [PubMed]
24. Gil, L.H.V.G.; Van Olphen, A.L.; Mittal, S.K.; Donis, R.O. Modulation of PKR activity in cells infected by bovine viral diarrhea virus. *Virus Res.* **2006**, *116*, 69–77. [CrossRef] [PubMed]
25. Magouras, I.; Mätzener, P.; Rümenapf, T.; Peterhans, E.; Schweizer, M. RNase-dependent inhibition of extracellular, but not intracellular, dsRNA-induced interferon synthesis by Erns of pestiviruses. *J. Gen. Virol.* **2008**, *89*, 2501–2506. [CrossRef]
26. Meyers, G.; Ege, A.; Fetzer, C.; Von Freyburg, M.; Elbers, K.; Carr, V.; Prentice, H.; Charleston, B.; Schürmann, E.-M. Bovine Viral Diarrhea Virus: Prevention of Persistent Fetal Infection by a Combination of Two Mutations Affecting Erns RNase and Npro Protease. *J. Virol.* **2007**, *81*, 3327–3338. [CrossRef]
27. Charleston, B.; Fray, M.D.; Baigent, S.; Carr, B.V.; Morrison, W.I. Establishment of persistent infection with non-cytopathic bovine viral diarrhoea virus in cattle is associated with a failure to induce type I interferon. *J. Gen. Virol.* **2001**, *82*, 1893–1897. [CrossRef]
28. Smirnova, N.P.; Webb, B.T.; Bielefeldt-Ohmann, H.; Van Campen, H.; Antoniazzi, A.Q.; Morarie, S.E.; Hansen, T.R. Development of fetal and placental innate immune responses during establishment of persistent infection with bovine viral diarrhea virus. *Virus Res.* **2012**, *167*, 329–336. [CrossRef]
29. Smirnova, N.P.; Ptitsyn, A.; Austin, K.J.; Bielefeldt-Ohmann, H.; Van Campen, H.; Han, H.; Van Olphen, A.L.; Hansen, T.R. Persistent fetal infection with bovine viral diarrhea virus differentially affects maternal blood cell signal transduction pathways. *Physiol. Genom.* **2008**, *36*, 129–139. [CrossRef]
30. Ohmann, H.B.; Rønsholt, L.; Bloch, B. Demonstration of Bovine Viral Diarrhoea Virus in Peripheral Blood Mononuclear Cells of Persistently Infected, Clinically Normal Cattle. *J. Gen. Virol.* **1987**, *68*, 1971–1982. [CrossRef]
31. Shoemaker, M.L.; Smirnova, N.P.; Bielefeldt-Ohmann, H.; Austin, K.J.; Van Olphen, A.; Clapper, J.A.; Hansen, T.R. Differential Expression of the Type I Interferon Pathway during Persistent and Transient Bovine Viral Diarrhea Virus Infection. *J. Interf. Cytokine Res.* **2009**, *29*, 23–36. [CrossRef]
32. Palomares, R.A.; Walz, H.G.; Brock, K.V. Expression of type I interferon-induced antiviral state and pro-apoptosis markers during experimental infection with low or high virulence bovine viral diarrhea virus in beef calves. *Virus Res.* **2013**, *173*, 260–269. [CrossRef] [PubMed]
33. Charleston, B.; Brackenbury, L.S.; Carr, B.V.; Fray, M.D.; Hope, J.C.; Howard, C.J.; Morrison, W.I. Alpha/Beta and Gamma Interferons are Induced by Infection with Noncytopathic Bovine Viral Diarrhea Virus In Vivo. *J. Virol.* **2002**, *76*, 923–927. [CrossRef] [PubMed]
34. Smirnova, N.P.; Webb, B.; McGill, J.L.; Schaut, R.G.; Bielefeldt-Ohmann, H.; Van Campen, H.; Sacco, R.E.; Hansen, T.R. Induction of interferon-gamma and downstream pathways during establishment of fetal persistent infection with bovine viral diarrhea virus. *Virus Res.* **2014**, *183*, 95–106. [CrossRef] [PubMed]
35. Georges, H.M.; Knapek, K.J.; Bielefeldt-Ohmann, H.; Van Campen, H.; Hansen, T.R. Attenuated lymphocyte activation leads to the development of immunotolerance in bovine fetuses persistently infected with BVDV†. *Biol. Reprod.* **2020**. [CrossRef]

36. Bustin, S.A.; Benes, V.; Garson, J.A.; Hellemans, J.; Huggett, J.F.; Kubista, M.; Mueller, R.; Nolan, T.; Pfaffl, M.W.; Shipley, G.L.; et al. The MIQE Guidelines: Minimum Information for Publication of Quantitative Real-Time PCR Experiments. *Clin. Chem.* **2009**, *55*, 611–622. [CrossRef] [PubMed]
37. Livak, K.J.; Schmittgen, T.D. Analysis of Relative Gene Expression Data Using Real-Time Quantitative PCR and the $2^{-\Delta\Delta CT}$ Method. *Methods* **2001**, *25*, 402–408. [CrossRef]
38. Smirnova, N.P.; Bielefeldt-Ohmann, H.; Van Campen, H.; Austin, K.J.; Han, H.; Montgomery, D.L.; Shoemaker, M.L.; Van Olphen, A.L.; Hansen, T.R. Acute non-cytopathic bovine viral diarrhea virus infection induces pronounced type I interferon response in pregnant cows and fetuses. *Virus Res.* **2008**, *132*, 49–58. [CrossRef]
39. Goddeeris, B.M.; Morrison, W.I. *Cell-Mediated Immunity in Ruminants*; CRC Press: Boca Raton, FL, USA, 1994.
40. Schultz, R.D.; Dunne, H.W.; Heist, C.E. Ontogeny of the Bovine Immune Response 1. *Infect. Immun.* **1973**, *7*, 981–991. [CrossRef]
41. Haynes, B.F. The Human Thymic Microenvironment. *Adv. Immunol.* **1984**, *36*, 87–142. [CrossRef]
42. Lobach, D.F.; Haynes, B.F. Ontogeny of the human thymus during fetal development. *J. Clin. Immunol.* **1987**, *7*, 81–97. [CrossRef]
43. Ohmann, H.B. Experimental fetal infection with bovine viral diarrhea virus. II. Morphological reactions and distribution of viral antigen. *Can. J. Comp. Med. Rev. Can. Med. Comp.* **1982**, *46*, 363–369.
44. Done, J.; Terlecki, S.; Richardson, C.; Harkness, J.; Sands, J.; Patterson, D.; Sweasey, D.; Shaw, I.; Winkler, C.; Duffell, S. Bovine virus diarrhoea-mucosal disease virus: Pathogenicity for the fetal calf following maternal infection. *Vet. Rec.* **1980**, *106*, 473–479. [CrossRef]
45. Falkenberg, S.M.; Bauermann, F.V.; Ridpath, J.F. Characterization of thymus-associated lymphoid depletion in bovine calves acutely or persistently infected with bovine viral diarrhea virus 1, bovine viral diarrhea virus 2 or HoBi-like pestivirus. *Arch. Virol.* **2017**, *162*, 3473–3480. [CrossRef] [PubMed]
46. Golub, R.; Tan, J.; Watanabe, T.; Brendolan, A. Origin and Immunological Functions of Spleen Stromal Cells. *Trends Immunol.* **2018**, *39*, 503–514. [CrossRef] [PubMed]
47. Ellis, J.A.; Davis, W.C.; Belden, E.L.; Pratt, D.L. Flow Cytofluorimetric Analysis of Lymphocyte Subset Alterations in Cattle Infected with Bovine Viral Diarrhea Virus. *Vet. Pathol.* **1988**, *25*, 231–236. [CrossRef] [PubMed]
48. Bolin, S.R.; McClurkin, A.W.; Coria, M.F. Effects of bovine viral diarrhea virus on the percentages and absolute num- bers of circulating B and T lymphocytes in cattle. *Am. J. Vet. Res.* **1988**, *46*, 884–886.
49. Burt, T.D. Fetal regulatory T cells and peripheral immune tolerance in utero: Implications for development and disease. *Am. J. Reprod. Immunol.* **2013**, *69*, 346–358. [CrossRef]
50. Mold, J.E.; Venkatasubrahmanyam, S.; Burt, T.D.; Michaëlsson, J.; Rivera, J.M.; Galkina, S.A.; Weinberg, K.; Stoddart, C.A.; McCune, J.M. Fetal and Adult Hematopoietic Stem Cells Give Rise to Distinct T Cell Lineages in Humans. *Science* **2010**, *330*, 1695–1699. [CrossRef]
51. Collen, T.; Douglas, A.J.; Paton, D.J.; Zhang, G.; Morrison, W. Single Amino Acid Differences are Sufficient for CD4+ T-Cell Recognition of a Heterologous Virus by Cattle Persistently Infected with Bovine Viral Diarrhea Virus. *Virology* **2000**, *276*, 70–82. [CrossRef]
52. Zhu, M.; Fu, Y. The complicated role of NF-kappaB in T-cell selection. *Cell Mol. Immunol.* **2010**, *7*, 89–93. [CrossRef]
53. Leonidas, C.P. Mechanisms of type-I- and type-II-interferon-mediated signalling. *Nat. Rev. Immunol.* **2005**, *5*, 375–386.
54. Thompson, M.R.; Sharma, S.; Atianand, M.; Jensen, S.B.; Carpenter, S.; Knipe, D.M.; Fitzgerald, K.A.; Kurt-Jones, E.A. Interferon γ-inducible Protein (IFI) 16 Transcriptionally Regulates Type I Interferons and Other Interferon-stimulated Genes and Controls the Interferon Response to both DNA and RNA Viruses*. *J. Biol. Chem.* **2014**, *289*, 23568–23581. [CrossRef] [PubMed]
55. Harwig, A.; Landick, R.; Berkhout, B. The Battle of RNA Synthesis: Virus versus Host. *Viruses* **2017**, *9*, 309. [CrossRef] [PubMed]
56. Benedictus, L.; Luteijn, R.D.; Otten, H.; Lebbink, R.J.; Van Kooten, P.J.S.; Wiertz, E.J.H.J.; Rutten, V.P.M.G.; Koets, A. Pathogenicity of Bovine Neonatal Pancytopenia-associated vaccine-induced alloantibodies correlates with Major Histocompatibility Complex class I expression. *Sci. Rep.* **2015**, *5*, 12748. [CrossRef]
57. Cyster, J.G. Chemokines and Cell Migration in Secondary Lymphoid Organs. *Science* **1999**, *286*, 2098–2102. [CrossRef] [PubMed]

58. Bishop, G.A.; Haxhinasto, S.A.; Stunz, L.L.; Hostager, B.S. Antigen-specific B-lymphocyte activation. *Crit. Rev. Immunol.* **2003**, *23*, 149–197. [CrossRef]
59. Maurer, K.; Krey, T.; Moennig, V.; Thiel, H.-J.; Rümenapf, T. CD46 Is a Cellular Receptor for Bovine Viral Diarrhea Virus. *J. Virol.* **2004**, *78*, 1792–1799. [CrossRef]
60. Krey, T.; Himmelreich, A.; Heimann, M.; Menge, C.; Thiel, H.-J.; Maurer, K.; Rümenapf, T. Function of Bovine CD46 as a Cellular Receptor for Bovine Viral Diarrhea Virus Is Determined by Complement Control Protein 1. *J. Virol.* **2006**, *80*, 3912–3922. [CrossRef]
61. Neill, J.D.; Ridpath, J.F. Gene expression changes in BVDV2-infected MDBK cells. *Biology* **2003**, *31*, 97–102. [CrossRef]
62. Alzamel, N.; Bayrou, C.; Decreux, A.; Desmecht, D. Soluble forms of CD46 are detected in Bos taurus plasma and neutralize BVDV, the bovine pestivirus. *Comp. Immunol. Microbiol. Infect. Dis.* **2016**, *49*, 39–46. [CrossRef]

Mycoplasma bovis in Spanish Cattle Herds: Two Groups of Multiresistant Isolates Predominate with One Remaining Susceptible to Fluoroquinolones

Ana García-Galán [1], Laurent-Xavier Nouvel [2], Eric Baranowski [2], Ángel Gómez-Martín [1,3], Antonio Sánchez [1], Christine Citti [2] and Christian de la Fe [1,*]

1 Ruminant Health Research Group, Department of Animal Health, Faculty of Veterinary Sciences, Regional Campus of International Excellence "*Campus Mare Nostrum*", University of Murcia, 30100 Murcia, Spain; ana.garcia25@um.es (A.G.-G.); angel.gomezmartin@uchceu.es (A.G.-M.); asanlope@um.es (A.S.)

2 IHAP, ENVT, INRAE, Université de Toulouse, 31300 Toulouse, France; xavier.nouvel@envt.fr (L.-X.N.); eric.baranowski@envt.fr (E.B.); christine.citti@envt.fr (C.C.)

3 Microbiological Agents associated with Reproduction (*ProVaginBio*) Research Group, Department of Animal Health and Public Health, Faculty of Veterinary Sciences, University CEU Cardenal Herrera of Valencia, CEU Universities, 46113 Valencia, Spain

* Correspondence: cdelafe@um.es;

Abstract: *Mycoplasma bovis* is an important bovine pathogen causing pneumonia, mastitis, and arthritis and is responsible for major economic losses worldwide. In the absence of an efficient vaccine, control of *M. bovis* infections mainly relies on antimicrobial treatments, but resistance is reported in an increasing number of countries. To address the situation in Spain, *M. bovis* was searched in 436 samples collected from beef and dairy cattle (2016–2019) and 28% were positive. Single-locus typing using *polC* sequences further revealed that two subtypes ST2 and ST3, circulate in Spain both in beef and dairy cattle, regardless of the regions or the clinical signs. Monitoring of ST2 and ST3 isolates minimum inhibitory concentration (MIC) to a panel of antimicrobials revealed one major difference when using fluoroquinolones (FQL): ST2 is more susceptible than ST3. Accordingly, whole-genome sequencing (WGS) further identified mutations in the *gyrA* and *parC* regions, encoding quinolone resistance-determining regions (QRDR) only in ST3 isolates. This situation shows the capacity of ST3 to accumulate mutations in QRDR and might reflect the selective pressure imposed by the extensive use of these antimicrobials. MIC values and detection of mutations by WGS also showed that most Spanish isolates are resistant to macrolides, lincosamides, and tetracyclines. Valnemulin was the only one effective, at least in vitro, against both STs.

Keywords: *Mycoplasma bovis*; minimum inhibitory concentration; antimicrobial resistance; mutations; Spain

---

1. Introduction

Isolated in the early 60s, *Mycoplasma bovis* is an important bovine pathogen that has a major economic impact on the global cattle industry [1,2]. *M. bovis* is usually associated with a variety of clinical manifestations, including pneumonia, mastitis, arthritis, keratoconjunctivitis, otitis media, and genital disorders [2,3]. In the absence of an efficient vaccine, the control of *M. bovis* infections mainly relies on antimicrobial treatments [4]. However, many countries have reported that the in vitro antimicrobial sensitivity of *M. bovis* isolates has been dramatically reduced [5–14].

M. bovis belongs to the class *Mollicutes*, a large group of wall-less bacteria with reduced genome and limited metabolic capacities, but a remarkable adaptive potential [15,16]. Treatment with ß-lactams, glycopeptides, cycloserines, or fosfomycin is ineffective against *Mollicutes* infections since they all target cell-wall synthesis [17,18]. Similarly, polymyxins and sulfonamides/trimethoprim, whose primary targets are respectively membrane lipopolysaccharides and folic acid, are not effective against these organisms [17,18]. Finally, *Mollicutes* are also resistant to rifampicin due to a natural mutation in the *rpoB* gene of the RNA polymerase β subunit, which prevents the antibiotic from binding to its target [19–21]. Antimicrobials active against *Mycoplasmas* include macrolides, lincosamides, tetracyclines, amphenicols, and pleuromutilins, which are all interfering with the synthesis of proteins, and fluoroquinolones (FLQ), which are DNA synthesis inhibitors [22].

General guidelines for antimicrobial testing of veterinary mycoplasmas are available, although no standard or interpretative breakpoint has been formally published [23]. Hence, current minimum inhibitory concentration (MIC) data are supported by molecular evidence of genetic mutations associated with antimicrobial resistance [22,24]. Hot spot mutations in 16S rRNA genes, *rrs3* and *rrs4*, are related to resistance against tetracyclines, while those in 23S rRNA genes, *rrl3* and *rrl4*, are associated with resistance to macrolides, lincosamides, phenicols, and pleuromutilins. Mutations in *rplD* and *rplV* genes encoding ribosomal proteins L4 and L22 and *rplC* gene encoding L3 are also linked to resistance against macrolides and pleuromutilins, respectively. Finally, FLQ resistance is mainly associated with mutations in the quinolone resistance-determining regions (QRDR) of *gyrA* and *gyrB* genes encoding DNA-gyrase, and in *parC* and *parE* genes encoding topoisomerase IV [22,24].

In Europe, *M. bovis* is particularly damaging to the beef industry due to its contribution towards the bovine respiratory disease complex (BRD) that affects calves raised in feedlots [25–27]. This pathogen often acts in co-infection with other viruses and bacteria, although it is the only etiological agent found in the chronic forms of the disease [28]. Regarding the dairy industry, sporadic *M. bovis* outbreaks have been notified in Austria, Denmark, Switzerland, and The Netherlands. Based on field data from the analysis of bulk tank milk, the prevalence of the infection in France and the UK is less than 1%, and that in Belgium and Greece it is 1.5% and 5.4%, respectively [29–36].

The beef and dairy industry is crucial to Spain, yet little is known about the epidemiological situation of *M. bovis* infections in this country. The antimicrobial susceptibility of *M. bovis* isolates was recently monitored in different European countries, including Spain [37,38]. However, these studies only considered isolates collected from young animals with respiratory disease and did not provide complete, epidemiological background information regarding the isolates.

The spread of *M. bovis* infection in animals, herds, regions, or countries is usually associated with animal movements and the introduction of asymptomatic carriers, which are occasionally shedding the pathogen in milk, nasal, or genital secretions [2,3]. Animal exchanges between farms are common in the Spanish beef industry, which also imports a large number of animals from other European countries, with France being the main supplier, followed by Ireland and Germany [39]. Animal movements between dairy farms are less common since the replacement of dairy cows is usually performed with animals born in the same herd. Nevertheless, when the replacement rate is not sufficient to maintain milk production levels, external animals may be introduced to the herd, especially in larger farms. Interestingly, a study showed that infected semen was also at the origin of *M. bovis* mastitis outbreaks in two closed dairy herds in Finland [40].

Recently, a large molecular study, including *M. bovis* strains isolated in France from 1977 to 2012, revealed that two groups emerged after 2000 [41]. Based on their partial *polC* sequences, these corresponded to subtypes (STs) 2 and 3. Another study further observed a difference between the two STs in their ability to acquire FLQ resistance in vitro. While ST3 isolates are more likely to acquire mutations in their QRDR and become resistant under selective pressure, the genetic context of ST2 isolates appears to hinder the development of resistance [42]. Field isolates from both STs were found to be resistant to the macrolides tylosin and tilmicosin and the tetracycline, oxytetracycline, regardless of the associated clinical signs (respiratory disease, mastitis, otitis, or arthritis) [43]. Interestingly, the first multiresistant ST3 isolate reported in France was collected in 2011 from a calf born in Spain and raised in a veal-calf herd in Southwest France [41]. This raised the question of how the two STs were distributed in Spanish herds when considering a large number of field isolates, and whether their antimicrobial susceptibility profiles were congruent with *polC* typing. Spain, which allowed unrestricted use of FLQ until very recently, may serve as a clear in vivo model to study the effects of the indiscriminate use of these antimicrobials.

The present study objectives were (i) to assess the circulation of *M. bovis* in Spanish cattle herds using a large collection of isolates collected from beef and dairy cattle and from different sample sources (nasal, auricular, conjunctival, synovial fluid and tissues swabs, and mastitic milk); (ii) to subtype this collection by single-locus sequencing of *polC* [41]; (iii) to determine the antimicrobial susceptibility of *M. bovis* isolates studying differences between STs, with a focus on antimicrobial agents approved to treat bovine respiratory disease and/or mastitis in Spain; and (iv) to assess the occurrence of genetic mutations conferring antimicrobial resistance in a selection of isolates representative of each ST.

2. Results

2.1. *M. bovis Circulating in Spanish Beef and Dairy Herds Belongs to STs 2 and 3*

In this study, 93 (35.7%) of the 260 analyzed animals were infected with *M. bovis*. Among the 436 analyzed samples, a total of 165 tested positive for *Mycoplasma* spp. and *M. bovis* was the most commonly found species, with 122 PCR-positive samples.

Among beef cattle, *M. bovis* was detected in 84 (40.9%) of the 205 analyzed animals. Specifically, the pathogen was detected in 81 (44.3%) of the 183 feedlots calves and 3 (13.6%) of the 22 pasture-raised animals. The pathogen was detected in 40 (32%) of the 125 healthy animals and 44 (55%) of the 80 animals with clinical signs of respiratory disease or arthritis. Within the 331 analyzed samples, 102 were tested positive. Most positive samples were obtained from nasal swabs (85/278) and the remaining were identified in auricular swabs (5/27) and tissues swabs from lung (9/16), spleen (1/1), liver (1/2), and mediastinal lymph nodes (1/1). However, the pathogen was not found in conjunctival swabs (n = 3) nor synovial fluid (n = 3). The positive samples were obtained from 26 of the 30 analyzed farms and 5 of the 8 analyzed regions (Figure S1). Among dairy cattle, *M. bovis* was detected in 9 (16.36%) of the 55 analyzed animals. Specifically, the pathogen was detected in 9 (23.1%) of the 39 dairy cows with mastitis but was not detected in any of the 5 dairy calves with clinical signs of respiratory disease nor any of the 11 asymptomatic calves. Within the 105 analyzed samples, positive samples were only detected in mastitic milk (20/66), while any positive results were detected in BTM (n = 9), or nasal (n = 27), auricular (n = 1), or conjunctival (n = 2) swabs. The positive samples were obtained from 2 of the 7 farms and the milk analysis laboratory, and 3 of the 5 analyzed regions (Figure S1).

Globally, *M. bovis* was successfully isolated from 112 PCR-positive samples. Based on their origin, 95 representative isolates were chosen for further characterization (epidemiological background provided in Table S1 and illustrated in Figure 1). Briefly, the collection included isolates from beef (n = 75) and dairy cattle (n = 20). Beef cattle isolates were obtained from nasal (62/75), auricular (6/75), lung (6/75) and spleen swabs (1/75), asymptomatic (35/75) or with clinical signs of respiratory disease (33/75), arthritis (6/75), or both (1/75). Dairy cattle isolates were obtained from mastitic milk. Single-locus sequence analysis of *polC* revealed two ST profiles: ST2 (n = 37) and ST3 (n = 58). Both STs were found in beef and dairy cattle, in healthy or diseased animals and in different sample sources. Both STs were found concomitantly in animals from the same farm, or even in different samples from the same animal (Figure 1, Table S1). For example, isolates J96 and J102 (ST3) and J103 (ST2) were collected from spleen, nasal, and lung swabs of the same animal respectively (Table S1). Sequences corresponding to ST2 and ST3 are provided in Table S2.

Hence, no other STs than ST2 or ST3 were found in Spanish herds. Both STs were present in asymptomatic beef cattle or with clinical signs of respiratory disease or arthritis and in dairy cows with mastitis.

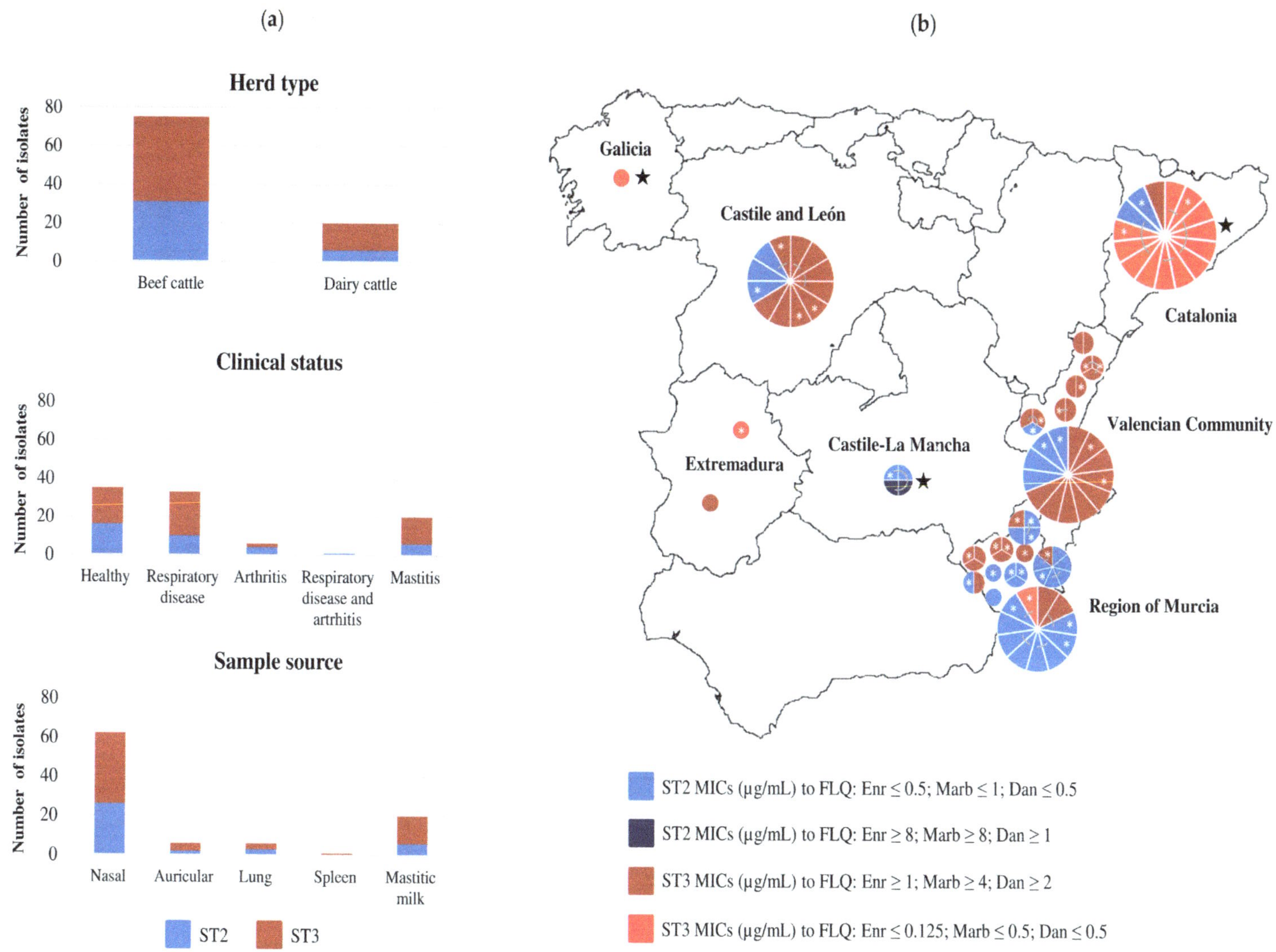

Figure 1. Epidemiological background of the 95 *Mycoplasma bovis* isolates included in this study: (**a**) Number of isolates of each subtype (ST) depending on the herd type, clinical status, and sample source; (**b**) Geographical origin of each isolate. Each circle represents a farm except in Catalonia, where a milk analysis laboratory provided samples. The radius of each circle is proportional to the number of isolates collected from the farm. Isolates collected from mastitic milk are indicated with a black star. Isolates linked with a grey line were obtained from the same animal. Isolates selected for whole-genome sequencing are indicated with a white asterisk. Enr = Enrofloxacin; Marb = Marbofloxacin; Dan = Danofloxacin.

2.2. The Antimicrobial Susceptibility Profiles of The Spanish Isolates to FLQ Differ Between PolC ST2 and ST3

The MIC values for the reference strain PG45 are shown in Table 1. Individual MIC values for each isolate are listed in Table S1. Statistical analyses revealed a significant difference in antimicrobial susceptibility to FLQ between ST2 and ST3 isolates ($p < 0.01$). No significant changes between STs were observed for macrolides, lincomycin, doxycycline, or valnemulin. The antimicrobial susceptibility profile of these two STs is illustrated in Table 1, Figures 1 and 2.

MIC values indicated a global decrease of *M. bovis* susceptibility to macrolides and lincomycin (MIC_{90} > 128), and to a lesser extent, doxycycline (MIC_{90} = 4 µg/mL). The majority of ST2 isolates (35/37) had low MIC values for FLQ (≤0.5 µg/mL for enrofloxacin and danofloxacin, and ≤ 1 µg/mL for marbofloxacin) (Figure 1, Table S1). Among the few exceptions were the isolates J320 and J323, obtained from mastitic milk of the same cow. The MIC of J320 was 16 µg/mL for enrofloxacin and marbofloxacin, and 1 µg/mL for danofloxacin and the MIC of J323 was 8 µg/mL for enrofloxacin and marbofloxacin, and 2 µg/mL for danofloxacin (Table S1). Interestingly, 4 ST2 isolates with different MIC profiles were obtained from the cranial quarters of that cow in different days: the isolates J319 (low MIC, left side) and J320 (high MIC, right side) one day, and the isolates J323 (high MIC, left side) and J324 (low MIC, right side) two days later (Figure 1, Table S1). On the contrary, most ST3 (43/58) isolates had high MIC values for FLQ (≥1, ≥4, and ≥2 µg/mL for enrofloxacin, marbofloxacin, and danofloxacin respectively). The remaining ST3 isolates (15/58) were collected from dairy cows with mastitis (13/15) and a few (2/15) from beef cattle with arthritis or asymptomatic (MIC ≤ 0.125 µg/mL for enrofloxacin, and ≤0.5 µg/mL for marbofloxacin and danofloxacin (Figure 1, Table S1). Finally, valnemulin was the only molecule that demonstrated activity against both STs.

Therefore, most of the *M. bovis* Spanish field isolates have a similar antimicrobial susceptibility profile against macrolides, lincomycin, and doxycycline with high MIC values and for valnemulin with low MIC values. On the contrary, antimicrobial susceptibility profiles against FLQ differed between ST2 and ST3, with high MIC values mainly associated with ST3 (Table 1).

Table 1. Minimum inhibitory concentration (MIC) ranges, MIC_{50} and MIC_{90} of *Mycoplasma bovis* isolates.

polC [a] ST	MIC Parameter	Macrolides			Lincosamide	Fluoroquinolones			Tetracycline	Pleuromutilin
		Tul	Gam	Tild	Lin	Enr	Marb	Dan	Dox	Val
1 PG45	MIC	1	8	1	1	0.125	0.5	0.125	0.0625	0.025
2 (n = 37)	MIC Range	16–>128	>128	>128	1–>128	0.125–16	0.25–16	0.125–2	0.25–4	0.025–0.2
	MIC_{50}	>128	>128	>128	>128	0.25	0.5	0.25	2	0.1
	MIC_{90}	>128	>128	>128	>128	0.5	1	0.5	4	0.1
3 (n = 58)	MIC Range	8–>128	>128	>128	1–>128	<0.0625–32	0.125–64	0.125–8	0.5–8	0.025–0.2
	MIC_{50}	>128	>128	>128	>128	16	32	4	2	0.1
	MIC_{90}	>128	>128	>128	>128	32	64	8	4	0.2

MIC values are given in µg/mL. Values are presented separately for each subtype (ST). The reference strain PG45 was used as control. Tul = Tulathromycin; Gam = Gamithromycin; Tild = Tildipirosin; Lin = Lincomycin; Enr = Enrofloxacin; Marb = Marbofloxacin; Dan = Danofloxacin; Dox = Doxycycline; Val = Valnemulin. [a] ST based on the single-locus sequence analysis of a region of the gene *polC* [41].

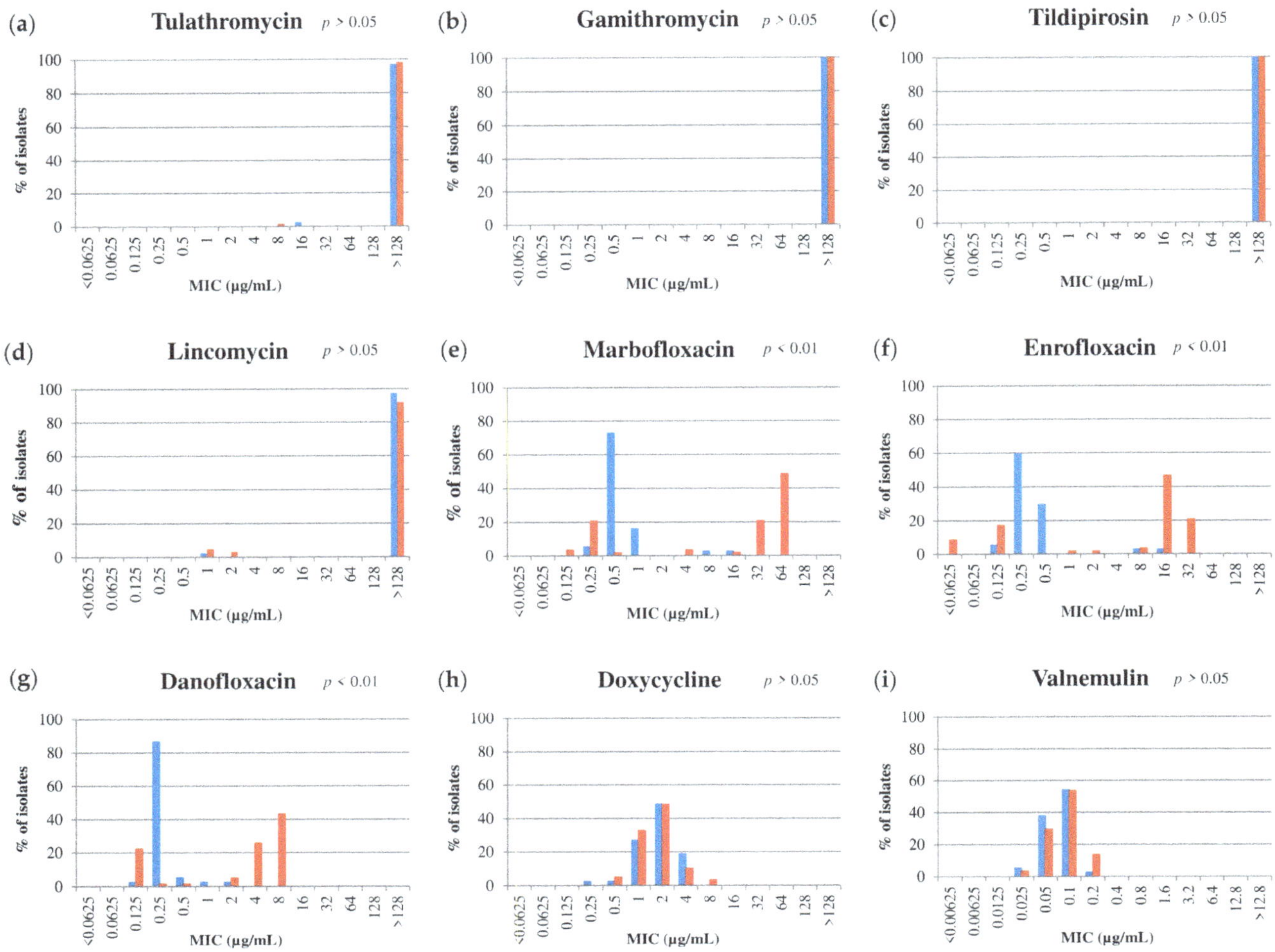

Figure 2. Minimum inhibitory concentration (MIC) distribution (%) of the 95 *Mycoplasma bovis* isolates for each antimicrobial included in this study: (**a**) Tulathromycin; (**b**) Gamithromycin; (**c**) Tildipirosin; (**d**) Lincomycin; (**e**) Marbofloxacin; (**f**) Enrofloxacin; (**g**) Danofloxacin; (**h**) Doxycycline; (**i**) Valnemulin. Blue bars correspond to subtype (ST) 2 and red bars to ST3. *P* values were obtained by comparing the log2MIC means between STs.

2.3. Analysis of Point Mutations Conferring Resistance to Antimicrobials: The Main Differences between ST2 and ST3 Are Found in The QRDR of GyrA and ParC Genes

A total of 36 *M. bovis* isolates belonging to ST2 (n = 16) and ST3 (n = 20) were subjected to whole-genome sequencing to compare nucleotide changes at QRDR, and rRNA (16S and 23S) and protein (L3, L4, and L22) genes (Tables 2–4). The epidemiological background of these isolates is provided in Table S1 and illustrated in Figure 1.

Nucleotide changes at QRDR revealed important differences between each ST, mainly located in *gyrA* and *parC*. While sequence analysis did not reveal any non-synonymous mutations in *gyrA* or *parC* for ST2 isolates, ST3 isolates were all characterized by at least one non-synonymous mutation in one or both genes. ST3 isolates were all characterized by a *parC* non-synonymous mutation at codon 10 (Gln10Arg). This mutation was associated with a substitution from serine to phenylalanine at *gyrA* codon 83 (Ser83Phe) and serine to isoleucine at *parC* codon 80 (Ser80Ile) in isolates with MIC values ≥ 1 µg/mL for FLQ. Among the few exceptions were the isolates J28, J228, and J279 having no mutation at *parC* codon 80, but a non-synonymous mutation at codon 116 (Ala116Pro in J228 and J279) or codons 81 and 84 (Ser81Pro; Asp84Asn in J28). Interestingly, while most of the ST2 and ST3 isolates showed a *gyrB* non-synonymous mutation associated with a substitution Asp362Asn, ST3 isolates J479, and J482 (MIC values ≥ 8 µg/mL for FLQ) were characterized by a substitution at *gyrB* codon 323

(Val323Ala) in combination with mutations Ser83Phe in *gyrA*, and Gln10Arg, Ser80Ile, and Val156Ile in *parC*.

Table 2. List of point mutations in the *gyrA*, *gyrB*, and *parC* quinolone resistance-determining regions (QRDR) identified in *Mycoplasma bovis* isolates and associated minimum inhibitory concentration (MIC) values for fluoroquinolones (FLQ).

Isolate	*polC* [a] ST	*gyrA*	*gyrB*		*parC*						MIC (µg/mL) [b]		
		83 [c]	362	323	10	80 [c]	81 [c]	84 [c]	116	156	Enr	Marb	Dan
PG45	1	Ser	Asp	Val	Gln	Ser	Ser	Asp	Ala	Val	0.125	0.5	0.125
J335	3	-	Asn	-	Arg	-	-	-	-	-	<0.0625	0.25	0.125
J403	3	-	Asn	-	Arg	-	-	-	-	-	<0.0625	0.25	0.125
J414	3	-	Asn	-	Arg	-	-	-	-	-	<0.0625	0.25	0.125
J433	3	-	Asn	-	Arg	-	-	-	-	-	0.125	0.25	0.125
J341	2	-	Asn	-	-	-	-	-	-	-	0.125	0.25	0.25
J6	2	-	Asn	-	-	-	-	-	-	-	0.25	0.5	0.25
J103	2	-	Asn	-	-	-	-	-	-	-	0.25	0.5	0.25
J175	2	-	Asn	-	-	-	-	-	-	-	0.25	0.5	0.25
J226	2	-	Asn	-	-	-	-	-	-	-	0.25	0.5	0.25
J276	2	-	Asn	-	-	-	-	-	-	-	0.25	0.5	0.25
J319	2	-	Asn	-	-	-	-	-	-	-	0.25	0.5	0.25
J330	2	-	Asn	-	-	-	-	-	-	-	0.25	0.5	0.25
J336	2	-	Asn	-	-	-	-	-	-	-	0.25	0.5	0.5
J356	2	-	Asn	-	-	-	-	-	-	-	0.25	0.5	0.25
J136	2	-	Asn	-	-	-	-	-	-	-	0.5	1	0.25
J137	2	-	Asn	-	-	-	-	-	-	-	0.5	0.5	0.125
J368	2	-	Asn	-	-	-	-	-	-	-	0.5	1	0.25
J377	2	-	Asn	-	-	-	-	-	-	-	0.5	1	0.25
J391	2	-	Asn	-	-	-	-	-	-	-	0.5	0.5	0.25
J410	2	-	Asn	-	-	-	-	-	-	-	0.5	0.5	0.25
J279	3	Phe	Asn	-	Arg	-	-	-	Pro	-	1	4	4
J228	3	Phe	Asn	-	Arg	-	-	-	Pro	-	2	4	2
J115	3	Phe	Asn	-	Arg	Ile	-	-	-	-	8	32	2
J28	3	Phe	Asn	-	Arg	-	Pro	Asn	-	-	16	64	8
J69	3	Phe	Asn	-	Arg	Ile	-	-	-	-	16	32	4
J72	3	Phe	Asn	-	Arg	Ile	-	-	-	-	16	64	8
J81	3	Phe	Asn	-	Arg	Ile	-	-	-	-	16	32	4
J96	3	Phe	Asn	-	Arg	Ile	-	-	-	-	16	32	4
J131	3	Phe	Asn	-	Arg	Ile	-	-	-	-	16	64	8
J305	3	Phe	Asn	-	Arg	Ile	-	-	-	-	16	64	8
J178	3	Phe	Asn	-	Arg	Ile	-	-	-	-	32	64	8
J233	3	Phe	Asn	-	Arg	Ile	-	-	-	-	32	64	8
J295	3	Phe	Asn	-	Arg	Ile	-	-	-	-	32	64	8
J388	3	Phe	Asn	-	Arg	Ile	-	-	-	-	32	64	8
J479	3	Phe	-	Ala	Arg	Ile	-	-	-	Ile	32	64	8
J482	3	Phe	-	Ala	Arg	Ile	-	-	-	Ile	32	64	8

Amino acid numbering refers to positions in *Escherichia coli* K12. [a] Subtype (ST) based on the single-locus sequence analysis of a region of the gene *polC* [41]. [b] Enr = Enrofloxacin; Marb = Marbofloxacin; Dan = Danofloxacin. [c] Mutations associated with FLQ resistance in previous studies [42,44–48].

Mutations in the 23S rRNA and 16S rRNA genes and the ribosomal proteins L3, L4, and L22 are listed in Table 3; Table 4. Regarding 23S rRNA, positions A534T, G748A were notably altered in both *rrl* alleles of all the isolates. Mutation A2058G affecting the majority of isolates (34/36) in one or both alleles was only absent in those with low MIC values for lincomycin (1 µg/mL). Mutations G954A in one or both alleles were altered in 31/36 isolates from both STs and the remaining five isolates had many compensatory non-synonymous mutations in L3, L4, and L22 proteins. Mutation T1249C in one allele was altered in 31/36 isolates from both STs. Mutations A1251T (1/36) and G2157A (5/36) in one allele and G2848T (2/36) in one allele were only found in ST3 isolates while G452A was present in one allele of a few number (5/36) of ST3 isolates. Some isolates from both STs (6/36) showed a single non-synonymous mutation in L4 or L22 (Table 3). Regarding 16S rRNA, mutations A965T and A967T were altered in both *rrs* alleles of all the isolates (MIC ≥ 1 μg/mL for doxycycline). Mutations C1192A in both alleles and T1199C in one or both alleles were altered in 31/36 isolates from both STs. Mutations C335T and C859T were present in one *rrs* allele of five isolates (from both STs) and one isolate (ST2) respectively (Table 4).

Hence, the main differences between ST2 and ST3 are found in the QRDR of *gyrA* and *parC* genes. None of the ST2 isolates have any amino acid substitution in either *gyrA* or *parC* while ST3 isolates with MIC values ≥ 1 μg/mL for FLQ have the mutation Ser83Phe in *gyrA* in combination with at least non-synonymous mutation in *parC* (positions 80, 81, 84, 116, and156).

Table 3. List of point mutations in 23S rRNA alleles of *Mycoplasma bovis* isolates and associated minimum inhibitory concentration (MIC) values for macrolides, lincomycin, and valnemulin.

Isolate	*polC* [a] ST	23S rRNA, *rrl* alleles [b]									L3 [c]	L4 [c]												L22 [c]		MIC (µg/mL) [d]				
		452	534	748 [e]	954	1249	1251	2058 [e,f]	2157	2848	265	11	24	36	44	62	63	68	79	94	178	178	178	5	93 [e]	Tul	Gam	Tild	Lin	Val
PG45	1	G	A	G	G	T	A	A	G	G	Ala	Ser	Thr	Thr	Ala	Val	Ala	Glu	Ala	Ala	Gly	Gly	Gly	Gln	Gln	1	8	1	1	0.025
J137	2	-	T **	A **	-	C *	-	-	-	-	Val	Thr	-	Ala	Thr	Ala	Thr	Ala	Thr	Thr	-	-	Val	-	His	16	>128	>128	1	0.1
J28	3	-	T **	A **	-	C *	-	-	-	-	Val	Thr	-	Ala	Thr	Ala	Thr	Ala	Thr	Thr	-	Leu	-	-	His	>128	>128	>128	1	0.05
J403	3	-	T **	A **	-	C *	-	G *	-	-	Val	Thr	-	-	Thr	Ala	Thr	Ala	Thr	Thr	Arg	-	-	-	His	>128	>128	>128	>128	0.1
J414	3	-	T **	A **	-	C *	-	G *	-	-	Val	Thr	-	Ala	Thr	Ala	Thr	Ala	Thr	Thr	Arg	-	-	-	His	>128	>128	>128	>128	0.1
J433	3	-	T **	A **	-	C *	-	G *	-	-	Val	Thr	-	Ala	Thr	Ala	Thr	Ala	Thr	Thr	Arg	-	-	-	His	>128	>128	>128	>128	0.1
J6	2	-	T **	A **	A *	C *	-	G **	-	-	-	-	-	-	-	-	-	-	-	-	-	-	-	-	-	>128	>128	>128	>128	0.1
J103	2	-	T **	A **	A *	C *	-	G **	-	-	-	-	Arg	-	-	-	-	-	-	-	-	-	-	-	-	>128	>128	>128	>128	0.025
J136	2	-	T **	A **	A *	C *	-	G **	-	-	-	-	-	-	-	-	-	-	-	-	-	-	-	Lys	-	>128	>128	>128	>128	0.05
J175	2	-	T **	A **	A *	C *	-	G **	-	-	-	-	-	-	-	-	-	-	-	-	-	-	-	-	-	>128	>128	>128	>128	0.05
J226	2	-	T **	A **	A *	C *	-	G **	-	-	-	-	-	-	-	-	-	-	-	-	-	-	-	-	-	>128	>128	>128	>128	0.1
J276	2	-	T **	A **	A *	C *	-	G **	-	-	-	-	-	-	-	-	-	-	-	-	-	-	-	-	-	>128	>128	>128	>128	0.05
J319	2	-	T **	A **	A *	C *	-	G **	-	-	-	-	-	-	-	-	-	-	-	-	-	-	-	-	-	>128	>128	>128	>128	0.05
J330	2	-	T **	A **	A *	C *	-	G **	-	-	-	-	-	-	-	-	-	-	-	-	-	-	-	-	-	>128	>128	>128	>128	0.1
J336	2	-	T **	A **	A *	C *	-	G **	-	-	-	-	-	-	-	-	-	-	-	-	-	-	-	-	-	>128	>128	>128	>128	0.05
J341	2	-	T **	A **	A *	C *	-	G **	-	-	-	-	-	-	-	-	-	-	-	-	-	-	-	-	-	>128	>128	>128	>128	0.05
J356	2	-	T **	A **	A *	C *	-	G **	-	-	-	-	-	-	-	-	-	-	-	-	-	-	-	-	-	>128	>128	>128	>128	0.1
J368	2	-	T **	A **	A *	C *	-	G **	-	-	-	-	-	-	-	-	-	-	-	-	-	-	-	-	-	>128	>128	>128	>128	0.1
J377	2	-	T **	A **	A *	C *	-	G **	-	-	-	-	-	-	-	-	-	-	-	-	-	-	-	-	-	>128	>128	>128	>128	0.05
J391	2	-	T **	A **	A *	C *	-	G **	-	-	-	-	-	-	-	-	-	-	-	-	-	-	-	-	-	>128	>128	>128	>128	0.2
J410	2	-	T **	A **	A *	C *	-	G **	-	-	-	-	-	-	-	-	-	-	-	-	-	-	-	-	-	>128	>128	>128	>128	0.1
J96	3	-	T **	A **	A *	C *	-	G **	A *	-	-	-	-	-	-	-	-	-	-	-	-	-	-	-	-	>128	>128	>128	>128	0.1
J178	3	-	T **	A **	A *	C *	-	G **	-	-	-	-	-	-	-	-	-	-	-	-	-	-	-	-	-	>128	>128	>128	>128	0.05
J228	3	-	T **	A **	A *	C *	-	G **	-	-	-	-	-	-	Thr	-	-	-	-	-	-	-	-	-	-	>128	>128	>128	>128	0.1
J233	3	-	T **	A **	A *	C *	-	G **	A *	-	-	-	-	-	-	-	-	-	-	-	-	-	-	-	-	>128	>128	>128	>128	0.1
J279	3	-	T **	A **	A *	C *	-	G **	-	-	-	-	-	-	-	-	-	-	-	-	-	-	-	-	-	>128	>128	>128	>128	0.1
J295	3	-	T **	A **	A *	C *	-	G **	A *	-	-	-	-	-	-	-	-	-	-	-	-	-	-	-	-	>128	>128	>128	>128	0.1

Table 3. *Cont.*

Isolate	*polC* [a] ST	23S rRNA, *rrl* alleles [b]									L3 [c]	L4 [c]												L22 [c]		MIC (μg/mL) [d]				
		452	534	748 [e]	954	1249	1251	2058 [e,f]	2157	2848	265	11	24	36	44	62	63	68	79	94	178	178	178	5	93 [e]	Tul	Gam	Tild	Lin	Val
J305	3	-	T **	A **	A *	C *	-	G **	A *	-	-	-	-	-	-	-	-	-	-	-	-	-	-	-	-	>128	>128	>128	>128	0.1
J335	3	-	T **	A **	A *	C *	T*	G **	-	-	-	-	-	-	-	-	-	-	-	-	-	-	-	-	-	>128	>128	>128	>128	0.05
J388	3	-	T **	A **	A *	C *	-	G **	A *	-	-	-	-	-	-	-	-	-	-	-	-	-	-	-	-	>128	>128	>128	>128	0.1
J479	3	-	T **	A **	A *	C *	-	G **	-	-	-	-	-	-	-	-	-	-	-	-	-	-	-	-	-	>128	>128	>128	>128	0.2
J482	3	-	T **	A **	A *	C *	-	G **	-	-	-	-	-	-	-	-	-	-	-	-	-	-	-	-	-	>128	>128	>128	>128	0.2
J69	3	A *	T **	A **	A **	-	-	G **	-	-	-	-	-	-	Thr	-	-	-	-	-	-	-	-	-	-	>128	>128	>128	>128	0.05
J72	3	A *	T **	A **	A **	-	-	G **	-	-	-	-	-	-	-	-	-	-	-	-	-	-	-	-	-	>128	>128	>128	>128	0.05
J81	3	A *	T **	A **	A **	-	-	G **	-	T *	-	-	-	-	-	-	-	-	-	-	-	-	-	-	-	>128	>128	>128	>128	0.1
J115	3	A *	T **	A **	A **	-	-	G **	-	T *	-	-	-	-	Thr	-	-	-	-	-	-	-	-	-	-	>128	>128	>128	>128	0.025
J131	3	A *	T **	A **	A **	-	-	G **	-	-	-	-	-	-	Thr	-	-	-	-	-	-	-	-	-	-	>128	>128	>128	>128	0.1

[a] Subtype (ST) based on the single-locus sequence analysis of a region of the gene *polC* [41]; [b] nucleotide numbering refers to *Escherichia coli* K12; a single * indicates mutation in one *rrl* allele and ** indicates mutation in both alleles; [c] amino acid numbering refers to positions in PG45; [d] Tul= Tulathromycin; Gam = Gamithromycin; Tild = Tildipirosin; Lin = Lincomycin; Val = Valnemulin. [e] Mutations associated with macrolides resistance in *M. bovis* [43,47,49]. [f] Mutation associated with lincomycin resistance in *Mycoplasma synoviae* [50].

Table 4. List of point mutations in 16S rRNA alleles of *Mycoplasma bovis* isolates and associated minimum inhibitory concentration (MIC) values for doxycycline.

Isolate	*polC* [a] ST	16S rRNA, *rrs* alleles [b]						MIC (µg/mL) [c]
		335	859	965 [d]	967 [d]	1192 [e]	1199	Dox
PG45	1	C	C	A	A	C	T	0.0625
J137	2	T *	T *	T **	T **	-	-	1
J28	3	T *	-	T **	T **	-	-	1
J403	3	T *	-	T **	T **	-	-	1
J414	3	T *	-	T **	T **	-	-	1
J433	3	T *	-	T **	T **	-	-	1
J276	2	-	-	T **	T **	A **	C **	1
J319	2	-	-	T **	T **	A **	C **	1
J341	2	-	-	T **	T **	A **	C **	1
J115	3	-	-	T **	T **	A **	C **	1
J335	3	-	-	T **	T **	A **	C **	1
J6	2	-	-	T **	T **	A **	C **	2
J103	2	-	-	T **	T **	A **	C **	2
J136	2	-	-	T **	T **	A **	C **	2
J175	2	-	-	T **	T **	A **	C **	2
J226	2	-	-	T **	T **	A **	C **	2
J336	2	-	-	T **	T **	A **	C **	2
J356	2	-	-	T **	T **	A **	C **	2
J377	2	-	-	T **	T **	A **	C **	2
J391	2	-	-	T **	T **	A **	C **	2
J410	2	-	-	T **	T **	A **	C **	2
J69	3	-	-	T **	T **	A **	C **	2
J72	3	-	-	T **	T **	A **	C **	2
J81	3	-	-	T **	T **	A **	C **	2
J178	3	-	-	T **	T **	A **	C **	2
J228	3	-	-	T **	T **	A **	C *	2
J279	3	-	-	T **	T **	A **	C *	2
J295	3	-	-	T **	T **	A **	C **	2
J305	3	-	-	T **	T **	A **	C **	2
J479	3	-	-	T **	T **	A **	C *	2
J482	3	-	-	T **	T **	A **	C *	2
J330	2	-	-	T **	T **	A **	C **	4
J368	2	-	-	T **	T **	A **	C **	4
J131	3	-	-	T **	T **	A **	C **	4
J233	3	-	-	T **	T **	A **	C **	4
J96	3	-	-	T **	T **	A **	C **	8
J388	3	-	-	T **	T **	A **	C **	8

[a] Subtype (ST) based on the single-locus sequence analysis of a region of the gene *polC* [41]; [b] nucleotide numbering refers to *Escherichia coli K12*; a single * indicates mutation in one *rrl* allele and ** indicates mutation in both alleles; [c] Dox = doxycycline. [d] Mutations associated with *M bovis* tetracyclines resistance in previous studies [43,51]. [e] Mutation associated with spectinomycin resistance in previous studies [47,48].

3. Discussion

M. bovis was found to be widely distributed in Spanish cattle herds. More specifically, *M. bovis* was mainly detected in feedlot calves (81/183) and to a lesser extent in pasture-raised animals (3/22) housed in 26 different farms from 5 Spanish regions. This pathogenic species was not only detected in animals suffering from respiratory infections and/or arthritis (44/80), but also in asymptomatic carriers (40/125). These results consolidate previous studies that reported the isolation of *M. bovis* from young cattle with respiratory disease in Spain between 2010–2012 and 2015–2016 [37,38]. Although the complete epidemiological background of those isolates was not provided, the authors indicated that each isolate was obtained from a different farm. Altogether, these data indicate that, at least among beef cattle, the infection may have already become endemic, as reported in other European countries [25–27]. The presence of asymptomatic carriers and the movement of cattle between beef cattle farms, which frequently involves the mix of animals of diverse origins [39], may explain the current situation in Spain. The isolation of *M. bovis* from clinical mastitis cases was unusual given the low prevalence of this infection in other European countries. Therefore, further studies are needed to confirm whether this particular situation only reflects a bias of the sampling procedure or indicates that Spain is facing an important increase in the number of mastitis cases associated with *M. bovis*.

M. bovis isolates circulating in Spain are divided into two *polC* STs, 2 and 3. These two STs are similar to recent French isolates [41–43]. Compared with France, where ST2 has been predominant since 2000 [41–43], almost two thirds (58/95) of the characterized Spanish isolates belong to ST3. Both STs are widely distributed among different farms and regions, and can be isolated from beef and dairy cattle, from animals with different clinical conditions, and even from different anatomic locations of the same animal. This argues in favor of an efficient circulation and transmission of both STs, as already suggested with French isolates. Thus, animal movement between farms, a common practice in the Spanish beef cattle industry, is likely contributing to the dissemination of *M. bovis* [39]. Animal movements between dairy farms is less common, but asymptomatic carriers can be introduced into the herd when the replacement rate of animals born in the same herd is insufficient to maintain milk production. Furthermore, artificial insemination may be another way of entry for *M. bovis*. This was recently documented in Finland, where semen was reported to be the source of *M. bovis* mastitis outbreaks in two dairy herds [40].

Antimicrobial susceptibility profiles against FLQ differed between ST2 and ST3 isolates. The analysis of the QRDR revealed that the main differences between these STs were located in *gyrA* and *parC*. Remarkably, ST3 isolates were all characterized by an unusual Gln10Arg mutation in *parC*. This mutation is unrelated to antimicrobial resistance, since it was found in ST3 isolates associated with high and low MIC values (≥ 1 and ≤ 1 μg/mL, respectively), and are likely to reflect phylogenetic evolution. ST3 isolates with MIC values ≥ 1 μg/mL were all characterized by mutation Ser83Phe in *gyrA* in combination with one or more amino acid substitution (Ser80Ile, Ser81Pro, Asp84Asn, Ala116Pro, or Val156Ile) in *parC*. Only three of these *parC* mutations, Ser80Ile, Ser81Pro, andAsp84Asn, have been previously described [42,45–48]. A point mutation Ser83Phe in *GyrA* is sufficient to reach an intermediate level of susceptibility to FLQ but additional substitutions in *parC* are required for resistance [42,44–48]. Interestingly, ST2 and a majority of ST3 (18/20) isolates had the mutation Asp362Asn in *gyrB*. This mutation also appears in recent French isolates and is related to phylogenetic evolution rather than drug resistance [41,42]. Two ST3 isolates harbor a Val323Ala mutation in *gyrB*, but its contribution to FLQ resistance is unknown.

Our results are consistent with in vitro studies showing that under selective pressure, ST3 isolates are more prone to accumulate QRDR mutations than ST2 isolates. Therefore, the widespread circulation of FLQ-resistant ST3 isolates in Spain might reflect the overuse of these antimicrobials in the field. Remarkably, two ST2 isolates were also found to be resistant to FLQ. They were isolated from a cow with clinical mastitis together with susceptible ST2 isolates. This may be the result of long-term treatment with FLQ, leading to the generation of resistant strains, and re-infection with susceptible strains. Globally, our results contrast with other countries where most *M. bovis* strains are susceptible to this family of antimicrobials [6,9–13].

MIC values confirmed the general decrease of *M. bovis* susceptibility to macrolides and lincomycin ($MIC_{90} > 128$) [5,9–13]. Analysis of 23S rRNA genes revealed that isolates with MIC values > 128 μg/mL for macrolides and lincomycin acquired mutations G748A (in both *rrl* alleles) and A2058G (in one or both *rrl* alleles). A combination of mutations in these hotspots is necessary and sufficient to achieve resistance to other macrolides, such as tylosin and tilmicosin, while mutation A2058G in one or both alleles has been linked to lincomycin resistance in *M. synoviae* [43,49,50]. Isolates J28 and J137 showed high MIC values (16–128 μg/mL) for macrolides but did not carry the mutation A2058G. Consistently, they are the only isolates with low MIC values for lincomycin (1 μg/mL). However, both isolates have several non-synonymous mutations in L4 and L22 proteins including Gln93His in L22, which is related to macrolide resistance and could explain the observed high MIC values for these antimicrobials [43]. No other point mutations related to antimicrobial resistance have been found in the *rrl* alleles or in L4 and L22 proteins. Since they appear together with other mutations conferring resistance, it is difficult to determine their importance.

As expected by the in vitro antimicrobial activity of pleuromutilins against a broad range of veterinary mycoplasmas [22], valnemulin was the only antimicrobial that demonstrated activity against both STs. Indeed, no mutation previously associated with pleuromutilin resistance [47] has been observed in any isolate. This is consistent with the fact that pleuromutilins are only registered for treatment in swine and poultry [52]. Valnemulin may thus be an interesting therapeutic alternative as it has been shown to be effective for the treatment of calves experimentally infected with *M. bovis* [53].

Overall, low in vitro susceptibility was observed for doxycycline (MIC_{90} = 4 μg/mL). Analysis of 16S rRNA genes revealed that isolates with MIC values ≥ 1 μg/mL were characterized by mutations A965T and A967T in both *rrs* alleles. Previous studies have concluded that this double mutation causes decreased susceptibility to other antimicrobials from the same group, such as oxytetracycline and tetracycline [43,51]. Mutations C1192A and T1199C were previously described in French isolates [43], although they did not further modify MIC values as it occurs with Spanish isolates. However, the mutation C1192A has been described both in Hungarian and Japanese isolates and was associated with high MIC values for spectinomycin [47,48]. As expected, mutations C335T and C859T, which have never been associated with antimicrobial resistance, had no influence on the susceptibility of the Spanish isolates. Finally, our results were also consistent with data suggesting that after macrolides, the highest resistances of the main veterinary mycoplasmas species are observed for tetracyclines [22].

In conclusion, our study revealed the extended circulation of *M. bovis* in Spanish beef cattle herds and its implication in mastitis cases. Circulating isolates are divided into two groups, ST2 and ST3, both being resistant to macrolides, lincosamides and tetracyclines. Most ST3 isolates circulating in Spain are resistant to FLQ, a situation which illustrates the remarkable capacity of ST3 to accumulate mutations in QRDR and the selective pressure imposed by the indiscriminate use of these antimicrobials. Valnemulin has been shown to be very effective against both STs in vitro, and its effectiveness in vivo should be further investigated.

4. Materials and Methods

4.1. Animal Sampling

All animal procedures were performed following the EU Directive 2010/63/EU for animal experimentation and had the authorization of the Ethics Committee on Animal Testing of the University of Murcia (Number: 307/2017).

In this study, 260 animals from 10 Spanish regions were sampled over a 4 year period (2016–2019). A total of 433 samples were collected from beef and dairy cattle.

Among beef cattle, 183 calves were raised in feedlots and 22 pasture-raised animals were sampled. Healthy animals (n = 125) and animals with clinical symptoms of respiratory disease or arthritis (n = 80) were both considered. In total, 331 samples were obtained from beef cattle. The sample collection was composed of nasal swabs (n = 278), auricular (n = 27) and conjunctival swabs (n = 3), synovial fluid (n = 3), as well as a number of swabs from tissues (lung, n = 16; liver, n = 2; spleen, n = 1; and mediastinal lymph node, n = 1). Those samples were obtained from 30 farms and 8 different regions (Figure S1).

Among dairy cattle, 39 cows with mastitis, and 16 calves with clinical signs of respiratory disease (n = 5) or asymptomatic (n = 11) were sampled. In total, 105 samples were obtained from dairy cattle. The sample collection was composed of mastitic milk (n = 66), bulk tank milk (BTM) (n = 9), and nasal (n = 27), auricular (n = 1), and conjunctival swabs (n = 2). Those samples were obtained from 7 farms and a milk analyses laboratory that provided samples and they were taken from 5 different regions (Figure S1).

4.2. Mycoplasma Isolation and Subtyping

For mycoplasma isolation from animal samples, swabs or mastitic milk samples (200 μL) were incubated at 37 °C for 24 h in 2 mL of SP4 medium [54] with modifications (Appendix A). Cultures were filtered through a 0.45 μm membrane filter (LLG-Labware, UK) and further incubated for 48 h before plating 5 μL onto solid SP4 medium. Agar plates were grown at 37 °C and examined daily under the microscope for the presence of mycoplasma colonies with the typical fried egg morphology.

The DNA extraction was performed from 200 μL of culture [55]. *M. bovis* detection was performed by PCR amplification of the membrane protein 81 gene [56]. *M. bovis* PCR positive cultures were three times cloned by picking single colonies and the identity of the final isolate was confirmed again by PCR.

M. bovis subtyping was performed by sequence analysis of a 520 bp region of the *polC* gene, as previously described [41]. Amplicon sequencing was performed at the molecular biology service of the University of Murcia and sequence analyses were conducted using MEGA 6 [57].

4.3. MIC Assays

Antimicrobials used for MIC assays included (i) the macrolides, tulathromycin (Carbosiynth, Compton, UK), gamithromycin (Sigma-Aldrich, St. Louis, MO, USA) and tildipirosin (Carbosiynth, Compton, UK), (ii) the lincosamide, lincomycin (Sigma-Aldrich, St. Louis, MO, USA), (iii) the FLQ, enrofloxacin (Fluka, Bio-Chemika, St. Louis, MO, USA), marbofloxacin (Tokio Chemical Industry, Chuo City, Japan) and danofloxacin (Fluka, Bio-Chemika, St. Louis, MO, USA), (iv) the tetracycline, doxycycline (Sigma-Aldrich, St. Louis, MO, USA), and (v) the pleuromutilin, valnemulin hydrochloride (Sigma-Aldrich, St. Louis, MO, USA). Stock solutions (1 mg/mL; 0.1 mg/mL for valnemulin hydrochloride) and two-fold dilutions were prepared in sterile distilled water. For preparing enrofloxacin, marbofloxacin, and danofloxacin, 0.1 M HCl was added dropwise until dissolution occurred and the volume was adjusted with sterile distilled water. A final range from 128 μg/mL to 0.0625 μg/mL was tested except for valnemulin, for which a final range from 12.8 μg/mL to 0.00625 μg/mL was studied.

Stationary-phase cultures of 95 *M. bovis* isolates and the reference strain PG45 were used for MIC assays. Mycoplasma cultures were carried out in PH medium [58] without antimicrobials, supplemented with sodium pyruvate (0.5%) and phenol red (0.005%), and mycoplasma titers were determined as previously described [59]. MIC assays were carried out in 96-well microtiter plates using the microbroth dilution method [23]. Briefly, 25.6 μL of each antimicrobial dilution and 25 μL of the diluted *M. bovis* inoculum (10^3–10^5 CFU/mL) were added to 150 μL of culture medium. Additionally, a positive control (well without antimicrobial) and a negative control (well without neither antimicrobial nor inoculum) were included in each essay. After 48 h of incubation at 37 °C, plates were examined for color change. MIC was defined as the lowest concentration of antimicrobial capable of completely inhibiting the growth of *M. bovis*. For each antimicrobial, the MIC range, MIC_{50} (lowest concentration of antimicrobial capable of inhibiting the growth of 50% of the isolates), and MIC_{90} (lowest concentration of antimicrobial capable of inhibiting the growth of 90% of the isolates) were calculated. All the assays were performed in duplicate. For accepting the results, MIC values of the duplicate tests had to be within one dilution, with the higher MIC value being used. If not, a third assay was performed, and the final MIC value was the mode of the three values.

4.4. Statistical Analysis

MIC values were transformed to a continuous variable by calculating their Log2 values. Log2MIC means values of ST2 and ST3 isolates were compared for each antimicrobial. Statistical analyses were run using the EpiInfo software [60] using ANOVA or Mann–Whitney/Wilcoxon Two-Sample Test (Kruskal–Wallis test for two groups) according to the inequality of population variances and with the significance level set at 0.01.

4.5. Whole-Genome Sequencing

Genomic DNA was extracted from a selection of 36 isolates (Table S1) from 15 mL of mycoplasma culture using a High Pure PCR Template Preparation Kit (Roche, Bâle, Suisse) according to the manufacturer's instructions. Whole-genome sequencing was performed using Illumina technology Hiseq (paired-end, 2 × 150pb) by Novogene Europe (Cambridge, UK). Bioinformatics analyses were performed on Galaxy platform (Genotoul, Toulouse, France). Quality controls of reads were performed using *FastQC* tool [61]. Alignments were carried out with *BWA-MEM* using PG45 as the reference [62], and alignments quality controls were checked with *QualiMap BamQC* [63]. SNP identification was done by alignment visualization with *Integrative Genomics Viewer* (IGV 2.7.0) [64] or by variant calling analysis with *breseq* [65]. All sequence files are available from the European Nucleotide Archive database (ENA), under study accession number PRJEB38707.

Author Contributions: Conceptualization, L.-X.N., and C.d.l.F.; methodology, A.G.-G., L.-X.N., Á.G.-M., A.S., and C.d.l.F.; software, A.G.-G., L.-X.N., and A.S.; validation, A.G.-G., L.-X.N., A.S., and C.d.l.F.; formal analysis, A.G.-G., L.-X.N., and C.d.l.F.; investigation, A.G.-G., L.-X.N., E.B., and C.d.l.F.; resources, C.d.l.F.; data curation, A.G.-G., L.-X.N., and C.d.l.F.; writing—original draft preparation, A.G.-G., L.-X.N., and E.B.; writing—review and editing, A.G.-G., L.-X.N., E.B., C.C., and C.d.l.F.; visualization, A.G.-G., L.-X.N., E.B., Á.G.-M., A.S., C.C., and C.d.l.F.; supervision, L.-X.N., Á.G.-M., and C.d.l.F.; project administration, C.d.l.F.; funding acquisition, C.d.l.F. All authors have read and agreed to the published version of the manuscript.

Acknowledgments: The authors are grateful to: Ángel García Muñoz, Juan Seva Alcaraz, and Juan Alcazar Triviño for providing us the contacts for taking samples; to Mercè Lazaro for providing us the mastitic milk samples received in her laboratory; to the veterinarians that collected samples in the field; to the farmers for allowing the collection of the samples; to the Genotoul bioinformatics platform Toulouse Midi-Pyrenees for providing help and storage resources.

Appendix A

The medium SP4 was prepared following previous recommendations [54] but with some modifications.The modified medium is composed of three parts (A, B, and C). Part A is composed of 4.2 g of Difco PPLO broth (BD), 6.4 g of Bacto Peptone (BD), 12 g of Bacto Tryptone (BD) and 724 mL of deionized water. The solid medium includes 7 g of European Bacteriological Agar (Conda-Pronadisa). The pH is adjusted to 7.8 and then part A is autoclaved at 121 °C for 20 min. Part B is composed of 60 mL of RPMI-1640 (Sigma-Aldrich), 21 mL of fresh yeast extract 50% *w*/*v*, 2.4 g of yeast extract (Conda-Pronadisa), 4.8 mL of phenol red 0.5%, (Sigma-Aldrich) and 0.642 g of ampicillin sodium salt (Fisher bioreagents). The pH is adjusted to 7.2 and then part B is filter-sterilized through a 0.2 µL pore size filter. Part C is composed of 251 mL of heat-inactivated horse serum (Hyclone) for 30 min at 56 °C.

References

1. Hale, H.H.; Helmboldt, C.F.; Plastridge, W.N.; Stula, E.F. Bovine mastitis caused by a Mycoplasma species. *Cornell Vet.* **1962**, *52*, 582–591. [PubMed]
2. Nicholas, R.A.J.; Ayling, R.D. *Mycoplasma bovis*: Disease, diagnosis, and control. *Res. Vet. Sci.* **2003**, *74*, 105–112. [CrossRef]
3. Maunsell, F.P.; Woolums, A.R.; Francoz, D.; Rosenbusch, R.F.; Step, D.L.; Wilson, D.J.; Janzen, E.D. *Mycoplasma bovis* infections in cattle. *J. Vet. Intern. Med.* **2011**, *25*, 772–783. [CrossRef] [PubMed]
4. Perez-Casal, J.; Prysliak, T.; Maina, T.; Suleman, M.; Jimbo, S. Status of the development of a vaccine against Mycoplasma bovis. *Vaccine* **2017**, *35*, 2902–2907. [CrossRef]

5. Gerchman, I.; Levisohn, S.; Mikula, I.; Lysnyansky, I. In vitro antimicrobial susceptibility of *Mycoplasma bovis* isolated in Israel from local and imported cattle. *Vet. Microbiol.* **2009**, *137*, 268–275. [CrossRef]
6. Soehnlen, M.K.; Kunze, M.E.; Karunathilake, K.E.; Henwood, B.M.; Kariyawasam, S.; Wolfgang, D.R.; Jayarao, B.M. In vitro antimicrobial inhibition of *Mycoplasma bovis* isolates submitted to the Pennsylvania Animal Diagnostic Laboratory using flow cytometry and a broth microdilution method. *J. Vet. Diagn.* **2011**, *23*, 547–551. [CrossRef]
7. Hendrick, S.H.; Bateman, K.G.; Rosengren, L.B. The effect of antimicrobial treatment and preventive strategies on bovine respiratory disease and genetic relatedness and antimicrobial resistance of *Mycoplasma bovis* isolates in a western Canadian feedlot. *Can. Vet. J. Rev. Vet. Can.* **2013**, *54*, 1146–1156.
8. Ayling, R.D.; Rosales, R.S.; Barden, G.; Gosney, F.L. Changes in antimicrobial susceptibility of *Mycoplasma bovis* isolates from Great Britain. *Vet. Rec.* **2014**, *175*, 486. [CrossRef]
9. Gautier-Bouchardon, A.V.; Ferré, S.; Le Grand, D.; Paoli, A.; Gay, E.; Poumarat, F. Overall decrease in the susceptibility of *Mycoplasma bovis* to antimicrobials over the past 30 years in France. *PLoS ONE* **2014**, *9*, e87672. [CrossRef]
10. Kawai, K.; Higuchi, H.; Iwano, H.; Iwakuma, A.; Onda, K.; Sato, R.; Hayashi, T.; Nagahata, H.; Oshida, T. Antimicrobial susceptibilities of Mycoplasma isolated from bovine mastitis in Japan. *Anim. Sci. J.* **2014**, *85*, 96–99. [CrossRef]
11. Sulyok, K.M.; Kreizinger, Z.; Fekete, L.; Hrivnák, V.; Magyar, T.; Jánosi, S.; Schweitzer, N.; Turcsányi, I.; Makrai, L.; Erdélyi, K.; et al. Antibiotic susceptibility profiles of *Mycoplasma bovis* strains isolated from cattle in Hungary, Central Europe. *BMC Vet. Res.* **2014**, *10*, 256. [CrossRef] [PubMed]
12. Heuvelink, A.; Reugebrink, C.; Mars, J. Antimicrobial susceptibility of *Mycoplasma bovis* isolates from veal calves and dairy cattle in the Netherlands. *Vet. Microbiol.* **2016**, *189*, 1–7. [CrossRef] [PubMed]
13. Kong, L.C.; Gao, D.; Jia, B.Y.; Wang, Z.; Gao, Y.-H.; Pei, Z.-H.; Liu, S.-M.; Xin, J.-Q.; Ma, H.-X. Antimicrobial susceptibility and molecular characterization of macrolide resistance of *Mycoplasma bovis* isolates from multiple provinces in China. *J. Vet. Med. Sci.* **2016**, *78*, 293–296. [CrossRef]
14. Jelinski, M.; Kinnear, A.; Gesy, K.; Andrés-Lasheras, S.; Zaheer, R.; Weese, S.; McAllister, T.A. Antimicrobial sensitivity testing of *Mycoplasma bovis* isolates derived from Western Canadian feedlot cattle. *Microorganisms* **2020**, *8*, 124. [CrossRef]
15. Citti, C.; Dordet-Frisoni, E.; Nouvel, L.X.; Kuo, C.; Baranowski, E. Horizontal gene transfers in mycoplasmas (Mollicutes). *Curr. Issues Mol. Biol.* **2018**, 3–22. [CrossRef] [PubMed]
16. Faucher, M.; Nouvel, L.-X.; Dordet-Frisoni, E.; Sagné, E.; Baranowski, E.; Hygonenq, M.-C.; Marenda, M.-S.; Tardy, F.; Citti, C. Mycoplasmas under experimental antimicrobial selection: The unpredicted contribution of horizontal chromosomal transfer. *PLoS Genet.* **2019**, *15*, e1007910. [CrossRef]
17. McCormack, W.M. Susceptibility of mycoplasmas to antimicrobial agents: Clinical implications. *Clin. Infect. Dis.* **1993**, *17* (Suppl. S1), S200–S201. [CrossRef] [PubMed]
18. Olaitan, A.O.; Morand, S.; Rolain, J.M. Mechanisms of polymyxin resistance: Acquired and intrinsic resistance in bacteria. *Front. Microbiol.* **2014**, *5*, 643. [CrossRef] [PubMed]
19. Gadeau, A.P.; Mouches, C.; Bove, J.M. Probable insensitivity of mollicutes to rifampin and characterization of spiroplasmal DNA-dependent RNA polymerase. *J. Bacteriol.* **1986**, *166*, 824–828. [CrossRef]
20. Pellegrin, J.L.; Maugein, J.; Clerc, M.T.; Leng, B.; Bové, J.M.; Bébéar, C. Activity of rifampin against Mollicutes, clostridia and L forms. Recent advances in mycoplasmology. *Zentralbl. Bakteriol. Suppl.* **1990**, *20*, 810–812.
21. Shepard, M.C.; Lunceford, C.D.; Ford, D.K.; Purcell, R.H.; Taylor-Robinson, D.; Razin, S.; Black, F.T. Ureaplasma urealyticum gen. nov., sp. nov.: Proposed nomenclature for the human T (T-Strain) mycoplasmas. *Int. J. Syst. Evol. Bacteriol.* **1974**, *24*, 160–171. [CrossRef]
22. Gautier-Bouchardon, A.V. Antimicrobial resistance in mycoplasma spp. *Microbiol. Spectr.* **2018**, *6*. [CrossRef]
23. Hannan, P.C. Guidelines and recommendations for antimicrobial minimum inhibitory concentration (MIC) testing against veterinary mycoplasma species. International research programme on comparative mycoplasmology. *Vet. Res.* **2000**, *31*, 373–395. [CrossRef] [PubMed]
24. Lysnyansky, I.; Ayling, R.D. Mycoplasma bovis: Mechanisms of resistance and trends in antimicrobial susceptibility. *Front. Microbiol.* **2016**, *7*. [CrossRef] [PubMed]
25. Arcangioli, M.-A.; Duet, A.; Meyer, G.; Dernburg, A.; Bézille, P.; Poumarat, F.; Le Grand, D. The role of *Mycoplasma bovis* in bovine respiratory disease outbreaks in veal calf feedlots. *Vet. J.* **2008**, *177*, 89–93. [CrossRef]
26. Nicholas, R.A.J. Bovine mycoplasmosis: Silent and deadly. *Vet. Rec.* **2011**, *168*, 459–462. [CrossRef]

27. Radaelli, E.; Luini, M.; Loria, G.R.; Nicholas, R.A.J.; Scanziani, E. Bacteriological, serological, pathological and immunohistochemical studies of *Mycoplasma bovis* respiratory infection in veal calves and adult cattle at slaughter. *Res. Vet. Sci.* **2008**, *85*, 282–290. [CrossRef]
28. Caswell, J.L.; Bateman, K.G.; Cai, H.Y.; Castillo-Alcala, F. *Mycoplasma bovis* in respiratory disease of feedlot cattle. *Vet. Clin. North Am. Food Anim. Pract.* **2010**, *26*, 365–379. [CrossRef]
29. Nielsen, P.K.; Petersen, M.B.; Nielsen, L.R.; Halasa, T.; Toft, N. Latent class analysis of bulk tank milk PCR and ELISA testing for herd level diagnosis of *Mycoplasma bovis*. *Prev. Vet. Med.* **2015**, *121*, 338–342. [CrossRef]
30. Spergser, J.; Macher, K.; Kargl, M.; Lysnyansky, I.; Rosengarten, R. Emergence, re-emergence, spread and host species crossing of *Mycoplasma bovis* in the Austrian Alps caused by a single endemic strain. *Vet. Microbiol.* **2013**, *164*, 299–306. [CrossRef]
31. Van Engelen, E.; Dijkman, R.; Holzhauer, M.; Junker, K.; Van Wuyckhuise, L.; Gonggrijp, M. Typing of *Mycoplasma bovis* from arthritis outbreaks in dairy herds. In Proceedings of the European Mycoplasma Meeting: Progress in Human and Animal Mycoplasmology, Pendik, Istanbul, Turkey, 3–5 June 2015.
32. Aebi, M.; van den Borne, B.H.P.; Raemy, A.; Steiner, A.; Pilo, P.; Bodmer, M. *Mycoplasma bovis* infections in Swiss dairy cattle: A clinical investigation. *Acta Vet. Scand.* **2015**, *57*, 10. [CrossRef] [PubMed]
33. Arcangioli, M.A.; Chazel, M.; Sellal, E.; Botrel, M.A.; Bezille, P.; Poumarat, F.; Calavas, D.; Le Grand, D. Prevalence of *Mycoplasma bovis* udder infection in dairy cattle: Preliminary field investigation in southeast France. *N. Z. Vet. J.* **2011**, *59*, 75–78. [CrossRef] [PubMed]
34. Filioussis, G.; Christodoulopoulos, G.; Thatcher, A.; Petridou, V.; Bourtzi-Chatzopoulou, E. Isolation of *Mycoplasma bovis* from bovine clinical mastitis cases in Northern Greece. *Vet. J.* **2007**, *173*, 215–218. [CrossRef] [PubMed]
35. Nicholas, R.A.J.; Fox, L.K.; Lysnyansky, I. Mycoplasma mastitis in cattle: To cull or not to cull. *Vet. J.* **2016**, *216*, 142–147. [CrossRef] [PubMed]
36. Passchyn, P.; Piepers, S.; De Meulemeester, L.; Boyen, F.; Haesebrouck, F.; De Vliegher, S. Between-herd prevalence of *Mycoplasma bovis* in bulk milk in Flanders, Belgium. *Res. Vet. Sci.* **2012**, *92*, 219–220. [CrossRef]
37. Klein, U.; de Jong, A.; Moyaert, H.; El Garch, F.; Leon, R.; Richard-Mazet, A.; Rose, M.; Maes, D.; Pridmore, A.; Thomson, J.R.; et al. Antimicrobial susceptibility monitoring of Mycoplasma hyopneumoniae and *Mycoplasma bovis* isolated in Europe. *Vet. Microbiol.* **2017**, *204*, 188–193. [CrossRef]
38. Klein, U.; de Jong, A.; Youala, M.; El Garch, F.; Stevenin, C.; Moyaert, H.; Rose, M.; Catania, S.; Gyuranecz, M.; Pridmore, A.; et al. New antimicrobial susceptibility data from monitoring of *Mycoplasma bovis* isolated in Europe. *Vet. Microbiol.* **2019**, *238*, 108432. [CrossRef]
39. Ministerio de Agricultura, Pesca y Alimentación. Available online: https://www.mapa.gob.es/ (accessed on 20 April 2020).
40. Haapala, V.; Pohjanvirta, T.; Vähänikkilä, N.; Halkilahti, J.; Simonen, H.; Pelkonen, S.; Soveri, T.; Simojoki, H.; Autio, T. Semen as a source of *Mycoplasma bovis* mastitis in dairy herds. *Vet. Microbiol.* **2018**, *216*, 60–66. [CrossRef]
41. Becker, C.A.M.; Thibault, F.M.; Arcangioli, M.-A.; Tardy, F. Loss of diversity within *Mycoplasma bovis* isolates collected in France from bovines with respiratory diseases over the last 35 years. *Infect. Genet. Evol.* **2015**, *33*, 118–126. [CrossRef]
42. Khalil, D.; Becker, C.A.M.; Tardy, F. Alterations in the quinolone resistance-determining regions and fluoroquinolone resistance in clinical isolates and laboratory-derived Mutants of *Mycoplasma bovis*: Not all genotypes may be equal. *Appl. Environ. Microbiol.* **2016**, *82*, 1060–1068. [CrossRef]
43. Khalil, D.; Becker, C.A.M.; Tardy, F. Monitoring the decrease in susceptibility to ribosomal RNAs targeting antimicrobials and its molecular basis in clinical *Mycoplasma bovis* isolates over time. *Microb. Drug Resist. Larchmt. N* **2017**, *23*, 799–811. [CrossRef] [PubMed]
44. Lysnyansky, I.; Mikula, I.; Gerchman, I.; Levisohn, S. Rapid detection of a point mutation in the parC gene associated with decreased susceptibility to fluoroquinolones in *Mycoplasma bovis*. *Antimicrob. Agents Chemother.* **2009**, *53*, 4911–4914. [CrossRef] [PubMed]
45. Mustafa, R.; Qi, J.; Ba, X.; Chen, Y.; Hu, C.; Liu, X.; Tu, L.; Peng, Q.; Chen, H.; Guo, A. In vitro quinolones susceptibility analysis of Chinese *Mycoplasma bovis* isolates and their phylogenetic scenarios based upon QRDRs of DNA topoisomerases revealing a unique transition in ParC. *Pak. Vet. J.* **2013**, *33*, 364–369.
46. Sato, T.; Okubo, T.; Usui, M.; Higuchi, H.; Tamura, Y. Amino acid substitutions in GyrA and ParC are associated with fluoroquinolone resistance in *Mycoplasma bovis* isolates from Japanese dairy calves. *J. Vet. Med. Sci.* **2013**, *75*, 1063–1065. [CrossRef]

47. Sulyok, K.M.; Kreizinger, Z.; Wehmann, E.; Lysnyansky, I.; Bányai, K.; Marton, S.; Jerzsele, Á.; Rónai, Z.; Turcsányi, I.; Makrai, L.; et al. Mutations associated with decreased susceptibility to seven antimicrobial families in field and laboratory-derived *Mycoplasma bovis* strains. *Antimicrob. Agents Chemother.* **2017**, *61*. [CrossRef]
48. Hata, E.; Harada, T.; Itoh, M. Relationship between antimicrobial susceptibility and multilocus sequence type of *Mycoplasma bovis* isolates and development of a method for rapid detection of point mutations involved in decreased susceptibility to macrolides, lincosamides, tetracyclines, and spectinomycin. *Appl. Environ. Microbiol.* **2019**, *85*. [CrossRef]
49. Lerner, U.; Amram, E.; Ayling, R.D.; Mikula, I.; Gerchman, I.; Harrus, S.; Teff, D.; Yogev, D.; Lysnyansky, I. Acquired resistance to the 16-membered macrolides tylosin and tilmicosin by *Mycoplasma bovis*. *Vet. Microbiol.* **2014**, *168*, 365–371. [CrossRef]
50. Lysnyansky, I.; Gerchman, I.; Flaminio, B.; Catania, S. Decreased susceptibility to macrolide-lincosamide in mycoplasma synoviae is associated with mutations in 23S ribosomal RNA. *Microb. Drug Resist.* **2015**, *21*, 581–589. [CrossRef]
51. Amram, E.; Mikula, I.; Schnee, C.; Ayling, R.D.; Nicholas, R.A.J.; Rosales, R.S.; Harrus, S.; Lysnyansky, I. 16S rRNA gene mutations associated with decreased susceptibility to tetracycline in *Mycoplasma bovis*. *Antimicrob. Agents Chemother.* **2015**, *59*, 796–802. [CrossRef]
52. CIMAVet. Centro de Información de Medicamentos para Veterinaria. Available online: https://cimavet.aemps.es/ (accessed on 20 April 2020).
53. Stipkovits, L.; Ripley, P.H.; Tenk, M.; Glávits, R.; Molnár, T.; Fodor, L. The efficacy of valnemulin (Econor) in the control of disease caused by experimental infection of calves with *Mycoplasma bovis*. *Res. Vet. Sci.* **2005**, *78*, 207–215. [CrossRef]
54. Waites, K.B.; Bébéar, C.M.; Robertson, J.A.; Talkington, D.F.; Kenny, G.E. *Cumitech 34: Laboratory Diagnosis of Mycoplasmal Infections*; American Society for Microbiology: Washington, WA, USA, 2001.
55. Tola, S.; Angioi, A.; Rocchigiani, A.M.; Idini, G.; Manunta, D.; Galleri, G.; Leori, G. Detection of *Mycoplasma agalactiae* in sheep milk samples by polymerase chain reaction. *Vet. Microbiol.* **1997**, *54*, 17–22. [CrossRef]
56. Foddai, A.; Idini, G.; Fusco, M.; Rosa, N.; De la Fe, C.; Zinellu, S.; Corona, L.; Tola, S. Rapid differential diagnosis of *Mycoplasma agalactiae* and *Mycoplasma bovis* based on a multiplex-PCR and a PCR-RFLP. *Mol. Cell. Probes* **2005**, *19*, 207–212. [CrossRef] [PubMed]
57. Tamura, K.; Stecher, G.; Peterson, D.; Filipski, A.; Kumar, S. MEGA6: Molecular evolutionary genetics analysis version 6.0. *Mol. Biol. Evol.* **2013**, *30*, 2725–2729. [CrossRef] [PubMed]
58. Gómez-Martín, A.; De la Fe, C.; Amores, J.; Sánchez, A.; Contreras, A.; Paterna, A.; Buendía, A.J.; Corrales, J.C. Anatomic location of *Mycoplasma mycoides* subsp. *capri* and *Mycoplasma agalactiae* in naturally infected goat male auricular carriers. *Vet. Microbiol.* **2012**, *157*, 355–362. [CrossRef]
59. Albers, A.C.; Fletcher, R.D. Simple method for quantitation of viable mycoplasmas. *Appl. Environ. Microbiol.* **1982**, *43*, 958–960. [CrossRef] [PubMed]
60. Epi Info^{TM}|CDC. Available online: https://www.cdc.gov/epiinfo/index.html (accessed on 20 April 2020).
61. Babraham Bioinformatics—FastQC A Quality Control Tool for High Throughput Sequence Data. Available online: https://www.bioinformatics.babraham.ac.uk/projects/fastqc/ (accessed on 20 April 2020).
62. Li, H.; Durbin, R. Fast and accurate short read alignment with Burrows-Wheeler transform. *Bioinformatics* **2009**, *25*, 1754–1760. [CrossRef]
63. Okonechnikov, K.; Conesa, A.; García-Alcalde, F. Qualimap 2: Advanced multi-sample quality control for high-throughput sequencing data. *Bioinformatics* **2016**, *32*, 292–294. [CrossRef]
64. Thorvaldsdóttir, H.; Robinson, J.T.; Mesirov, J.P. Integrative Genomics Viewer (IGV): High-performance genomics data visualization and exploration. *Brief. Bioinform.* **2013**, *14*, 178–192. [CrossRef]
65. Deatherage, D.E.; Barrick, J.E. Identification of mutations in laboratory-evolved microbes from next-generation sequencing data using breseq. In *Engineering and Analyzing Multicellular Systems*; Humana Press: New York, NY, USA, 2014; Volume 1151, pp. 165–188. [CrossRef]

10

Pestivirus K (Atypical Porcine Pestivirus): Update on the Virus, Viral Infection and the Association with Congenital Tremor in Newborn Piglets

Alais M. Dall Agnol [1,2,3], Alice F. Alfieri [1,2,3] and Amauri A. Alfieri [1,2,3,*]

1 Laboratory of Animal Virology, Department of Veterinary Preventive Medicine, Universidade Estadual de Londrina, Londrina, CEP 86057-970 Paraná, Brazil; alaisagnol@hotmail.com (A.M.D.A.); aalfieri@uel.br (A.F.A.)

2 Multi-User Animal Health Laboratory, Molecular Biology Unit, Department of Veterinary Preventive Medicine, Universidade Estadual de Londrina, CEP 86057-970 Paraná, Brazil

3 Rodovia Celso Garcia Cid Road-Campus Universitário, Londrina, PO Box 10011, CEP 86057-970 Paraná, Brazil

* Correspondence: alfieri@uel.br.

Abstract: The atypical porcine pestivirus (APPV) belongs to the species *Pestivirus K* of the genus *Pestivirus* and the family *Flaviviridae*, and it has been associated with congenital tremor (CT) type A-II in newborn piglets. Although APPV was discovered in 2015, evidence shows that APPV has circulated in pig herds for many years, at least since 1986. Due to the frequently reported outbreaks of CT on different continents, the importance of this virus for global pig production is notable. Since 2015, several studies have been conducted to clarify the association between APPV and CT. However, some findings regarding APPV infection and the measures taken to control and prevent the spread of this virus need to be contextualized to understand the infection better. This review attempts to highlight advances in the understanding of APPV associated with type A-II CT, such as etiology, epidemiology, diagnosis, and control and prevention measures, and also describes the pathophysiology of the infection and its consequences for pig production. Further research still needs to be conducted to elucidate the host's immune response to APPV infection, the control and prevention of this infection, and the possible development of vaccines.

Keywords: APPV; pestiviruses; congenital tremor type A-II; persistent infection; pigs

---

1. Introduction

In 2015, the atypical porcine pestivirus (APPV) was first described and identified by next-generation sequencing (NGS) in pig serum samples [1]. Initially, the virus was not believed to be associated with any clinical manifestations; later, an experimental inoculation study conducted in the United States (US) demonstrated that APPV was associated with the occurrence of congenital tremor (CT) in newborn piglets [2]. At present, the occurrence of APPV associated with CT is frequently reported by several studies on different continents, including the Americas (North and South), Europe, and Asia [3,4].

Since 2015, several studies have been conducted to clarify the association between APPV and CT. However, several findings regarding the infection and the measures taken to control and prevent the spread of the virus need to be contextualized to characterize the infection better. This review aims to address advances in understanding APPV associated with CT type A-II and further describe the pathophysiology of this virus and its consequences for pig production.

2. Congenital Tremor Syndrome

CT is a neurological disorder that affects newborn piglets and is characterized by muscle spasms in the head and body, which can be localized or generalized [5,6]. The intensity of the tremors is variable, and in more severe cases, they include generalized tremors that result in difficulty in standing or walking and, consequently, inability to suckle, resulting in death due to starvation. The clinical manifestation of CT is also called shaker pig syndrome, trembling pigs, or congenital myoclonus [6,7].

CT syndrome is classified into A and B according to the presence or absence of histopathological lesions in the central nervous system (CNS). In CT type A, histopathological changes are found in the brain or spinal cord. When histopathological lesions are not observed, it is classified as CT type B. Based on the etiology of CT type A, this type is subdivided into five subgroups (I-V) [5]. CT type A-I is characterized by cerebellar hypoplasia, dysplasia, hypomyelination of the spinal cord, and its etiology associated with other porcine pestivirus infections in the classical swine fever virus (CSFV) [8].

For a long time, the cause of CT A-II was not defined, although its infectious etiology has always been related to this type of tremor [9]. Since 2016, the etiology of CT A-II has been attributed to the newly described APPV, which has already been demonstrated by experimental infections [2,10]. Other viruses also were detected coinfection with APPV, such as porcine circovirus type 2 [11], astrovirus [12], porcine circovirus type 3 [13], linda virus [14], porcine circovirus-like virus P1 [15], and *Teschovirus A* [16], however, the role played by these three viruses as the primary cause of CT A-II is debatable.

CT type A-III is related to a genetic defect presented only by the Landrace breed, in which a lack of myelin is observed together with a reduction in the number of oligodendrocytes [17]. CT type A-IV is caused by a recessive genetic defect in the Saddleback swine and is characterized by hypomyelination of the brain and spinal cord [18,19]. Type A-V is caused by metrifonate (trichlorfon) intoxication. The occurrence of this type of CT may be associated with the use of metrifonate as an antiparasitic medication, and when administered during pregnancy, CT type A-V can cause cerebellar hypoplasia and cause piglets to be born with ataxia and tremor [20,21]. Finally, CT type B has no known specific cause, and changes in the CNS are not observed [5].

3. Atypical Porcine Pestivirus

3.1. Classification and Etiology

Until 2017, only four "classical" species belonged to the genus *Pestivirus*: bovine viral diarrhea virus 1 (BVDV-1); bovine viral diarrhea virus 2 (BVDV-2); border disease virus (BDV); and CSFV [22]. However, a large number of viruses linked to pestiviruses have been described [1,23–32], and Smith et al. [22] proposed that the study group of the *Flaviviridae* family of the International Committee on Viral Taxonomy (ICTV) revise the taxonomy of the genus *Pestivirus*. Thus, the genus *Pestivirus* was divided into 11 species, *Pestivirus A* (BVDV-1) [33], *Pestivirus B* (BVDV-2) [34], *Pestivirus C* (CSFV) [35], *Pestivirus D* (BDV) [36], *Pestivirus E* (pronghorn antelope pestivirus) [29], *Pestivirus F* (porcine pestivirus) [26], *Pestivirus G* (giraffe pestivirus) [23], *Pestivirus H* (HoBi-like pestivirus) [27], *Pestivirus I* (Aydin-like pestivirus) [24], *Pestivirus J* (rat pestivirus) [25], and *Pestivirus K* (atypical porcine pestivirus) [1], and one unclassified virus, bat pestivirus [30].

APPV is the single species of *Pestivirus K*, to the genus *Pestivirus*, and to the family *Flaviviridae* [37]. The viral particle is spherical, with a diameter of approximately 60 nm [38] and enveloped. Viral genomes are single-stranded, positive-sense RNA, exhibiting a genome size of approximately 11 to 11.6 kb. The genome comprises a 5′-noncoding region (NCR), one single open reading frame region encoding a single polyprotein with 3635 amino acids, and a 3′-NCR region [1,39]. The polyprotein is processed into 12 proteins, C (capsid protein), E^{rns}, E1, E2 (envelope proteins), and nonstructural proteins N^{pro}, p7, NS2, NS3, NS4A, NS4B, NS5A, and NS5B [40].

Phylogenic analyzes of the complete or partial genome of APPV strains detected in different countries and years, and in pigs from commercial farms and wild boars, demonstrate a high degree of genetic variability, subdividing into different clusters [3,41–44].

3.2. Pathogenesis and Clinical-Pathological Manifestation Associated with APPV

Two studies of experimental infection were carried out to associate APPV infection with CT and elucidate the pathogenesis. The first experimental inoculation was performed by Arruda et al. [2] and occurred in the US. Five pregnant sows, a group at 45 days and another at 62 days of gestation, were inoculated in the fetal amniotic vesicle, intranasally, and intravenously with known serum samples positive for APPV. In the period following the inoculation, no inoculated sow showed detectable viremia by qRT-PCR and no observation of clinical signs suggestive of CT. After birth, piglets were monitored for CT, and 57% to 100% of piglets showed signs of tremor. In the second experimental study carried out in the Netherlands by de Groof et al. [10], APPV-positive sera were inoculated intramuscularly in three gilts at 32 days of gestation. At 10 days postinfection, the sera from three gilts were RT-PCR-positive for the virus, and one of the gilts presented a relatively lower viral load than the other gilts. At birth, two of the three litters contained piglets showing clinical signs of CT, ranging from mild to severe signs in almost all piglets. No piglets born from the gilt that had low viremia showed signs of CT.

In both experimental studies, clinical signs were classified according to intensity; the most severe cases were characterized by intense tremors throughout the body, while the mild ones were characterized by muscle fasciculation in the limbs. Another clinical sign frequently observed was the presence of piglets with the splay leg [2,10]. This clinical manifestation is a syndrome characterized by temporary dysfunctionality of the posterior leg muscles, occurring shortly after birth, and resulting in difficulty or inability to stand and walk [45]. The presence of APPV RNA was detected in different organs of all piglets that showed signs of CT, and in some of the piglets not affected by CT [2,10]. These experiments were essential to elucidate the association of APPV with CT. However, Koch's postulate was not fulfilled by the two studies, probably due to the difficulty of viral isolation in cell cultures.

In the various studies that describe natural and experimental infections, the virus can be detected by conventional RT-PCR, qRT-PCR, and immunohistochemical in a wide variety of organs. The highest viral loads are observed primarily in the CNS and lymphoid tissues. In the CNS, the virus is found in greater quantities in the cerebellum and lymphoid tissues, mainly in the inguinal lymph nodes, submandibular lymph nodes, and thymus, suggesting that the cerebellum and lymph nodes are target organs of APPV [46,47]. In other organs, such as the brain, brain stem, spinal cord, heart, liver, spleen, lungs, and kidneys, the viral load is relatively lower [42,46,47].

To date, no significant macroscopic lesions have been described in piglets with CT [48–50]. Histopathological findings in APPV infections primarily include vacuolization of the white matter in the cerebellum [48,50,51]. Studies using Luxol® Fast Blue staining have shown a reduction in the intensity of myelin staining in the white matter of the spinal cord, cerebrum, cerebellum, and sciatic nerve, which implies a decrease in the amount of myelin in these tissues [16,48,50,52,53]. Gliosis has also been observed in the cerebral cortex and, to a lesser extent, in the spinal cord [16,49,50]. Other histopathological lesions observed in affected piglets were neuronal necrosis, neuronophagia with satellitosis, particularly at the cerebral cortex and spinal cord, Wallerian degeneration of the spinal cord, and necrosis of Purkinje cells of the cerebellum [49]. Transmission electron microscopy performed in two CNS tissues revealed not only hypomyelination of the cerebellar white matter but also more severe changes, such as interruption and breakdown of myelin, in animals affected by APPV [50]. These histopathological lesions described in piglets with CT, primary demyelination, and/or hypomyelination, can be considered a neuropathological characteristic associated with APPV infection [49]. The high viral loads of APPV in the CNS, along with the lesions observed in these tissues, explains the intensity of the neurological symptoms caused by APPV [46,47].

3.3. Viral Shedding and Transmission

Piglets that developed CT and recovered were monitored by some studies to assess the possibility of viral excretion and duration. Therefore, de Groof et al. [10] followed five pigs that presented CT and recovered at 8.5 months of age; these animals continued to shed APPV in their feces. Excretion in feces was also suggested by Postel et al. [53] since high viral loads were detected in the duodenum, pancreas, and colon. APPV is found in salivary glands; therefore, the virus is shedding by saliva until at least the sixth month of life [50]. In these same animals, the virus was also found in semen. Another study evaluated semen collection from three commercial boar herds and detected the presence of the viral genome in swab and fluid preputial and in the semen from 15% of boars from a commercial boar stud, suggesting that artificial insemination may be an important form of transmission [54].

Regarding transmission, the horizontal and vertical forms of transmission were described, with the latter being the most important and responsible for the development of CT in newborn piglets from naturally infected sows. Transplacental transmission was demonstrated by experimental inoculation. Pregnant sows were infected with serum samples known to be positive for APPV, and the birth of piglets with CT of different levels of severity was observed [2,10].

In a controlled exposure, using fetal fluid from litters that had exhibited CT, a batch of 91 gilts was submitted to oral exposure to the antigen approximately 54 days before breeding. Signs of CT were observed in 45.0% of the litters and 30.8% of all piglets born [51]. These data suggest probable horizontal transmission, due to oral exposure, and the development of CT cases.

In piglets, horizontal transmission was described after the monitoring of piglets that showed signs of CT and obtained a confirmed diagnosis for APPV. After weaning, naive piglets were mixed with APPV-positive piglets. Due to close contact, infection of susceptible piglets occurred, suggesting that transmission occurs after mixing infected with susceptible piglets. No manifestation of disease was observed in this type of late infection; moreover, these animals were transiently infected [55]. It is likely that this type of transmission is related to environmental contamination and implies the spread of the virus. However, little is known about the forms of transmission and their possible effects; therefore, further investigations are necessary for a satisfactory clarification on this topic.

3.4. *Epidemiology and Implications in Pig Production*

In the United States, APPV was first identified by NGS in pig serum samples collected in 2014 from five different states [1]. In subsequent years, several studies from different countries reported the circulation of APPV in the US [1,2,51,54,56], Germany [53,55,57–61], Netherlands [10], Sweden [62], Austria [50], England [63], China [38,42,44,46,47,61,64–73], Spain [41,74], South Korea [75], Brazil [16,48,49,76], Great Britain [61], Italy [43,61], Serbia [61], Switzerland [61,77], Taiwan [61], Canada [52], and Hungary [78].

Epidemiological surveys demonstrate a high number of the pigs positive for APPV, depending on the region evaluated and the assay used. Postel and colleagues [61] used qRT-PCR to analyze 1460 serum samples from asymptomatic pigs from Germany, Italy, Serbia, Great Britain, Switzerland, China, and Taiwan and found a prevalence of 8.9% (130/1460) of APPV-positive samples. Additionally, in this same study, the highest (17.5%; 35/200) prevalence of positive samples was in Italy. Michelitsch et al. [59], by indirect immunofluorescence test (IFI), found an antibody prevalence of 16.3% (182/1115) in pig serum samples in Germany. In Switzerland, 1080 sera from pigs for slaughter, which were obtained between 1986 and 2018, were evaluated by qRT-PCR, and the APPV genome was detected in 13% [77].

Although this virus was discovered recently, some studies have shown that APPV has been circulating in pig herds for a long time. A study conducted in Spain detected the presence of the viral genome in pig serum samples collected in 1997 [41]. In Switzerland, another investigation analyzed 1080 pig sera collected between 1986 and 2018 and revealed that 7% (6/87) of the samples collected in slaughter pigs in 1986 were APPV-positive [77]. These findings correspond to reports of the long-term presence of APPV in the world.

The presence of APPV in wild boars has been demonstrated in Germany, Spain, and Italy, and the prevalence of the virus varies according to the country. In Germany, 456 wild boar serum samples were analyzed, and 19% of samples revealed the presence of the viral genome, while 52% of the serum samples had antibodies against the E^{rns} protein [50]. In Spain and Italy, the prevalence observed was lower, 0.23% (1/437), and 0.69% (3/430) of the evaluated sera had the virus genome, respectively [43,74]. Transmission of APPV from wild boars to pigs or vice versa has not been demonstrated to date. However, wild boars are sources of various pathogens that infect domestic pigs, including other pestiviruses, such as CSFV [79], and can contribute to their transmission. Due to the importance of the transmission of viral pathogens, these wild animals are a challenge for pig health and must be considered for effective control plans to be devised.

Regarding the occurrence of CT, the litters from first parity sows are most affected by APPV infection, and this infection rarely occurs in higher birth order [10,48,49]. During an outbreak on a farm in the Netherlands, 48 litters with CT were born from gilts and were monitored, the number of piglets affected within each litter ranged from <10 to 100%. Furthermore, the total mortality of piglets, reached 26%, with 60% of these deaths being attributed to CT [10]. In Brazil, an outbreak of CT observed in piglets born to gilts, lasted for three weeks, and the mortality rate reached 30% [49].

3.5. *APPV Infection and Immunity*

The dynamics of APPV infection can be hypothesized in two ways: persistently infected and transiently infected animals. These forms of infection are known to other pestiviruses, as is the case with CSFV [79] and BVDV in cattle [80]. In APPV infection, the dynamics have not been fully elucidated; however, this phenomenon can be explained by two studies [50,55]. Schwarz et al. [50] monitored the health status of two piglets (one female and one male) aged up to six months; shortly after birth, these two animals showed CT. Specific antibodies to APPV NS3 were detected at birth and at up to eight weeks of age. The tremor symptoms decreased and disappeared completely until 14 weeks; however, both piglets still presented viremia, antibody titer, and shedding of the virus by saliva. At six months the male piglet reached sexual maturity, and a high viral load was detected in saliva and semen; on the other hand, viremia was reduced.

Cagatay et al. [55], using direct and indirect tests, monitored 20 piglets from unaffected and affected litters by CT from birth to slaughter. In the vertically infected and symptomatic piglets, viremia was detected from the first days of life until slaughter. For the presence of antibodies, these piglets showed high levels of antibodies at six days of age, and these antibodies were undetectable at 21 and/or 48 days of age. It is possible that these antibodies came from the sows and disappeared with the drop in passive immunity. On the other hand, piglets infected horizontally after being mixed at weaning with those infected vertically showed viremia at 48 days of age and high titers of specific antibodies to E2 when evaluated at 69 and 161 days of life, suggesting the induction of protective immunity against infection.

Based on piglets infected horizontally, the immune response was higher for the E2 protein, and neutralizing antibody titers correlated with the presence of E2-specific antibodies, while a correlation with E^{rns}-specific antibodies was not observed [58].

Due to the longevity of viral shedding, detectable viremia, together with the disappearance of specific antibodies over time, may suggest that persistent infection (PI) can be attributed to piglets that are intrauterine-infected. Soon after birth, these piglets can show signs of CT, which usually regresses over time [41,50,61]. On the other hand, piglets infected horizontally, through contact with persistently infected animals, develop a transient infection, with viremia detected for several weeks, but over time the piglet develops active immunity against APPV, and the virus becomes undetectable [55]. These studies provide evidence of the dynamics of infections and the immune response; however, the studies examine a small number of animals, meaning that further studies are required for complete elucidation.

3.6. *Diagnostic Methods of APPV*

Currently, a wide variety of diagnostic techniques are available for use in elucidating APPV infection in pigs. Due to practicality, speed, sensitivity, and specificity, molecular tests are the most commonly used. Among these tests, both conventional RT-PCR [16,48,49] and qRT-PCR [2] have been described in viral detection in several studies. Different clinical samples can be subjected to viral detection. In clinically affected animals, the CNS and the lymphoid organs are specimens of choice, since higher viral loads are found in these tissues, especially the cerebellum and lymph nodes [46,47]. Another available technique is NGS [2,10,51], which has been used since the first viral description in 2015 [1], and NGS is still employed as a diagnostic tool, assisting in the detection of the viral genome. In addition, NGS provides data on possible coinfections and primarily obtains larger fragments of the viral genome, which favors the phylogenetic study of circulating strains.

Histological tests performed from tissues fixed in paraffin are of great diagnostic importance, enabling the visualization of lesions caused by APPV. Luxol®® Fast Blue staining helps to observe the demyelination caused by the APPV in the CNS, primarily located in the cerebellum and spinal cord [16,48,50,52,53]. Histopathology, together with an immunohistochemical technique [46], and in situ hybridization [53,60] enables the detection of the viral agent (protein or nucleic acid) at the lesion site.

Other important methods that are used to assist in the diagnosis of infectious diseases are serological tests. The tests described for APPV infection are IFI [59], virus neutralization [55], and indirect enzyme-linked immunosorbent assay (ELISA) to the NS3, E2, and E^{rns} proteins [50,55,58,61]. These tests have many important applications, and they can be used for population-based epidemiological studies and monitoring of infection in the herd; the tests also feature easy execution and low cost.

3.7. Control and Prevention

To date, there are no effective drugs or vaccines available to treat or prevent APPV infection. Zhang et al. [81] constructed a recombinant baculovirus of APPV glycoprotein E2, which induced a robust humoral and cellular immune response in mice. Based on these studies and knowing that the E2 protein is responsible for inducing neutralizing antibodies [55], this vaccine appears to be a promising tool as likely prevention of APPV in pigs. However, further viral challenge studies are needed to demonstrate an effective immune response.

As litters of gilts are most affected by APPV infection [10,49], it is probable that the introduction of naive gilts in the herd is an important issue in the epidemiology of the disease [49,55]. Therefore, preventive measures are necessary to address this issue. The use of acclimatization for replacement gilts is an interesting tool that can be used in diseases that do not have vaccines and/or when available are not completely effective for prevention. Gatto et al. [3] suggest the protocol similar to what is used for the control of enzootic pneumonia caused by *Mycoplasma hyopneumoniae*. However, once horizontal transmission in gilts after oral exposure to fetal fluid antigen positive for APPV has been demonstrated, followed by the induction of CT in the litters of these gilts [51], this measure needs to be considered carefully. There is a need to conduct studies focused on this tool and, therefore, the development of protocols aimed at infection by APPV.

Another important point to be considered when designing control programs is the possibility of PI animals. Sensitive diagnostic methods that are able to detect PI animals, such as qRT-PCR, especially in the case of breeders, are highly important. After identifying these animals, they must be removed from the herd due to viral shedding by semen, feces, and oral fluid, which favors viral transmission. Another issue to be monitored is the semen used in the practice of artificial insemination; one possible measure is to include testing for APPV in the routine tests performed on these boars and their semen.

Despite specific measures to control APPV, biosecurity measures cannot be overlooked. When replacing breeders, animals from herds with a good health strategy must be purchased, and quarantining must be performed before introduction on the farm. Traffic control of people and vehicles on farms must be considered in addition to the execution of adequate cleaning and disinfection programs in the facilities. Finally, the control of wild animals, rodents, and insects contributes to the health of the herd in general.

4. Conclusions and Perspectives

The new porcine pestivirus (APPV) is strongly related to cases of CT type A-II, which until 2016, had an undefined etiology. Despite the recent discovery of APPV, evidence has shown that this virus has been circulating in pig herds for many years, since at least 1986, along with longstanding reports of CT, and the importance of this virus for global pig production is notable. In addition, APPV belongs to the genus *Pestivirus*, presenting important biological characteristics for the epidemiology of the disease, such as viral persistence, which can represent viral maintenance and a constant source of both horizontally and vertically transmitted infection in pig herds. These points are highly important for viral prevention. However, these issues and others regarding this disease still need to be elucidated, and further research should investigate the host's immune response, the control and prevention of APPV infection, and the development of vaccines.

Author Contributions: Conceptualization, A.M.D.A. and A.A.A.; Writing Original Draft Preparation, A.M.D.A.; Writing Review and Editing, A.F.A. and A.A.A. All authors have read and agreed to the published version of the manuscript.

Acknowledgments: The authors thank the following Brazilian Institutes for financial support: the National Council of Technological and Scientific Development (CNPq), the Brazilian Federal Agency for Support and Evaluation of Graduate Education (CAPES), the Financing of Studies and Projects (FINEP), and the Araucaria Foundation (FAP/PR). A.A.A. and A.F.A. are recipients of CNPq fellowships. A.M.D.A. is recipients of INCT-Leite/CAPES fellowship (grant number 88887.495081/2020-00).

References

1. Hause, B.M.; Collin, E.A.; Peddireddi, L.; Yuan, F.; Chen, Z.; Hesse, R.A.; Gauger, P.C.; Clement, T.; Fang, Y.; Anderson, G. Discovery of a novel putative atypical porcine pestivirus in pigs in the USA. *J. Gen. Virol.* **2015**, *96*, 2994–2998. [CrossRef]
2. Arruda, B.L.; Arruda, P.H.; Magstadt, D.R.; Schwartz, K.J.; Dohlman, T.; Schleining, J.A.; Patterson, A.R.; Visek, C.A.; Victoria, J.G. Identification of a divergent lineage porcine pestivirus in nursing piglets with congenital tremors and reproduction of disease following experimental inoculation. *PLoS ONE* **2016**, *11*, e0150104. [CrossRef]
3. Gatto, I.R.H.; Sonálio, K.; de Oliveira, L.G. Atypical Porcine Pestivirus (APPV) as a new species of pestivirus in pig production. *Front. Vet. Sci.* **2019**, *6*, 35. [CrossRef]
4. Pan, S.; Mou, C.; Chen, Z. An emerging novel virus: Atypical porcine pestivirus (APPV). *Rev. Med. Virol.* **2019**, *29*, 2018. [CrossRef]
5. Done, J.T. Congenital nervous diseases of pigs: A review. *Lab. Anim.* **1968**, *2*, 207–218. [CrossRef]
6. Stenberg, H.; Jacobson, M.; Malmberg, M. A review of congenital tremor type A-II in piglets. *Anim. Health Res. Rev.* **2020**, 1–5. [CrossRef] [PubMed]
7. Leman, A.D.; Hurtgen, J.P.; Hilley, H.D. Influence of intrauterine events on postnatal survival in the pig. *J. Anim. Sci.* **1979**, *49*, 221–224. [CrossRef] [PubMed]
8. Done, J.T.; Harding, J.D. The relationship of maternal swine fever infection to cerebellar hypoplasia in piglets. *Proc. R. Soc. Med.* **1966**, *59*, 1083–1084. [PubMed]
9. Vandekerckhove, P.; Maenhout, D.; Curvers, P.; Hoorens, J.; Ducatelle, R. Type A2 congenital tremor in piglets. *Zentralbl. Veterinarmed. A* **1989**, *36*, 763–771. [CrossRef] [PubMed]
10. de Groof, A.; Deijs, M.; Guelen, L.; van Grinsven, L.; van Os-Galdos, L.; Vogels, W.; Derks, C.; Cruijsen, T.; Geurts, V.; Vrijenhoek, M.; et al. Atypical Porcine Pestivirus: A possible cause of congenital tremor type A-II in newborn piglets. *Viruses* **2016**, *8*, 271. [CrossRef]
11. Stevenson, G.W.; Kiupel, M.; Mittal, S.K.; Choi, J.; Latimer, K.S.; Kanitz, C.L. Tissue distribution and genetic typing of porcine circoviruses in pigs with naturally occurring congenital tremors. *J. Vet. Diagn. Investig.* **2001**, *13*, 57–62. [CrossRef]
12. Blomström, A.L.; Ley, C.; Jacobson, M. Astrovirus as a possible cause of congenital tremor type AII in piglets? *Acta Vet. Scand.* **2014**, *56*, 82. [CrossRef] [PubMed]
13. Chen, G.H.; Mai, K.J.; Zhou, L.; Wu, R.T.; Tang, X.Y.; Wu, J.L.; He, L.L.; Lan, T.; Xie, Q.M.; Sun, Y.; et al. Detection and genome sequencing of porcine circovirus 3 in neonatal pigs with congenital tremors in South China. *Transbound. Emerg. Dis.* **2017**, *64*, 1650–1654. [CrossRef] [PubMed]

14. Lamp, B.; Schwarz, L.; Högler, S.; Riedel, C.; Sinn, L.; Rebel-Bauder, B.; Weissenböck, H.; Ladinig, A.; Rümenapf, T. Novel pestivirus species in pigs, Austria, 2015. *Emerg. Infect. Dis.* **2017**, *23*, 1176–1179. [CrossRef] [PubMed]
15. Wen, L.; Mao, A.; Jiao, F.; Zhang, D.; Xie, J.; He, K. Evidence of porcine circovirus-like virus P1 in piglets with an unusual congenital tremor. *Transbound. Emerg. Dis.* **2018**, *65*, e501–e504. [CrossRef]
16. Possatti, F.; Headley, S.A.; Leme, R.A.; Dall Agnol, A.M.; Zotti, E.; de Oliveira, T.E.S.; Alfieri, A.F.; Alfieri, A.A. Viruses associated with congenital tremor and high lethality in piglets. *Transbound. Emerg. Dis.* **2018**, *65*, 331–337. [CrossRef]
17. Blakemore, W.F.; Harding, J.D.; Done, J.T. Ultrastructural observations on the spinal cord of a Landrace pig with congenital tremor type AIII. *Res. Vet. Sci.* **1974**, *17*, 174–178. [CrossRef]
18. Patterson, D.S.; Sweasey, D.; Brush, P.J.; Harding, J.D. Neurochemistry of the spinal cord in British Saddleback piglets affected with congenital tremor, type A-IV, a second form of hereditary cerebrospinal hypomyelinogenesis. *J. Neurochem.* **1973**, *21*, 397–406. [CrossRef]
19. Patterson, D.S.; Sweasey, D.; Harding, J.D. Lipid deficiency in the central nervous system of Landrace piglets affected with congenital tremor A3. A form of cerebrospinal hypomyelinogenesis. *J. Neurochem.* **1972**, *19*, 2791–2799. [CrossRef]
20. Bölske, G.; Kronevi, T.; Lindgren, N.O. Congenital tremor in pigs in Sweden. A case report. *Nord. Vet. Med.* **1978**, *30*, 534–537.
21. Knox, B.; Askaa, J.; Basse, A.; Bitsch, V.; Eskildsen, M.; Mandrup, M.; Ottosen, H.E.; Overby, E.; Pedersen, K.B.; Rasmussen, F. Congenital ataxia and tremor with cerebellar hypoplasia in piglets borne by sows treated with Neguvon vet. (metrifonate, trichlorfon) during pregnancy. *Nord. Vet. Med.* **1978**, *30*, 538–545. [PubMed]
22. Smith, D.B.; Meyers, G.; Bukh, J.; Gould, E.A.; Monath, T.; Scott Muerhoff, A.; Pletnev, A.; Rico-Hesse, R.; Stapleton, J.T.; Simmonds, P.; et al. Proposed revision to the taxonomy of the genus Pestivirus, family Flaviviridae. *J. Gen. Virol.* **2017**, *98*, 2106–2112. [CrossRef] [PubMed]
23. Avalos-Ramirez, R.; Orlich, M.; Thiel, H.J.; Becher, P. Evidence for the presence of two novel pestivirus species. *Virology* **2001**, *286*, 456–465. [CrossRef]
24. Becher, P.; Schmeiser, S.; Oguzoglu, T.C.; Postel, A. Complete genome sequence of a novel pestivirus from sheep. *J. Virol.* **2012**, *86*, 11412. [CrossRef] [PubMed]
25. Firth, C.; Bhat, M.; Firth, M.A.; Williams, S.H.; Frye, M.J.; Simmonds, P.; Conte, J.M.; Ng, J.; Garcia, J.; Bhuva, N.P.; et al. Detection of zoonotic pathogens and characterization of novel viruses carried by commensal Rattus norvegicus in New York City. *mBio* **2014**, *5*, e01933-14. [CrossRef] [PubMed]
26. Kirkland, P.D.; Frost, M.J.; Finlaison, D.S.; King, K.R.; Ridpath, J.F.; Gu, X. Identification of a novel virus in pigs—Bungowannah virus: A possible new species of pestivirus. *Virus Res.* **2007**, *129*, 26–34. [CrossRef]
27. Liu, L.; Kampa, J.; Belák, S.; Baule, C. Virus recovery and full-length sequence analysis of atypical bovine pestivirus Th/04_KhonKaen. *Vet. Microbiol.* **2009**, *138*, 62–68. [CrossRef]
28. Neill, J.D.; Ridpath, J.F.; Fischer, N.; Grundhoff, A.; Postel, A.; Becher, P. Complete genome sequence of pronghorn virus, a pestivirus. *Genome Announc.* **2014**, *2*. [CrossRef]
29. Vilcek, S.; Ridpath, J.F.; Van Campen, H.; Cavender, J.L.; Warg, J. Characterization of a novel pestivirus originating from a pronghorn antelope. *Virus Res.* **2005**, *108*, 187–193. [CrossRef]
30. Wu, Z.; Ren, X.; Yang, L.; Hu, Y.; Yang, J.; He, G.; Zhang, J.; Dong, J.; Sun, L.; Du, J.; et al. Virome analysis for identification of novel mammalian viruses in bat species from Chinese provinces. *J. Virol.* **2012**, *86*, 10999–11012. [CrossRef]
31. Sozzi, E.; Lavazza, A.; Gaffuri, A.; Bencetti, F.C.; Prosperi, A.; Lelli, D.; Chiapponi, C.; Moreno, A. Isolation and full-length sequence analysis of a pestivirus from aborted lamb fetuses in Italy. *Viruses* **2019**, *11*, 744. [CrossRef]
32. Hurtado, A.; Aduriz, G.; Gómez, N.; Oporto, B.; Juste, R.A.; Lavin, S.; Lopez-Olvera, J.R.; Marco, I. Molecular identification of a new pestivirus associated with increased mortality in the Pyrenean Chamois (Rupicapra pyrenaica pyrenaica) in Spain. *J. Wildl. Dis.* **2004**, *40*, 796–800. [CrossRef] [PubMed]
33. Colett, M.S.; Larson, R.; Gold, C.; Strick, D.; Anderson, D.K.; Purchio, A.F. Molecular cloning and nucleotide sequence of the pestivirus bovine viral diarrhea virus. *Virology* **1988**, *165*, 191–199. [CrossRef]
34. Ridpath, J.F.; Bolin, S.R. The genomic sequence of a virulent bovine viral diarrhea virus (BVDV) from the type 2 genotype: Detection of a large genomic insertion in a noncytopathic BVDV. *Virology* **1995**, *212*, 39–46. [CrossRef] [PubMed]

35. Ruggli, N.; Moser, C.; Mitchell, D.; Hofmann, M.; Tratschin, J.D. Baculovirus expression and affinity purification of protein E2 of classical swine fever virus strain Alfort/187. *Virus Genes* **1995**, *10*, 115–126. [CrossRef] [PubMed]
36. Becher, P.; Shannon, A.D.; Tautz, N.; Thiel, H.J. Molecular characterization of border disease virus, a pestivirus from sheep. *Virology* **1994**, *198*, 542–551. [CrossRef] [PubMed]
37. International Committee on Taxonomy of Viruses. Virus Taxonomy: 2019 Release. Available online: https://talk.ictvonline.org/taxonomy/ (accessed on 26 May 2020).
38. Liu, J.; Ren, X.; Li, H.; Yu, X.; Zhao, B.; Liu, B.; Ning, Z. Development of the reverse genetics system for emerging atypical porcine pestivirus using in vitro and intracellular transcription systems. *Virus Res.* **2020**, *283*, 197975. [CrossRef] [PubMed]
39. Simmonds, P.; Becher, P.; Bukh, J.; Gould, E.A.; Meyers, G.; Monath, T.; Muerhoff, S.; Pletnev, A.; Rico-Hesse, R.; Smith, D.B.; et al. ICTV virus taxonomy profile: Flaviviridae. *J. Gen. Virol.* **2017**, *98*, 2–3. [CrossRef]
40. Blome, S.; Beer, M.; Wernike, K. New leaves in the growing tree of Pestiviruses. *Adv. Virus Res.* **2017**, *99*, 139–160.
41. Muñoz-González, S.; Canturri, A.; Pérez-Simó, M.; Bohórquez, J.A.; Rosell, R.; Cabezón, O.; Segalés, J.; Domingo, M.; Ganges, L. First report of the novel atypical porcine pestivirus in Spain and a retrospective study. *Transbound. Emerg. Dis.* **2017**, *64*, 1645–1649. [CrossRef]
42. Shen, H.; Liu, X.; Zhang, P.; Wang, L.; Liu, Y.; Zhang, L.; Liang, P.; Song, C. Identification and characterization of atypical porcine pestivirus genomes in newborn piglets with congenital tremor in China. *J. Vet. Sci.* **2018**, *19*, 468–471. [CrossRef] [PubMed]
43. Sozzi, E.; Salogni, C.; Lelli, D.; Barbieri, I.; Moreno, A.; Alborali, G.L.; Lavazza, A. Molecular survey and phylogenetic analysis of Atypical Porcine Pestivirus (APPV) identified in swine and wild boar from Northern Italy. *Viruses* **2019**, *11*, 1142. [CrossRef]
44. Yan, X.L.; Li, Y.Y.; He, L.L.; Wu, J.L.; Tang, X.Y.; Chen, G.H.; Mai, K.J.; Wu, R.T.; Li, Q.N.; Chen, Y.H.; et al. 12 novel atypical porcine pestivirus genomes from neonatal piglets with congenital tremors: A newly emerging branch and high prevalence in China. *Virology* **2019**, *533*, 50–58. [CrossRef] [PubMed]
45. Papatsiros, V.G. The splay leg syndrome in piglets: A review. *American J. Anim. Vet. Sci.* **2012**, *7*, 80–83.
46. Liu, J.; Li, Z.; Ren, X.; Li, H.; Lu, R.; Zhang, Y.; Ning, Z. Viral load and histological distribution of atypical porcine pestivirus in different tissues of naturally infected piglets. *Arch. Virol.* **2019**, *164*, 2519–2523. [CrossRef]
47. Yuan, J.; Han, Z.; Li, J.; Huang, Y.; Yang, J.; Ding, H.; Zhang, J.; Zhu, M.; Zhang, Y.; Liao, J.; et al. Atypical Porcine Pestivirus as a novel type of pestivirus in pigs in China. *Front. Microbiol.* **2017**, *8*, 862. [CrossRef]
48. Mósena, A.C.S.; Weber, M.N.; da Cruz, R.A.S.; Cibulski, S.P.; da Silva, M.S.; Puhl, D.E.; Hammerschmitt, M.E.; Takeuti, K.L.; Driemeier, D.; de Barcellos, D.; et al. Presence of atypical porcine pestivirus (APPV) in Brazilian pigs. *Transbound. Emerg. Dis.* **2018**, *65*, 22–26. [CrossRef]
49. Possatti, F.; de Oliveira, T.E.S.; Leme, R.A.; Zotti, E.; Dall Agnol, A.M.; Alfieri, A.F.; Headley, S.A.; Alfieri, A.A. Pathologic and molecular findings associated with atypical porcine pestivirus infection in newborn piglets. *Vet. Microbiol.* **2018**, *227*, 41–44. [CrossRef]
50. Schwarz, L.; Riedel, C.; Högler, S.; Sinn, L.J.; Voglmayr, T.; Wöchtl, B.; Dinhopl, N.; Rebel-Bauder, B.; Weissenböck, H.; Ladinig, A.; et al. Congenital infection with atypical porcine pestivirus (APPV) is associated with disease and viral persistence. *Vet. Res.* **2017**, *48*, 1. [CrossRef]
51. Sutton, K.M.; Lahmers, K.K.; Harris, S.P.; Wijesena, H.R.; Mote, B.E.; Kachman, S.D.; Borza, T.; Ciobanu, D.C. Detection of atypical porcine pestivirus genome in newborn piglets affected by congenital tremor and high preweaning mortality. *J. Anim. Sci.* **2019**, *97*, 4093–4100. [CrossRef]
52. Dessureault, F.G.; Choinière, M.; Provost, C.; Gagnon, C.A. First report of atypical porcine pestivirus in piglets with congenital tremor in Canada. *Can. Vet. J.* **2018**, *59*, 429–432. [PubMed]
53. Postel, A.; Hansmann, F.; Baechlein, C.; Fischer, N.; Alawi, M.; Grundhoff, A.; Derking, S.; Tenhündfeld, J.; Pfankuche, V.M.; Herder, V.; et al. Presence of atypical porcine pestivirus (APPV) genomes in newborn piglets correlates with congenital tremor. *Sci. Rep.* **2016**, *6*, 27735. [CrossRef] [PubMed]
54. Gatto, I.R.H.; Arruda, P.H.; Visek, C.A.; Victoria, J.G.; Patterson, A.R.; Krull, A.C.; Schwartz, K.J.; de Oliveira, L.G.; Arruda, B.L. Detection of atypical porcine pestivirus in semen from commercial boar studs in the United States. *Transbound. Emerg. Dis.* **2018**, *65*, e339–e343. [CrossRef]

55. Cagatay, G.N.; Meyer, D.; Wendt, M.; Becher, P.; Postel, A. Characterization of the humoral immune response induced after infection with Atypical Porcine Pestivirus (APPV). *Viruses* **2019**, *11*, 880. [CrossRef] [PubMed]
56. Chen, F.; Knutson, T.P.; Braun, E.; Jiang, Y.; Rossow, S.; Marthaler, D.G. Semi-quantitative duplex RT-PCR reveals the low occurrence of Porcine Pegivirus and Atypical Porcine Pestivirus in diagnostic samples from the United States. *Transbound. Emerg. Dis.* **2019**, *66*, 1420–1425. [CrossRef]
57. Beer, M.; Wernike, K.; Dräger, C.; Höper, D.; Pohlmann, A.; Bergermann, C.; Schröder, C.; Klinkhammer, S.; Blome, S.; Hoffmann, B. High prevalence of highly variable atypical porcine pestiviruses found in Germany. *Transbound. Emerg. Dis.* **2017**, *64*, e22–e26. [CrossRef]
58. Cagatay, G.N.; Antos, A.; Meyer, D.; Maistrelli, C.; Keuling, O.; Becher, P.; Postel, A. Frequent infection of wild boar with atypical porcine pestivirus (APPV). *Transbound. Emerg. Dis.* **2018**, *65*, 1087–1093. [CrossRef]
59. Michelitsch, A.; Dalmann, A.; Wernike, K.; Reimann, I.; Beer, M. Seroprevalences of newly discovered porcine pestiviruses in German pig farms. *Vet. Sci.* **2019**, *6*, 86. [CrossRef]
60. Pfankuche, V.M.; Hahn, K.; Bodewes, R.; Hansmann, F.; Habierski, A.; Haverkamp, A.K.; Pfaender, S.; Walter, S.; Baechlein, C.; Postel, A.; et al. Comparison of different In Situ Hybridization techniques for the detection of various RNA and DNA viruses. *Viruses* **2018**, *10*, 384. [CrossRef]
61. Postel, A.; Meyer, D.; Cagatay, G.N.; Feliziani, F.; De Mia, G.M.; Fischer, N.; Grundhoff, A.; Milićević, V.; Deng, M.C.; Chang, C.Y.; et al. High abundance and genetic variability of Atypical Porcine Pestivirus in pigs from Europe and Asia. *Emerg. Infect. Dis.* **2017**, *23*, 2104–2107. [CrossRef]
62. Blomström, A.L.; Fossum, C.; Wallgren, P.; Berg, M. Viral metagenomic analysis displays the co-infection situation in healthy and PMWS affected pigs. *PLoS ONE* **2016**, *11*, e0166863. [CrossRef]
63. Williamson, S. Congenital tremor associated with atypical porcine pestivirus. *Vet. Rec.* **2017**, *180*, 42–43.
64. Zhang, K.; Wu, K.; Liu, J.; Ge, S.; Xiao, Y.; Shang, Y.; Ning, Z. Identification of atypical porcine pestivirus infection in swine herds in China. *Transbound. Emerg. Dis.* **2017**, *64*, 1020–1023. [CrossRef]
65. Guo, Z.; Wang, L.; Qiao, S.; Deng, R.; Zhang, G. Genetic characterization and recombination analysis of atypical porcine pestivirus. *Infect. Genet. Evol.* **2020**, *81*, 104259. [CrossRef]
66. Pan, S.; Yan, Y.; Shi, K.; Wang, M.; Mou, C.; Chen, Z. Molecular characterization of two novel atypical porcine pestivirus (APPV) strains from piglets with congenital tremor in China. *Transbound. Emerg. Dis.* **2019**, *66*, 35–42. [CrossRef]
67. Wang, X.; Xie, Y.; He, D.; Yan, H. Near-complete genome sequence of a newly emerging subgenotype of Atypical porcine pestivirus. *Microbiol. Resour. Announc.* **2020**, *9*. [CrossRef]
68. Wu, Z.; Liu, B.; Du, J.; Zhang, J.; Lu, L.; Zhu, G.; Han, Y.; Su, H.; Yang, L.; Zhang, S.; et al. Discovery of diverse rodent and bat pestiviruses with distinct genomic and phylogenetic characteristics in several Chinese provinces. *Front. Microbiol.* **2018**, *9*, 2562. [CrossRef]
69. Xie, Y.; Wang, X.; Su, D.; Feng, J.; Wei, L.; Cai, W.; Li, J.; Lin, S.; Yan, H.; He, D. Detection and genetic characterization of Atypical Porcine Pestivirus in Piglets with congenital tremors in Southern China. *Front. Microbiol.* **2019**, *10*, 1406. [CrossRef]
70. Yin, Y.; Shi, K.; Sun, W.; Mo, S. Complete genome sequence of an Atypical Porcine Pestivirus strain, GX01-2018, from Guangxi Province, China. *Microbiol. Resour. Announc.* **2019**, *8*. [CrossRef]
71. Zhang, H.; Wen, W.; Hao, G.; Hu, Y.; Chen, H.; Qian, P.; Li, X. Phylogenetic and genomic characterization of a novel atypical porcine pestivirus in China. *Transbound. Emerg. Dis.* **2018**, *65*, e202–e204. [CrossRef]
72. Zhang, X.; Dai, R.; Li, Q.; Zhou, Q.; Luo, Y.; Lin, L.; Bi, Y.; Chen, F. Detection of three novel atypical porcine pestivirus strains in newborn piglets with congenital tremor in southern China. *Infect. Genet. Evol.* **2019**, *68*, 54–57. [CrossRef] [PubMed]
73. Zhou, K.; Yue, H.; Tang, C.; Ruan, W.; Zhou, Q.; Zhang, B. Prevalence and genome characteristics of atypical porcine pestivirus in southwest China. *J. Gen. Virol.* **2019**, *100*, 84–88. [CrossRef]
74. Colom-Cadena, A.; Ganges, L.; Muñoz-González, S.; Castillo-Contreras, R.; Bohórquez, J.A.; Rosell, R.; Segalés, J.; Marco, I.; Cabezon, O. Atypical porcine pestivirus in wild boar (Sus scrofa), Spain. *Vet. Rec.* **2018**, *183*, 569. [CrossRef] [PubMed]
75. Kim, S.; Jeong, C.; Yoon, S.; Lee, K.; Yang, M.; Kim, B.; Lee, S.; Kang, S.; Kim, W. Detection of atypical porcine pestivirus (APPV) from a case of congenital tremor in Korea. *Korean J. Vet. Serv.* **2017**, *40*, 209–213.
76. Gatto, I.R.H.; Harmon, K.; Bradner, L.; Silva, P.; Linhares, D.C.L.; Arruda, P.H.; de Oliveira, L.G.; Arruda, B.L. Detection of atypical porcine pestivirus in Brazil in the central nervous system of suckling piglets with congenital tremor. *Transbound. Emerg. Dis.* **2018**, *65*, 375–380. [CrossRef] [PubMed]

77. Kaufmann, C.; Stalder, H.; Sidler, X.; Renzullo, S.; Gurtner, C.; Grahofer, A.; Schweizer, M. Long-term circulation of Atypical Porcine Pestivirus (APPV) within Switzerland. *Viruses* **2019**, *11*, 653. [CrossRef]
78. Dénes, L.; Biksi, I.; Albert, M.; Szeredi, L.; Knapp, D.G.; Szilasi, A.; Bálint, Á.; Balka, G. Detection and phylogenetic characterization of atypical porcine pestivirus strains in Hungary. *Transbound. Emerg. Dis.* **2018**, *65*, 2039–2042. [CrossRef]
79. Moennig, V. The control of classical swine fever in wild boar. *Front. Microbiol.* **2015**, *6*, 1211. [CrossRef]
80. Ridpath, J. Preventive strategy for BVDV infection in North America. *Jpn. J. Vet. Res.* **2012**, *60*, S41–S49.
81. Zhang, H.; Wen, W.; Hao, G.; Chen, H.; Qian, P.; Li, X. A subunit vaccine based on E2 protein of atypical porcine pestivirus induces Th2-type immune response in mice. *Viruses* **2018**, *10*, 673. [CrossRef]

11

Infection of Ruminants, Including Pregnant Cattle, with Bungowannah Virus

Andrew J. Read, Deborah S. Finlaison and Peter D. Kirkland *

Virology Laboratory, Elizabeth Macarthur Agriculture Institute, Woodbridge Road, Menangle, New South Wales 2568, Australia; andrew.j.read@dpi.nsw.gov.au (A.J.R.); deborah.finlaison@dpi.nsw.gov.au (D.S.F.)

* Correspondence: peter.kirkland@dpi.nsw.gov.au.

Abstract: Bungowannah virus is a pestivirus known to cause reproductive losses in pigs. The virus has not been found in other species, nor is it known if it has the capacity to cause disease in other animals. Eight sheep, eight calves and seven pregnant cows were experimentally infected with Bungowannah virus. It was found that sheep and calves could be infected. Furthermore, it was shown that the virus is able to cross the bovine placenta and cause infection of the foetus. These findings demonstrate the potential for species other than pigs to become infected with Bungowannah virus and the need to prevent them from becoming infected.

Keywords: Bungowannah virus; pestivirus F; ruminant infection

1. Introduction

In June 2003 a syndrome of sudden death in sucker pigs, followed by a marked increase in stillborn foetuses and pre-weaning losses, occurred on a large farm in NSW, Australia [1]. Myocarditis and myonecrosis were also observed in affected pigs. A novel pestivirus, known as Bungowannah virus, was subsequently identified [2]. A series of field and laboratory studies have provided strong evidence that Bungowannah virus is the aetiological agent in this disease [2–8]. Bungowannah virus contains all of the genomic and structural elements of classically described pestiviruses, yet phylogenetic analysis demonstrates that it is genetically remote from any of the other pestivirus species [9,10]. Bungowannah virus is the only extant isolate of *pestivirus F* species [10].

Pestiviruses were initially classified according to their host specificity. Whilst this classification was originally appropriate for classical swine fever virus (CSFV), it was soon shown that bovine viral diarrhea virus (BVDV) and border disease virus (BDV) could naturally infect a variety of ruminants, pigs and other mammals. Recently, CSFV has also been shown to naturally infect cattle [11]. In contrast, Bungowannah virus has only ever been detected in pigs. The origin of this virus is not known, nor what threat it may pose to other species. Bungowannah virus has been shown to replicate in ovine and bovine cells in vitro [12] and so the possibility that it may infect ruminants has been raised. This paper documents the outcome of experimental infections of sheep and cattle with Bungowannah virus. Patterns of virus shedding and pathology are described.

2. Materials and Methods

A series of inoculation experiments were conducted in both sheep and cattle. Cattle were either directly inoculated using intranasal instillation or by co-housing with pigs that were chronically infected with Bungowannah virus. Sheep were either directly inoculated using intranasal instillation or subcutaneous injection or by co-housing with pigs that were chronically infected with Bungowannah virus. The specific details are as follows:

2.1. *Virus Amplification*

The inoculum used for each of the direct inoculation experiments was derived from pooled pig foetal tissues that were passaged once in PK-15 cells (RIE5–1, Collection of Cell Lines in Veterinary Medicine, Friedrich-Loeffler-Institut, Insel Riems, Germany). The titre of infectious virus was also determined by titration in PK-15 cells using standard methods.

2.2. *Viral Transport Medium*

Swabs were collected into 3 mL of sterile phosphate buffered saline (137 mM NaCl, 8 mM Na_2HPO_4, 2.7 mM KCl and 1.5 mM KH_2PO_4, pH 7.4) containing 0.5% gelatin (*w*/*v*), 5000 IU penicillin/mL, 95,000 IU streptomycin, 50 µg/mL amphotericin B and 0.1% (*w*/*v*) phenol red (PBGS).

2.3. *Bungowannah Virus Real-Time Polymerase Chain Reaction (qRT-PCR)*

Bungowannah virus RNA was identified from samples using a real-time, reverse transcription PCR (qRT-PCR). The method has been previously described [3]. The fluorescence threshold was set manually at 0.05 and the background was automatically adjusted. qRT-PCR results were expressed as cycle threshold (Ct) values and classified as negative if no amplification was observed after the 45 cycles. For quantification, a 10-fold dilution series of Bungowannah virus RNA standards ranging from 10^7 to 10^2 RNA copies/5 µL [6] was included in the assay and the quantity of Bungowannah virus RNA in a sample was determined from the standard curve.

2.4. *Bungowannah Virus Neutralisation Test*

Antibody titres against Bungowannah virus were measured by virus neutralisation test (VNT). The VNT was performed as described previously [5]. Selected serum samples were tested in the VNT in a two-fold dilution series commencing at 1/4.

2.5. *Infection of Sheep*

Sheep used in these trials were obtained from a flock that was free of infection with ruminant pestiviruses and had not been vaccinated against pestiviruses. All sheep were tested for anti-pestivirus antibodies using a bovine viral diarrhea virus agarose gel immunodiffusion assay [13] and were found to be negative.

2.5.1. Direct Inoculation

Six 3-month-old Merino lambs were infected intranasally with 2 mL of cell culture amplified Bungowannah virus (5.6 $\log_{10}$ $TCID_{50}$/mL). Two other sheep were inoculated with the same dose subcutaneously while another two other sheep were held as uninfected controls. The inoculated sheep were held in two 11 m^2 rooms (four intranasally infected sheep in one room, the remaining four infected sheep in the other room). The two uninfected sheep were held in a similar 11 m^2 room and were not challenged.

Conjunctival, nasal, oral and rectal swabs, along with serum samples, were collected from all sheep prior to exposure to Bungowannah virus and daily for 14 days. Blood samples were subsequently collected approximately weekly until 6 weeks post-exposure. Clinical signs, including rectal temperatures, were also recorded daily for the first 14 days. The swabs and sera were tested for the presence of Bungowannah virus using real-time PCR (qRT-PCR). Serum samples were tested for the presence of antibodies against Bungowannah virus using a VNT.

2.5.2. Exposure to Chronically Infected Pigs

Four 3-month-old Merino lambs were held in a small room (16 m^2) with three pigs that were chronically infected with Bungowannah virus. The pigs (08-01, 08-05 and 10-01) had been infected in utero and were shown to be shedding Bungowannah virus (oropharyngeal secretions—6.9, 7.0 and

3.4 log_{10} copies/swab, respectively) 7 days prior to the trial [7]. The sheep and the pigs were co-housed for 48 h. During this time there were two periods of six hours of direct physical contact between the sheep and pigs. During the remainder of the time the pigs were separated from the sheep by a mesh partition which allowed for limited direct contact. The clinical examination and sampling were conducted as described above.

2.6. Infection of Calves

Calves used in the following trials were obtained from a herd that was free of infection with ruminant pestiviruses and had not been vaccinated against pestiviruses. All calves were tested for anti-pestivirus antibodies using a bovine viral diarrhea virus agarose gel immunodiffusion assay [13] and were found to be negative.

2.6.1. Direct Inoculation

Eight 10-week-old Holstein–Friesian calves were infected intranasally with 2 mL of cell culture-amplified Bungowannah virus (5.6 log_{10} $TCID_{50}$/mL). Two additional calves were held as uninfected controls and did not receive a challenge. The conditions under which they were held, the clinical examination and sampling were conducted as described above for the sheep.

2.6.2. Exposure to Chronically Infected Pigs

Four 5-week-old Holstein–Friesian calves were held with two pigs (08-01 and 08-05; oropharyngeal secretions 5.5 and 7.1 log_{10} copies/swab respectively, 6 days prior to trial) [7] chronically infected with Bungowannah virus. The conditions under which they were held, the clinical examination and sampling were conducted as described above for the sheep.

2.7. Infection of Pregnant Cows

Five pregnant Holstein-Friesian and two Illawarra-Shorthorn cows were chosen for the trial. They were obtained from a herd known to be free of infection with ruminant pestiviruses and had not been vaccinated against pestiviruses. All cows were tested for anti-pestivirus antibodies using a bovine viral diarrhea virus agarose gel immunodiffusion assay [13] and found to be negative. They were infected by intranasal instillation of 2 mL of the cell culture amplified Bungowannah virus (4.5 log_{10} TCID/mL). Cows were between 53 and 65 days of pregnancy at the time of inoculation. Nasal and conjunctival swabs and serum samples were collected daily for 14 days following inoculation. The swabs and sera were tested for the presence of Bungowannah virus using qRT-PCR. Serum samples were then collected monthly until calving and were tested for antibodies against Bungowannah virus using a VNT. Pregnancy was monitored by ultrasound examination on a monthly basis. Cows were induced to calve between 255 and 276 days of pregnancy. Serum samples were collected from each calf after birth and prior to suckling. Conjunctival, nasal, oral and rectal swabs and serum samples were collected from calves every 48–72 h for 14 days. Vaginal swabs were also collected from the cows post-partum. A post-mortem examination of the calves was performed between 2 and 4 weeks of age. A wide range of tissues including brain, myocardium and skin (and testicle from a male) were tested for the presence of Bungowannah virus by qRT-PCR. Samples for qRT-PCR were collected by firmly rubbing a swab across the freshly cut surface of a section of the tissue and placed into 3 mL of PBGS. Skin biopsies were stored in 3 mL PBGS. All samples were stored at 4 °C until tested by qRT-PCR and virus isolation.

2.8. Animal Ethics Approval

The trials described in this paper were approved by the Elizabeth Macarthur Agricultural Institute Animal Ethics Committee. The specific approvals were AEC M09/17 "Studies of the biology of Bungowannah virus infections (PMC) in sheep and cattle" (7 December 2009) and AEC M10/16 "Effects of Bungowannah virus infection in pregnant cattle" (22 December 2010).

3. Results

3.1. Infection of Sheep

3.1.1. Direct Inoculation

Bungowannah virus RNA was detected between days four and 11 in the nasal swabs of five of the six sheep exposed by intranasal instillation. Ct values ranged between 27.9 and 39.9 (Table 1). Low levels of Bungowannah virus RNA were sporadically detected between days three and 13 of infection in serum samples from four of the six intranasally inoculated sheep. Ct values ranged between 36.5 and 38.1. Two of these sheep had Bungowannah virus RNA detected in serum on three occasions (Table 1).

Table 1. Bungowannah virus qRT-PCR results from sheep intranasally and subcutaneously inoculated.

		Days Post Inoculation														
Sheep	**Sample**	**0**	**1**	**2**	**3**	**4**	**5**	**6**	**7**	**8**	**9**	**10**	**11**	**12**	**13**	**14**
1N	Nasal	-	-	-	-	36.8	-	-	33.3	-	37.6	34.3	34.1	-	-	-
	Serum	-	-	-	-	-	-	37.1	-	37.8	-	-	36.5	-	-	-
2N	Nasal	-	-	-	-	36.0	36.6	32.6	-	34.5	32.2	37.4	37.5	-	-	-
	Serum	-	-	-	-	-	-	-	-	37.7	-	-	-	-	-	-
3N	Nasal	-	-	-	-	30.0	32.3	27.9	29.1	29.6	34.2	39.9	-	-	-	-
	Serum	-	-	-	37.2	-	-	-	-	-	-	-	-	-	-	-
4N	Nasal	-	-	-	-	29.4	-	34.2	31.1	-	30.5	-	38.4	-	-	-
	Serum	-	-	-	-	-	-	-	38.1	-	36.6	-	-	-	37.1	-
5N	Nasal	-	-	-	-	-	33.2	-	-	-	-	-	-	-	-	-
	Serum	-	-	-	-	-	-	-	-	-	-	-	-	-	-	-
6N	Nasal	-	-	-	-	-	-	-	-	-	-	-	-	-	-	-
	Serum	-	-	-	-	-	-	-	-	-	-	-	-	-	-	-
7S	Nasal	-	-	-	-	-	-	-	-	-	-	-	-	-	-	-
	Serum	-	-	-	-	-	-	-	-	-	-	-	-	-	-	-
8S	Nasal	-	-	-	-	-	-	-	-	-	-	-	-	-	-	-
	Serum	-	-	-	-	-	-	-	-	-	-	-	-	-	-	-
9C	Nasal	-	-	-	-	-	-	-	-	-	-	-	-	-	-	-
	Serum	-	-	-	-	-	-	-	-	-	-	-	-	-	-	-
10C	Nasal	-	-	-	-	-	-	-	-	-	-	-	-	-	-	-
	Serum	-	-	-	-	-	-	-	-	-	-	-	-	-	-	-

A dash indicates that Bungowannah virus RNA was not detected.

Bungowannah viral RNA was not detected in oral, conjunctival or rectal swabs of any of the inoculated or control sheep, nor in serum or nasal swabs for the control sheep or those inoculated subcutaneously. None of the infected sheep developed clinical signs during the course of the infection. The rectal temperatures remained within normal limits. All eight sheep directly inoculated (either intranasally or subcutaneously) developed Bungowannah virus-specific antibodies (Table 2).

Table 2. Bungowannah VN titres from sheep intranasally and subcutaneously inoculated.

Sheep	Route of Infection	Days Post Inoculation 0	9	15	21	29	36	43
1N	Intranasal	-	-	256	128	256	256	256
2N	Intranasal	-	-	-	32	32	32	64
3N	Intranasal	-	-	64	64	128	128	128
4N	Intranasal	-	-	-	64	128	64	256
5N	Intranasal	-	-	-	64	256	512	256
6N	Intranasal	-	-	-	32	128	128	64
7S	Subcutaneous	-	-	-	128	256	256	256
8S	Subcutaneous	-	-	64	256	256	256	256
9C	Uninfected	-	-	-	-	-	-	-
10C	Uninfected	-	-	-	-	-	-	-

A dash indicates that neutralising anti-Bungowannah virus antibodies were not detected.

3.1.2. Exposure to Chronically Infected Pigs

Viral RNA was detected only in the nasal swabs of three of the four sheep during the period of co-mingling with the chronically infected pigs. The Ct values ranged from 36.1 to 36.4. Bungowannah virus RNA was not detected in serum or any other swabs during this time and was not detected in serum or any swabs after the pigs were removed from the room. None of the sheep developed Bungowannah virus-specific antibodies.

3.2. *Infection of Calves*

3.2.1. Direct Inoculation

Bungowannah virus RNA was detected in nasal swabs of all eight calves on at least three occasions between days two and 11 (Table 3). Viral RNA was detected sporadically in serum samples from six of these eight calves between days five and 10 of infection and intermittently in the oral swabs from four calves between days four and eight. Bungowannah virus was not detected in any rectal swabs. All eight directly inoculated calves developed antibodies directed against Bungowannah virus by 14 days post-inoculation (Table 4). A very mild nasal discharge was observed in five of the challenged calves. The rectal temperatures remained within normal limits.

Table 3. Bungowannah virus qRT-PCR results from calves intranasally inoculated.

Calf	Sample	Days Post Inoculation 0	1	2	3	4	5	6	7	8	9	10	11	12	13	14
1N	Nasal	-	-	-	-	-	-	27.5	34.5	32.5	-	-	-	-	-	-
	Oral	-	-	-	-	-	-	37.6	37.7	-	-	-	-	-	-	-
	Serum	-	-	-	-	-	-	-	-	-	-	-	-	-	-	-
2N	Nasal	-	-	34.5	30.4	31.8	31.5	28.1	28.4	-	-	-	-	-	-	-
	Oral	-	-	-	-	-	-	-	-	-	-	-	-	-	-	-
	Serum	-	-	-	-	-	-	-	35.9	-	-	-	-	-	-	-
3N	Nasal	-	-	-	-	-	33.9	30.5	31.2	-	37.9	-	-	-	-	-
	Oral	-	-	-	-	-	-	-	-	-	-	-	-	-	-	-
	Serum	-	-	-	-	-	-	-	37.7	-	-	-	-	-	-	-
4N	Nasal	-	-	37.0	32.1	-	-	33.0	30.0	32.8	31.2	-	-	-	-	-
	Oral	-	-	-	-	-	-	-	-	-	-	-	-	-	-	-
	Serum	-	-	-	-	-	35.7	-	-	37.5	35.7	-	-	-	-	-
5N	Nasal	-	-	33.9	30.2	31.4	27.6	27.1	28.4	29.3	35.2	-	-	-	-	-
	Oral	-	-	-	-	-	-	36.7	-	-	-	-	-	-	-	-
	Serum	-	-	-	-	-	-	-	-	-	-	-	-	-	-	-

Table 3. *Cont.*

Calf	Sample	Days Post Inoculation 0	1	2	3	4	5	6	7	8	9	10	11	12	13	14
6N	Nasal	-	-	36.2	34.1	-	31.0	29.7	30.7	27.6	33.6	-	37.4	-	-	-
	Oral	-	-	-	-	-	-	-	-	-	-	-	-	-	-	-
	Serum	-	-	-	-	-	36.3	-	36.3	36.0	37.6	-	-	-	-	-
7N	Nasal	-	-		33.1	31.4	32.5	30.1	29.2	29.7	-	-	-	-	-	-
	Oral	-	-	-	-	36.6		36.6	-	-	-	-	-	-	-	-
	Serum	-	-	-	-	-	-	37.3	36.4		36.5	37.7	-	-	-	-
8N	Nasal	-	-	-	-	31.7	31.6	30.3	31.4	33.4	-	-	-	-	-	-
	Oral	-	-	-	-	-	-	-	-	37.5	-	-	-	-	-	-
	Serum	-	-	-	-	-	37.3	-	-	-	-	-	-	-	-	-
9C	Nasal	-	-	-	-	-	-	-	-	-	-	-	-	-	-	-
	Oral	-	-	-	-	-	-	-	-	-	-	-	-	-	-	-
	Serum	-	-	-	-	-	-	-	-	-	-	-	-	-	-	-
10C	Nasal	-	-	-	-	-	-	-	-	-	-	-	-	-	-	-
	Oral	-	-	-	-	-	-	-	-	-	-	-	-	-	-	-
	Serum	-	-	-	-	-	-	-	-	-	-	-	-	-	-	-

A dash indicates that Bungowannah virus RNA was not detected. Calves 9C and 10C were uninfected.

Table 4. Bungowannah VN titres from calves intranasally inoculated.

Calf	Route of Infection	Days Post Inoculation 0	7	14	21	28	35	42	49
1N	Intranasal	-	-	16	512	1024	2048	2048	4096
2N	Intranasal	-	-	64	256	1024	2048	2048	2048
3N	Intranasal	-	-	32	256	1024	4096	8192	4096
4N	Intranasal	-	-	64	2048	2048	16,384	8192	2048
5N	Intranasal	-	-	32	128	512	2048	1024	4096
6N	Intranasal	-	-	16	1024	256	2048	8192	4096
7N	Intranasal	-	-	128	1024	4096	16,384	32,768	32,768
8N	Intranasal	-	-	16	128	1024	2048	4096	8192
9C	Uninfected	-	-	-	-	-	-	-	-
10C	Uninfected	-	-	-	-	-	-	-	-

A dash indicates that neutralising anti-Bungowannah virus antibodies were not detected. Calves 9C and 10C were uninfected.

3.2.2. Exposure to Chronically Infected Pigs

Viral RNA was detected in the nasal swabs of two of the four calves during the 48 h that they were housed in contact with chronically infected pigs. The virus was detected in the oral swab of another calf on day two and the nasal swab of this same calf on day eight. This calf was the only one of the four to develop antibodies against Bungowannah virus. Neutralising antibodies were first detected 16 days post-exposure. The antibody titre in this calf peaked at 2048 between 63 and 84 days post-inoculation. Bungowannah viral RNA was not detected in any other samples collected. Calves remained healthy throughout the study.

3.3. Infection of Pregnant Cows

Each of the seven cows inoculated with Bungowannah virus were found to shed Bungowannah virus RNA in nasal secretions. Shedding began in most cows at day three, with peak virus shedding between days seven and 10. One cow was still shedding viral RNA in nasal secretions on day 14 (Table 5). Bungowannah virus RNA was not detected in conjunctival swabs but was detected in the serum of four of the seven cows for a period of one to three days. No signs of respiratory disease or pyrexia were observed in the cows.

Table 5. qRT-PCR results for pregnant cows infected with Bungowannah virus.

Cow		Days Post Inoculation														
		0	1	2	3	4	5	6	7	8	9	10	11	12	13	14
1	Nasal	-	-	-	36.6	-	31.8	33.9	33.6	30.2	31.0	31.6	32.7	-	-	
	Serum	-	-	-	-	-	-	-	-	-	33.4	35.5	35.0	-	-	-
2	Nasal	-	-	-	30.5	35.6	30.9	36.2	28.7	29.3	27.8	31.8	34.0	34.3	-	-
	Serum	-	-	-	-	-	-	-	-	-	-	-	-	-	-	-
3	Nasal	-	-	-	35.6	36.0	-	37.4	35.4	33.2	33.6	31.8	34.6	35.4	-	-
	Serum	-	-	-	-	-	-	-	-	36.8	-	-	-	-	-	-
4	Nasal	-	-	-	-	34.3	34.0	29.8	28.5	28.5	33.1	-	37.4	-	-	-
	Serum	-	-	-	-	-	-	37.9	27.2	34.0	37.5	-	-	-	-	-
5	Nasal	-	-	-	-	-	-	37.4	36.3	-	-	-	37.8	36.4	34.7	32.2
	Serum	-	-	-	-	-	-	-	-	-	-	-	-	-	-	-
6	Nasal	-	-	-	37.3	31.8	36.7	35.8	31.1	32.1	-	-	-	-	-	-
	Serum	-	-	-	-	-	-	-	-	-	-	-	-	-	-	36.5
7	Nasal	-	37.4	35.4	36.2	-	33.4	32.2	29.7	30.5	27.2	31.8	35.6	-	-	-
	Serum	-	-	-	-	-	-	-	-	-	-	-	-	-	-	-

A dash indicates that Bungowannah virus RNA was not detected.

All cows developed neutralising antibodies against Bungowannah virus (Table 6). One cow had developed antibodies by day 11, and the remainder by day 14. Titres peaked on day 44 post infection. Neutralising antibody was detected for the duration of the pregnancy for all cows. A biphasic antibody titre developed in Cow 3 with a peak of 2048 on days 37 and 44, a decline to 512 on days 66 and 100, and then a rise to 1024 on day 128 and 2048 on day 163.

Table 6. Bungowannah VN titres from pregnant cows intranasally inoculated.

Cow	Days Post Inoculation												
	0	7	11	14	21	31	37	44	52	66	100	128	163
1	-	-	-	32	1024	2048	4096	4096	2048	1024	1024	512	1024
2	-	-	-	32	128	512	512	1024	256	512	512	256	128
3	-	-	-	8	256	512	2048	2048	1024	512	512	1024	2048
4	-	-	-	8	128	512	1024	2048	512	512	512	512	256
5	-	-	8	8	128	512	256	256	128	512	128	256	64
6	-	-	-	8	128	512	512	1024	512	NT	2048	512	1024
7	-	-	-	16	16	64	64	64	64	64	64	64	32

A dash indicates that neutralising anti-Bungowannah virus antibodies were not detected.

Pregnancies in the cows were unremarkable with no abnormalities were detected by ultrasound. At birth and before suckling three of the seven calves were found to have antibodies against Bungowannah virus. Bungowannah virus RNA was also detected in ear skin biopsy samples from these same three calves, with Ct values of 26.0, 32.7 and 33.6. The calf with the highest RNA concentration (lowest Ct value) was the progeny of Cow 3. Bungowannah virus RNA was also detected in the serum of this calf. Viral RNA was not detected in conjunctival, oral, nasal or rectal swabs. All calves appeared normal at birth and displayed normal behaviour. The virus was detected in the vaginal swabs from dams of the three positive calves, but not from the other cows. Cow 3 had a Ct value of 30.4, while the other two were 35.8 and 36.6.

Post-mortem examination of all calves was unremarkable, with no gross abnormalities detected. The three calves found to have Bungowannah virus RNA in the skin at birth were euthanased and necropsied at four weeks of age. Viral RNA was again detected in the skin of these calves, and also detected in the testicle of the single male calf among these three (Table 7). Viral RNA was not detected in any other tissues (oesophagus, stomach, duodenum, jejunum, ileum, caecum, colon, liver, bile, mesenteric lymph node, tracheobronchial lymph node, prescapular lymph node, tonsil, thymus, spleen, trachea, lung, thyroid, adrenal gland, kidney, urine, epididymis, ovary, uterus, skeletal muscle, bone marrow, myocardium, cortex, cerebellum or medulla). Virus isolation was attempted on all qRT-PCR positive samples but was not successful.

Table 7. Summary of laboratory results for progeny of cows infected with Bungowannah virus.

Calf	Gestational Age at Infection (Days)	Gestational Age at Birth (Days)	Skin (Copies/mL)	Serum (Copies/mL)	Testicle (Copies/mL)	VNT
1	63	274	1.5×10^6	-	Female	>512
2	65	276	8.1×10^4	-	Female	>512
3	65	276	2.4×10^7	5.0×10^2	6.4×10^5	>512
4	65	274	-	-	-	-
5	65	276	-	-	-	-
6	63	274	-	-	-	-
7	53	255	-	-	Female	-

A dash indicates that a result was undetected. Calf numbers correspond to cow numbers.

4. Discussion

In this study we have demonstrated that Bungowannah virus can infect a proportion of both cattle and sheep after intranasal or subcutaneous inoculation, although infection was less efficient by the intra-nasal route when compared to pigs [5]. Additionally, viral RNA was detected sporadically at low levels in the serum of a proportion of infected sheep and cattle. These results suggest that following intra-nasal or subcutaneous exposure, the infection is predominantly localized. Systemic infection, as determined by the detection of viraemia, only occurred in a proportion of infections.

No significant disease was observed in the infected sheep and cattle, despite all the intranasally infected cattle shedding Bungowannah virus RNA in nasal swabs for up to two weeks after infection. The qRT-PCR results indicated that only low levels of virus were shed. The pattern of detection of RNA was consistent with virus replication rather than residual inoculum as there was a short period after inoculation when no RNA was detected. Similarly, viral RNA was detected in the nasal swabs of five of the six sheep infected intranasally, yet no disease was observed. It is interesting to note that the development of the humoral immune response in the two subcutaneously inoculated sheep occurred over a similar period as the intranasally inoculated sheep. We speculate the infection was localised at the injection site in these two animals and, in the absence of a viraemia, shedding via the upper respiratory tract did not occur. The low level of viral RNA detection in nasal secretions of sheep and cattle would suggest that ruminants are unlikely to play a significant role in transmission of the virus.

It was also possible to infect a calf through co-habitation with a chronically infected pig for 48 h. Interestingly, this calf was the most curious of the four calves in the trial and interacted the most with the pigs. It is possible that if given longer exposure to the infected pigs the other calves may have become infected.

Although all cows became infected, transplacental infection of the calf only occurred in less than half of the cases. Viraemia was associated with in utero infection in two of the four cows in which it was detected. It is noteworthy that Cow 3 developed a rising anti-Bungowannah virus antibody titre during the last trimester of pregnancy. The progeny of this cow was the calf with the highest levels of Bungowannah RNA at birth. We speculate that the dam's immune system may have been stimulated by transplacental transfer of Bungowannah virus antigen during the last trimester of pregnancy.

Each of the three calves that became infected had seroconverted by the time of birth. Persistent infections were not established, despite the cow being infected at a stage of gestation where immunotolerance and persistent infections would be expected, as usually occurs with BVDV infection. These three calves had significant levels of Bungowannah virus RNA present in skin samples at birth, over 210 days after their dams were infected. We hypothesise that these calves did develop a generalised infection in utero, but subsequently cleared the infection some time prior to birth. The skin and testes were the only sites where the viral RNA was not cleared. The testes are an immunoprivileged site, and so it may be that the infection continued at this site for a longer period of time, perhaps much closer to birth. It has also been suggested that skin is also immunoprivileged [14]. It has been shown that a live BVDV vaccine is able to cross the bovine placenta, cause a prolonged transient infection in the foetus and result in detection of viral RNA in the skin for many weeks after birth [15]. It appears a similar mechanism of infection has occurred in these calves with prolonged detection in the skin. The detection of viral RNA in the post-partum vaginal swabs of the three dams provides further evidence for a prolonged infection in these calves and is comparable to what was observed following infection in pregnant pigs [9].

The timing of infection of pregnant cows was designed to maximise the likelihood of producing persistently infected calves. Infection of cattle with BVDV during the first 90 days of gestation will generally produce calves that are immunotolerant to BVDV [16,17]. The results of this trial indicate that Bungowannah virus and BVDV infections in cattle behave differently, with Bungowannah failing to establish immunotolerance and persistence in the bovine foetus.

Understanding why Bungowannah virus resulted in a humoral response in these calves may lead to a deeper understanding of the functional differences between specific proteins in BVDV and Bungowannah virus and how they do or do not affect evasion of the host innate immune response in the bovine or porcine foetus [18].

In conclusion, while cattle and sheep can be infected with Bungowannah virus, they appear to be less susceptible to infection compared to pigs when challenged with a similar dose of virus. When compared to the infection of pigs [9], ruminant species appear to shed less virus and for a shorter period of time. As a result, transmission of Bungowannah virus is likely to be inefficient in ruminants and, without further host adaptation, it will probably not be able to be sustained in these species.

Author Contributions: Conceptualization, A.J.R., D.S.F. and P.D.K.; methodology, A.J.R., D.S.F. and P.D.K.; investigation, A.J.R.; data curation, A.J.R.; writing—original draft preparation, A.J.R.; writing—review and editing, A.J.R., D.S.F. and P.D.K. All authors have read and agreed to the published version of the manuscript.

Acknowledgments: We wish to acknowledge Bob Rheinberger for his generosity and expertise while conducting the ultrasound examinations of the cattle fetuses. We are indebted to the staff of the Virology Laboratory at EMAI (in particular Katherine King and Melinda Frost) for their invaluable assistance during the testing of the samples described in this study, and to Xingnian Gu for his veterinary assistance during sample collection.

References

1. McOrist, S.; Thornton, E.; Peake, A.; Walker, R.; Robson, S.; Finlaison, D.; Kirkland, P.; Reece, R.; Ross, A.; Walker, K.; et al. An infectious myocarditis syndrome affecting late-term and neonatal piglets. *Aust. Vet. J.* **2004**, *82*, 509–511. [CrossRef]
2. Kirkland, P.D.; Frost, M.; Finlaison, D.S.; King, K.R.; Ridpath, J.F.; Gu, X. Identification of a novel virus in pigs-Bungowannah virus: A possible new species of pestivirus. *Virus Res.* **2007**, *129*, 26–34. [CrossRef] [PubMed]
3. Finlaison, D.S.; King, K.R.; Frost, M.J.; Kirkland, P.D. Field and laboratory evidence that Bungowannah virus, a recently recognised pestivirus, is the causative agent of the porcine myocarditis syndrome (PMC). *Vet. Microbiol.* **2009**, *136*, 259–265. [CrossRef] [PubMed]
4. Kirkland, P.D.; Read, A.J.; Frost, M.J.; Finlaison, D.S. Bungowannah virus—A probable new species of pestivirus—What have we found in the last 10 years? *Anim. Health Res. Rev.* **2015**, *16*, 60–63. [CrossRef] [PubMed]
5. Finlaison, D.S.; King, K.R.; Gabor, M.; Kirkland, P.D. An experimental study of Bungowannah virus infection in weaner aged pigs. *Vet. Microbiol.* **2012**, *160*, 245–250. [CrossRef] [PubMed]

6. Finlaison, D.S.; Cook, R.W.; Srivastava, M.; Frost, M.J.; King, K.R.; Kirkland, P.D. Experimental infections of the porcine foetus with Bungowannah virus, a novel pestivirus. *Vet. Microbiol.* **2010**, *144*, 32–40. [CrossRef] [PubMed]
7. Finlaison, D.S.; Kirkland, P.D. The outcome of porcine foetal infection with Bungowannah virus is dependent on the stage of gestation at which infection occurs. Part 1: Serology and virology. *Viruses* **2020**, *12*, 691.
8. Finlaison, D.S.; Kirkland, P.D. The outcome of porcine foetal infection with Bungowannah virus is dependent on the stage of gestation at which infection occurs. Part 2: Clinical signs and gross pathology. *Viruses*, under review.
9. Kirkland, P.D.; Frost, M.J.; King, K.R.; Finlaison, D.S.; Hornitzky, C.L.; Gu, X.; Richter, M.; Reimann, I.; Dauber, M.; Schirrmeier, H.; et al. Genetic and antigenic characterization of Bungowannah virus, a novel pestivirus. *Vet. Microbiol.* **2015**, *178*, 252–259. [CrossRef] [PubMed]
10. Smith, D.B.; Meyers, G.; Bukh, J.; Gould, E.A.; Monath, T.; Scott Muerhoff, A.; Pletnev, A.; Rico-Hesse, R.; Stapleton, J.T.; Simmonds, P.; et al. Proposed revision to the taxonomy of the genus Pestivirus, family Flaviviridae. *J. Gen. Virol.* **2017**, *98*, 2106–2112. [CrossRef] [PubMed]
11. Chakraborty, A.K.; Karam, A.; Mukherjee, P.; Barkalita, L.; Borah, P.; Das, S.; Sanjukta, R.; Puro, K.; Ghatak, S.; Shakuntala, I.; et al. Detection of classical swine fever virus E2 gene in cattle serum samples from cattle herds of Meghalaya. *Virus Dis.* **2018**, *29*, 89–95. [CrossRef] [PubMed]
12. Richter, M.; Reimann, I.; Wegelt, A.; Kirkland, P.D.; Beer, M. Complementation studies with the novel "Bungowannah" virus provide new insights in the compatibility of pestivirus proteins. *Virology* **2011**, *418*, 113–122. [CrossRef] [PubMed]
13. Kirkland, P.D.; MacKintosh, S.G. Ruminant Pestivirus Infections. In *Australia and New Zealand Standard Diagnostic Procedures*; Elizabeth Macarthur Agricultural Institute: Camden, Australia, 2006; pp. 1–30.
14. Frazer, I.H.; Thomas, R.; Zhou, J.; Leggatt, G.R.; Dunn, L.; McMillan, N.; Tindle, R.W.; Filgueira, L.; Manders, P.; Barnard, P.; et al. Potential strategies utilised by papillomavirus to evade host immunity. *Immunol. Rev.* **1999**, *168*, 131–142. [CrossRef] [PubMed]
15. Wernike, K.; Michelitsch, A.; Aebischer, A.; Schaarschmidt, U.; Konrath, A.; Nieper, H.; Sehl, J.; Teifke, J.P.; Beer, M. The Occurrence of a Commercial N(pro) and E(rns) Double Mutant BVDV-1 Live-Vaccine Strain in Newborn Calves. *Viruses* **2018**, *10*, 274. [CrossRef] [PubMed]
16. Liess, B.; Orban, S.; Frey, H.R.; Trautwein, G.; Wiefel, W.; Blindow, H. Studies on transplacental transmissibility of a bovine virus diarrhoea (BVD) vaccine virus in cattle. II. Inoculation of pregnant cows without detectable neutralizing antibodies to BVD virus 90-229 days before parturition (51st to 190th day of gestation). *Zent. Vet. B* **1984**, *31*, 669–681. [CrossRef]
17. Duffell, S.J.; Harkness, J.W. Bovine virus diarrhoea-mucosal disease infection in cattle. *Vet. Rec.* **1985**, *117*, 240–245. [CrossRef] [PubMed]
18. Peterhans, E.; Schweizer, M. BVDV: A pestivirus inducing tolerance of the innate immune response. *Biologicals* **2013**, *41*, 39–51. [CrossRef] [PubMed]

12

Infection Dynamics of *Mycoplasma bovis* and other Respiratory Mycoplasmas in Newly Imported Bulls on Italian Fattening Farms

Salvatore Catania [1], Michele Gastaldelli [1], Eliana Schiavon [1], Andrea Matucci [1], Annalucia Tondo [1], Marianna Merenda [1] and Robin A. J. Nicholas [2,*]

1 Istituto Zooprofilattico Sperimentale delle Venezie, viale Dell'Università 10, 371735 Legnaro, PD, Italy; scatania@izsvenezie.it (S.C.); mgastaldelli@izsvenezie.it (M.G.); eschiavon@izsvenezie.it (E.S.); amatucci@izsvenezie.it (A.M.); atondo@izsvenezie.it (A.T.); mmerenda@izsvenezie.it (M.M.)

2 The Oaks, Nutshell Lane, Farnham, Surrey GU9 0HG, UK

* Correspondence: robin.a.j.nicholas@gmail.com;

Abstract: Italian beef production is mainly based on a feedlot system where calves are housed with mixed aged cattle often in conditions favourable to bovine respiratory disease (BRD). In Veneto, an indoor system is also used for imported bulls around 300–350 kg. Mycoplasmas, in particular *Mycoplasma bovis* and *Mycoplasma dispar*, contribute to BRD in young calves, but their role in the disease in older cattle has not been investigated. In this study, ten heads of cattle were selected from each of the 24 groups kept in 13 different farms. Bulls were sampled by nasal swabbing at 0, 15, and 60 days after arrival for *Mycoplasma* isolation. Identification was carried out by 16S-rDNA PCR followed by denaturing gradient gel electrophoresis. *M. bovis*, *M. dispar*, and *M. bovirhinis* were identified, and prevalence was analysed by mixed-effects logistic regression models. This showed that most bulls arrived free of *M. bovis*, but within two weeks, approximately 40% became infected, decreasing to 13% by the last sampling. In contrast, the prevalence of *M. dispar* was not dependent on time or seasonality, while *M. bovirhinis* only showed a seasonality-dependent trend. The Italian fattening system creates an ideal environment for infection with *M. bovis*, probably originating from previously stabled animals.

Keywords: *Mycoplasma bovis*; bovine respiratory disease; cattle; prevalence

---

1. Introduction

Most European countries operate a feedlot system for male beef production where young calves, usually about one month old, are brought in mostly from dairy farms, then fattened to approximately 240 kg. In Italy, a mixed-age indoor system is also used, which involves the importation of bulls at 300–350 kg from other European countries. This system is mainly located in the Po Valley with the largest herds in the Veneto region [1] and accounts for approximately an 85% share of the beef market. On arrival, the bulls are placed indoors directly with cattle of different ages often sharing the same air space. The cattle are kept for approximately 6 months until they reach a target weight of approximately 650 kg. While relatively productive, the system is prone to severe outbreaks of bovine respiratory disease (BRD) caused by different pathogens, such as bovine viral diarrhoea (BVD) virus, para-influenza virus 3 (PI3), infectious bovine rhinotracheitis (IBR) virus, *Pasteurella*, *Mannheimia*, and mycoplasmas [2]. BRD is often exacerbated by overcrowding and poor ventilation and compounded by the heterogeneity of breeds and diverse origins of the cattle.

At least 30 different mycoplasmas have been isolated from cattle, of which only a few are considered pathogenic, notably *Mycoplasma bovis* and *M. dispar*, which can cause serious respiratory disease in young and adult animals, respectively [3]. Other mycoplasmas have a pathogenic impact on the reproductive system, such as *M. bovigenitalium* [4], while others, such as *M. bovis*, *M. californicum*, and *M. canadense*, are causes of or associated with mastitis [5]. *M. bovirhinis* is frequently isolated from the respiratory tract but is mostly considered to be non-pathogenic [6].

M. bovis has been identified as the major pathogen affecting young animals in northern Italy [2] and is suspected of being involved in disease in older livestock. For this reason, we decided to investigate the prevalence and epidemiology of *Mycoplasma* species in this specialised older cattle sector.

In this study, we used *Mycoplasma* isolation and species identification by 16S-rDNA PCR, followed by denaturing gradient gel electrophoresis (DGGE) to assess the prevalence of *M. bovis*, *M. dispar*, and *M. bovirhinis* in different batches of imported bulls stabled in Italian farms. Animals were sampled by nasal swabs at different times after arrival following a longitudinal experimental design. In addition to isolation, *M. bovis* presence was also determined by a specific PCR protocol.

2. Results

Of the 711 analysed nasal swabs, 485 (68.2%) were positive for species belonging to the *Mollicutes* class. The majority of the isolated organisms belonged to the species *M. bovirhinis* (283, 39.8%), *M. bovis* (136, 19.1%), *M. dispar* (86, 12.1%), and to species of the genus *Ureaplasma* (66, 9.3%) (Table S1). Approximately half of all isolated organisms were found in mixed cultures with other species of the *Mollicutes* class. In addition, *M. bovis* was detected in 276 swabs (approximately 39% of the total samples) by direct PCR in contrast to the 136 isolates (19% of the total samples) obtained by culture.

2.1. Analysis of Prevalence of Mollicutes Class Organisms

Isolates identified as belonging to the *Mollicutes* class largely varied in prevalence over time post-arrival and among the different bull batches and fattening farms (Figure 1a).

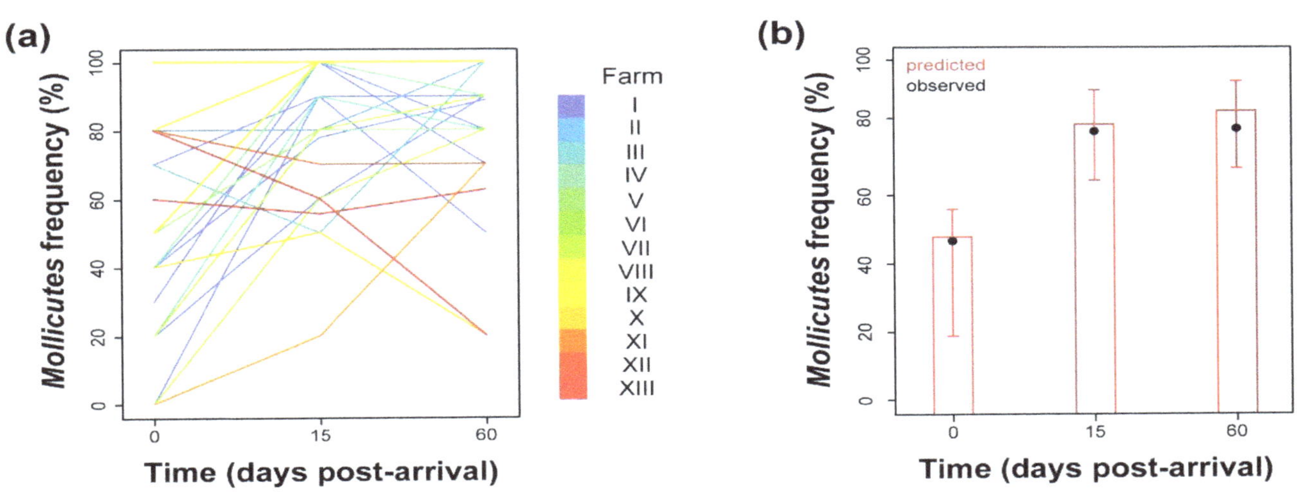

Figure 1. (**a**) Batch-related frequency of isolation of organisms belonging to the *Mollicutes* class analysed over time after arrival. Each line colour is depicted according to the identity of the stabling farm. (**b**) Model-predicted *Mollicutes* prevalence inferred at the population level over time post arrival (red). Observed mean prevalence values are depicted as solid black circles. Vertical lines correspond to the 95% CI of the predicted mean.

However, at the population level, we could identify a clear, significant time-dependent trend (Tables S2 and S3) characterised by an initial prevalence value of incoming animals of approximately 48%, with a 95% confidence interval (95% CI) ranging from 30% to 67%. At 15 days post-arrival (p.a.), the estimated frequency of *Mollicutes*-positive animals significantly increased with an odds ratio of 4.6 (95% CI, 2.2–10.5; adjusted $p = 0.003$) to reach a plateau at approximately 81% (Figure 1b). No effects of the environmental conditions (variable "season", see the paragraph in Materials and Methods) on predicted prevalence were observed (Table S3).

2.2. Analysis of Prevalence of M. bovis

The frequency of *M. bovis* isolation clearly varied in a time-dependent fashion (Figure 2a). At arrival, 18 of 24 batches (75%) were negative for *M. bovis*, and 21 (87.5%) showed a prevalence lower than 10%. Such results were confirmed by PCR (Figure 2b): 17 of 24 batches (71%) were negative at arrival, and 20 (83%) showed a prevalence lower than 10%.

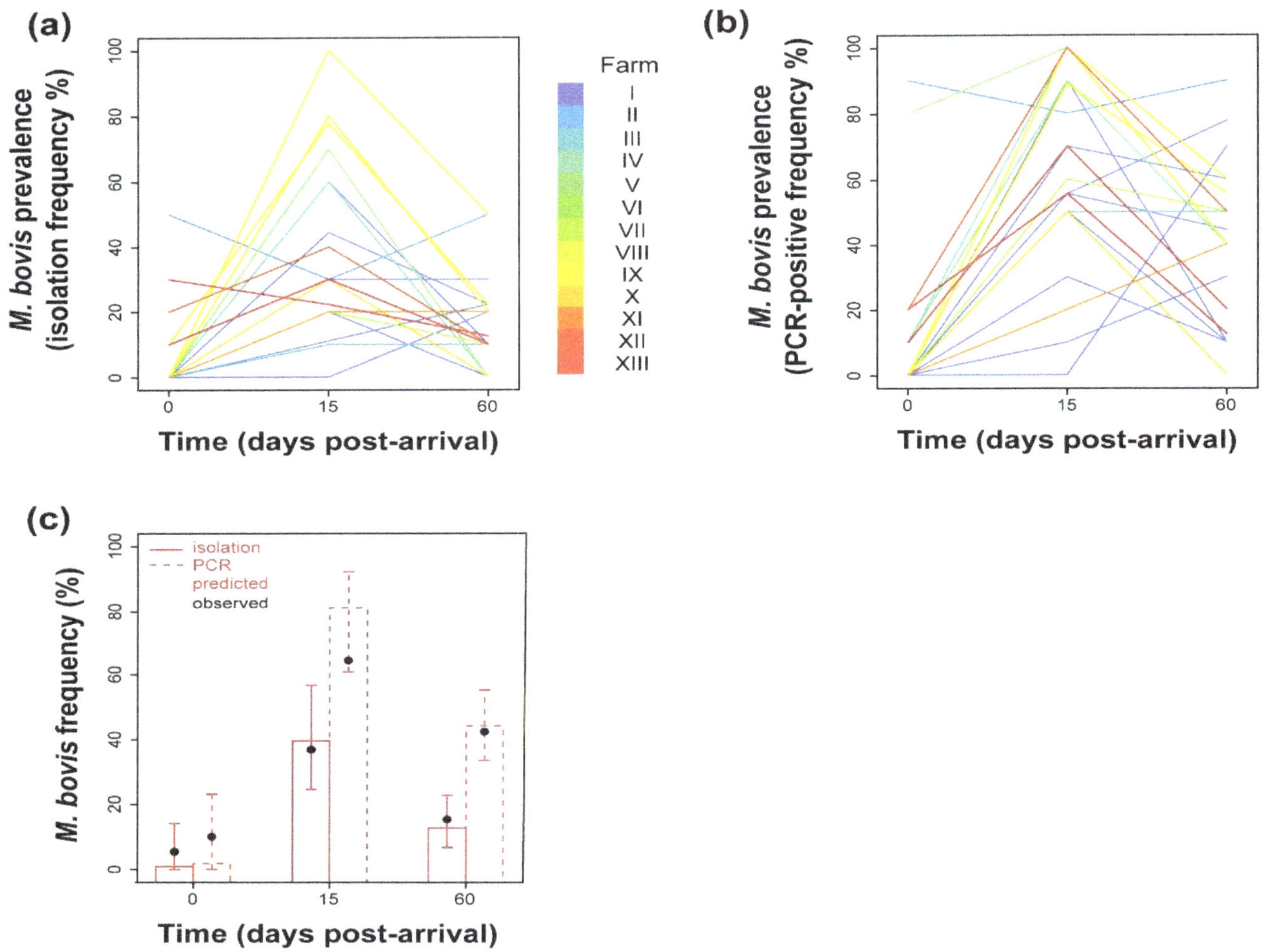

Figure 2. (**a**) Batch-related frequency of isolation of *M. bovis* analysed over time after arrival. Each line colour is depicted according to the identity of the stabling farm. (**b**) Batch-related frequency of *M. bovis*-specific PCR positives among bull batches analysed over time after arrival. (**c**) Model-predicted *M. bovis* prevalence, inferred at the population level and assessed from isolation (continuous line) and PCR (dashed line) data. Observed mean prevalence values from isolation and PCR data are depicted as solid black circles. Vertical lines correspond to the 95% CI of the predicted mean.

With both approaches, we could clearly observe an increase in frequency at 15 p.a., followed by a general decrease 45 days later, which however largely varied in rate among farms/batches. The logistic models constructed confirmed such observations (Tables S4 and S6). At the population level, the probability of isolating *M. bovis* or testing bulls positive by PCR significantly depended on the time of sampling (Tables S5 and S7). The mean predicted *M. bovis* prevalence among newly introduced animals was estimated in the range of 1–2%, with upper confidence limits of 14% (isolation) and 23% (PCR) (Figure 2c). Such prevalence dramatically increased 15 days after introduction into stables, with an odds ratio of 73.4 for isolation (95% CI, 6.7–750, adjusted $p = 0.015$) and 213 for PCR (95% CI, 35–1901, adjusted $p = 0.0001$), to reach an estimated prevalence of approximately 40% (95% CI, 25–57%) in case of isolation and 81% (95% CI, 61–92%) according to PCR. At 60 days p.a., the estimated prevalence dropped to a lower level that differed with respect to the preceding one only when considering PCR-based frequency (adjusted $p = 0.02$). Environmental conditions did not show any predictive role in *M. bovis* prevalence (Tables S5 and S7).

2.3. Analysis of Prevalence of *M. dispar*

Unlike *M. bovis*, the analysis of prevalence of *M. dispar* did not show any dependence on time, as shown by the batch trend lines (Figure 3) and the model we constructed (Tables S8 and S9). In fact, the mean predicted prevalence was estimated as constant with a value of 9.4% (95% CI, 6.7—13%). Similar to time, inclusion of seasonality did not increase the predictive power of the model (Table S9).

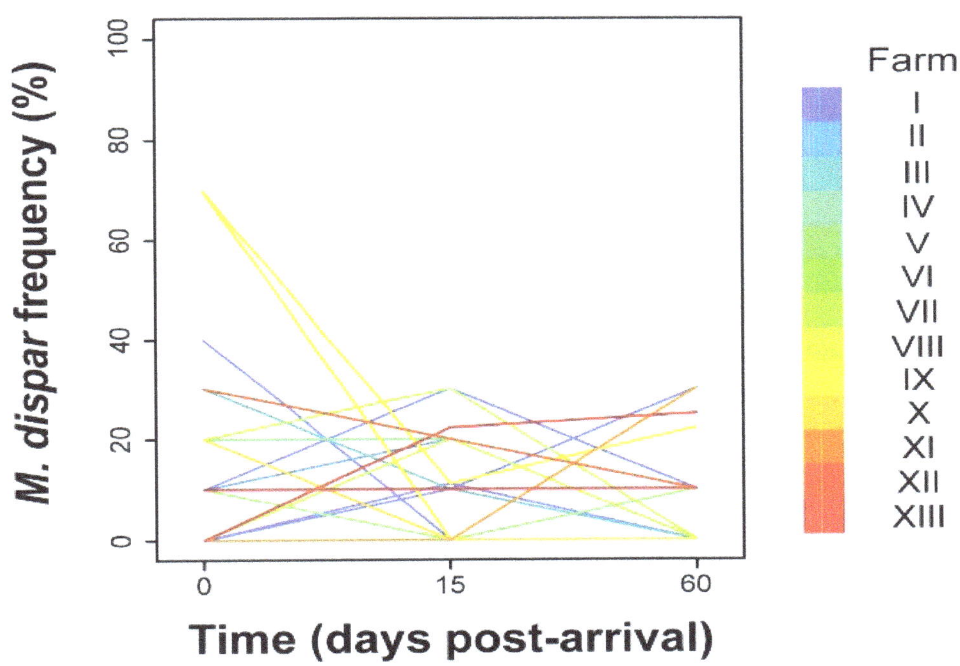

Figure 3. Batch-related frequency of isolation of *M. dispar* analysed over time after arrival. Each line colour is depicted according to the identity of the stabling farm.

2.4. Analysis of Prevalence of *M. bovirhinis*

As already observed especially in the case of *M. bovis*, trend analysis of *M. bovirhinis* isolation over time post-arrival showed high variability among the sampled batches/farms (Figure 4a). Although there appeared to be an increase in prevalence over time, this was not significant (Table S11). Instead, we found that *M. bovirhinis* isolation probability depended on the stabling environmental conditions described by the variable "season" (Tables S10 and S11). In fact, the estimated mean prevalence of *M. bovirhinis* passed from 21.6% (95% CI, 12.9–33.9%), observed in the cold months of the year, to 33.1% (95% CI, 20–49.4%) in the warm season (Figure 4b), with an odds ratio of 1.8 (95% CI, 1.08–2.77).

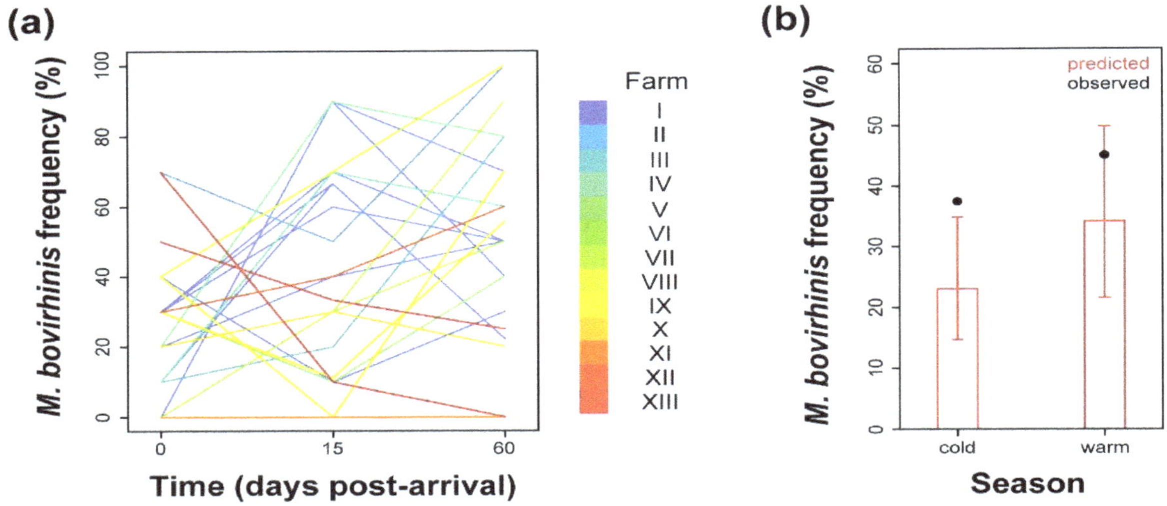

Figure 4. (**a**) Batch-related frequency of isolation of *M. bovirhinis* analysed over time after arrival. Each line colour is depicted according to the identity of the stabling farm. (**b**) Model-predicted *M. bovirhinis* prevalence inferred at the population level over arrival season (red). Observed mean prevalence values are depicted as solid black circles. Vertical lines correspond to the 95% CI of the predicted mean.

3. Discussion

The impact of BRD on cattle production is estimated to cause a decrease in mean carcass weight of at least 9 kg, leading to heavy losses of farmers' incomes [7]. A better understanding of the spread of bovine mycoplasmas, involved in the BRD complex, may thus benefit practitioners by providing them with more comprehensive advice on how to control this significant economic and welfare problem [8]. The Italian bull production system is based on a singular approach typical of northeastern Italy and is believed, by local practitioners, to be exceptionally susceptible to BRD with a significant role played by mycoplasmas. However, the problems of this type of farming have not been well studied, leading to a poor understanding of the causes and risk factors of BRD.

The results of the present study showed that most nasal samples taken from bulls throughout the testing period were positive for organisms belonging to the *Mollicutes* class. Amplification of a fragment of the 16s rRNA gene followed by DGGE and profile comparison with reference strains led to their identification at species level (Table S1). In 71% of the cases, swabs were positive to *M. bovis* (19.1%), *M. dispar* (12.1%), and/or *M. bovirhinis* (39.8%) species, as pure or mixed cultures. In a previous work on Danish cattle farms [9], similar proportions of *M. bovirhinis* and *M. dispar* were detected, but *M bovis* was surprisingly absent. Our results showed a significant presence of *M. bovis* in the Italian bull meat sector with nearly a fifth of samples being positive, confirming other reports on the high prevalence of this mycoplasma in Britain [6], Ireland [10], France [8], and Canada [11].

In the present study, it appears evident that the majority of bulls arrived at the farm free of *M. bovis*, but within 2 weeks, its prevalence dramatically increased up to approximately 40% and 81% when tested by culture and *M. bovis*-specific PCR, respectively. Although high variability was observed at farm/batch level, our results showed that there was a rapid spread of *M. bovis* to the newly arrived bulls most likely from infected cattle already on the farm and/or possibly from the small number of infected imported bulls. In this regard, the phylogenetical typing of isolated strains could be useful to better understand the mechanism whereby *M. bovis* spreads among imported bulls, and future studies on that are strongly advised. The decrease in the percentage of infected cattle at 60 days p.a. indicates that some bulls overcame the infection to a point where it was no longer detectable in individual animals probably as a result of the host immune response mounted against this pathogen. Such a trend was seen in whatever diagnostic method used to detect *M. bovis*-positive bulls.

In contrast to *M. bovis*, *M. dispar* prevalence did not follow a time-dependent behaviour. Much variability was observed among batches and farms (Figure 3), such that at the population level, it did not allow to reveal a common, statistically significant trend, suggesting a constant prevalence of 9.4%. Similarly, stabling animals in different seasons did not change the rate of spread of *M. dispar*. General unfavourable environmental conditions and/or the specific immune status of the bulls may account for the observed differences in the rate of spread between *M. bovis* and *M. dispar*. In our opinion, the low prevalence of *M. bovis* among incoming animals suggests the majority of these individuals may have been naïve to *M. bovis* infection, a condition that facilitated the spread of farm-resident *M. bovis* strains, exacerbated by the close contact with infected older bulls in overcrowded conditions. In contrast, the higher *M. dispar* prevalence observed already on arrival may indicate that the immune systems of the incoming animals were already primed to this mycoplasma species, providing a protective shield against *M. dispar* infection and spread. Alternatively, an unfavourable environment and breeding conditions may have limited the spread. It is also possible that the high prevalence of *M. bovis* may have competitively excluded the colonisation of *M dispar* although evidence is needed to support this.

Similarly to *M. dispar*, *M. bovirhinis* prevalence showed high variability among batches and farms, such that we could not statistically define a common trend over time. However, we observed a significant effect of environmental conditions brought about by seasonality, with higher prevalence associated with warmer conditions. This trait seems to be specific for this species as it was not observed with *M. bovis* and *M. dispar*. *M. bovirhinis* is not considered a primary pathogen and, although it is one of the most commonly occurring species in respiratory diseases [6], it can also be frequently isolated from healthy or asymptomatic animals, where it may be considered part of the natural bacterial flora. The decrease in prevalence of *M. bovirhinis* seen in the winter months may be due to the preferential colonisation of respiratory pathogens, including *M. bovis* and *M. dispar* [12–14], when cattle are more susceptible. Alternatively, such an association may derive from spurious effects given by hidden confounding variables.

In conclusion, our results showed that the Italian fattening bull system creates an ideal environment for the spread and diffusion of *Mollicutes* and, more specifically, of *M. bovis*. The spread of the latter did not seem to be related to the health status of the new bulls; in fact, the high circulation of *M. bovis* is localised during the first weeks after arrival. Most likely, the spread was related to the presence of older infected bulls that provided the source of infection, possibly a dominant farm-specific *M. bovis* strain, to the newly imported bulls as previously reported [8]. A similar situation is seen in other livestock sectors, such as multiage layers hens flocks where the spread of mycoplasma from older birds can cause economic losses in the newest flocks [15,16]. This kind of problem has been controlled in the poultry industry by "all in, all out" systems stocked with *Mycoplasma*-free or by vaccination and could be applied with specific modifications to the bull meat sector studied here. The newly acquired knowledge of *M. bovis* diffusion dynamics from this study will enable better management of BRD, focusing on the herd management, such as improving ventilation and other husbandry techniques.

4. Materials and Methods

4.1. Animals

In this study, we longitudinally analysed 24 different male cattle batches, imported in 2011–2013 and stabled into 13 different fattening farms (identified as I–XIII) of Northern Italy. Most batches consisted of 54 heads of cattle, in large part imported from France. The capacity of the selected farms differed among each other, ranging from 400 to 1500 bulls per farm. For each batch, 10 bulls were randomly selected and sampled for the entire period of the study, with the exception of 7 animals that were lost during the observational period due to mortality or slaughtering (Table S12). Two deep nasal swabs, one for *M. bovis* PCR and the other for *Mollicutes* isolation, were taken from each animal on arrival, and at 15 and 60 days after arrival. A total of 711 samples were collected: 240 on arrival, 238 at the second, and 233 at the third sampling.

4.2. Mollicute Cultivation

To ensure *Mollicutes* vitality, immediately after sampling, swabs were immersed into 2 mL of *Mycoplasma* liquid medium (ML; Mycoplasma Experience Ltd., Bletchingley, UK) and maintained at 4 °C until arrival at the laboratory. Mycoplasma cultivation and isolation were then performed in ML and PPLO (Pleuro-Pneumonia like Organisms) broth media. Briefly, the inoculated cultures were incubated at 37 °C with 5% CO_2 for at least 7 days. The broths were checked daily up to 14 days to detect any change in colour or turbidity. Broths that showed any change were immediately inoculated onto a plate of semisolid *Mycoplasma* agar medium (MS; Mycoplasma Experience). Alternatively, broths that did not show any change were plated onto agar medium at the end of the observation period. If no colonies grew after 14 days, the sample was considered negative.

4.3. Mycoplasma Identification

To identify the species of the different *Mollicutes* grown in broth media, DNA was extracted with the Maxwell 16 LEV Blood DNA kit and Maxwell 16 Instrument following the manufacturer's instructions (Promega), amplified by a 16S-rDNA-targeting PCR and analysed by denaturing gradient gel electrophoresis (DGGE), following a previously reported protocol [17]. Identification of the different *Mollicutes* genera and species was carried out by direct comparison of the lane of interest with the profile of reference strains. To investigate the presence of *M. bovis* DNA on the collected swabs, total DNA was extracted from an aliquot of the relative transport medium, amplified by a *M. bovis*-specific PCR protocol [18] and analysed by electrophoresis in 1% agar gel.

4.4. Statistical Analysis

The statistical analysis of this study was conducted under R environment [19]. The prevalence of organisms belonging to the *Mollicutes* class and to the species *M. bovis*, *M. dispar*, and *M. bovirhinis* was analysed according to a longitudinal framework, in which the same animals were repeatedly sampled along time post arrival. In addition, the potential correlation among observations from the same animals (coded by the variable "ID") and from bulls belonging to the same batch ("batch" variable) or farm ("farm" variable) was considered. For such reasons, we decided to construct logistic mixed effects (hierarchical) models to predict bulls' positivity to each of the 4 considered organisms. For all models, we first determined the correlation structure that best suited to the observed data. Random intercept models were constructed, assuming as random effects the covariates "ID", "farm", and "batch" alone or in nestling combinations. Random intercept and slope models were then evaluated, adding a random slope described by the categorical covariate "time" (time post arrival) to the previously selected random intercept model. In all cases, the best-fitting correlation structure was described by a random slope associated to the covariate "time" and a random intercept expressed by the grouping variable "farm". At the population level, in addition to the covariate "time", we tested the descriptive variable "season", coded as "cold" if the bulls were stabled between November and March and "warm" otherwise. The significance of both random and fixed effects variables was estimated by repeated likelihood ratio tests. All models but the ones predicting the probability of isolating *M. bovis* and *M. dispar* were estimated with the function *glmer* of the *lme4* package [20], applying a maximum likelihood with Laplace approximation and "bobyqa" optimisation for convergence. In the case of the models describing *M. bovis* and *M. dispar* prevalence from isolation, the aforementioned approach led to singular fits, in which some components of the variance–covariance matrix were estimated as zero. To overcome this problem, we employed the function *bglmer* of the package *blme* [21] that allows obtaining inferences based on a penalised maximum likelihood with priors for the covariance matrix of the random effects following a Wishart distribution. Multiple comparisons were performed with the function *pairs* of the package *emmeans*, applying Tukey's p value adjustment method [22].

Supplementary Materials:
Table S1: Species and genera of the *Mollicutes* class isolated from the analysed nasal swabs. Table S2: Parameter

estimates of the logistic mixed effects model analysing the isolation frequency of organisms of the *Mollicutes* class. Table S3: Analysis of deviance table (type II likelihood ratio tests) of the full model relating the isolation frequency of organisms of the *Mollicutes* class to the variables time and season.. Table S4: Parameter estimates of the logistic mixed effects model analyzing the frequency of *M. bovis* isolation. Table S5: Analysis of deviance table (type II likelihood ratio tests) of the full model relating the frequency of isolation of *M. bovis* to the variables time and season. Table S6: Parameter estimates of the logistic mixed effects model analyzing the frequency of *M. bovis*-specific PCR positives. Table S7: Analysis of deviance table (type II likelihood ratio tests) of the full model relating the frequency of *M. bovis*-specific PCR positives to the variables time and season. Table S8: Parameter estimates of the logistic mixed effects model analyzing the frequency of *M. dispar* isolation. Table S9: Analysis of deviance table (type II likelihood ratio tests) of the full model relating the frequency of isolation of *M. dispar* to the variables time and season. Table S10: Parameter estimates of the logistic mixed effects model analyzing the frequency of *M. bovirhinis* isolation. Table S11: Analysis of deviance table (type II likelihood ratio tests) of the full model relating the frequency of isolation of *M. bovirhinis* to the variables time and season. Table S12: Data structure description.

Author Contributions: Conceptualisation, S.C. and R.A.J.N.; *Mollicute* cultivation and identification, A.M. and A.T.; software, M.G.; formal analysis, M.G.; investigation, E.S. and M.M.; data curation, S.C., M.M., and M.G.; writing—original draft preparation, S.C.; writing—review and editing, M.G. and R.A.J.N.; visualisation, M.G.; supervision, S.C. and R.A.J.N.; project administration, S.C. and R.A.J.N.; funding acquisition, S.C. and R.A.J.N. All authors have read and agreed to the published version of the manuscript.

References

1. Cozzi, G. Present situation and future challenges of beef cattle production in Italy and the role of the research. *Ital. J. Anim. Sci.* **2007**, *6* (Suppl. 1), 389–396. [CrossRef]
2. Radaelli, E.; Luini, M.; Loria, G.R.; Nicholas, R.A.J.; Scanziani, E. Bacteriological, serological, pathological and immunohistochemical studies of *Mycoplasma bovis* respiratory infection in veal calves and adult cattle at slaughter. *Res. Vet. Sci.* **2008**, *85*, 282–290. [CrossRef] [PubMed]
3. Nicholas, R.A.J.; Ayling, R.D. *Mycoplasma bovis*: Disease, diagnosis, and control. *Res. Vet. Sci.* **2003**, *74*, 105–112. [CrossRef]
4. Nicholas, R.; Ayling, R.; McAuliffe, L. *Mycoplasma Diseases of Ruminants*; CABI Publishing: Wallingford, UK, 2008; ISBN 9780851990125.
5. Nicholas, R.A.J.; Fox, L.K.; Lysnyansky, I. Mycoplasma mastitis in cattle: To cull or not to cull. *Vet. J.* **2016**, *216*, 142–147. [CrossRef] [PubMed]
6. Ayling, R.D.; Bashiruddin, S.E.; Nicholas, R.A.J. *Mycoplasma* species and related organisms isolated from ruminants in Britain between 1990 and 2000. *Vet. Rec.* **2004**, *155*, 413–416. [CrossRef] [PubMed]
7. Pardon, B.; Hostens, M.; Duchateau, L.; Dewulf, J.; De Bleecker, K.; Deprez, P. Impact of respiratory disease, diarrhea, otitis and arthritis on mortality and carcass traits in white veal calves. *BMC Vet. Res.* **2013**, *9*, 79. [CrossRef] [PubMed]
8. Timsit, E.; Arcangioli, M.-A.; Bareille, N.; Seegers, H.; Assié, S. Transmission dynamics of *Mycoplasma bovis* in newly received beef bulls at fattening operations. *J. Vet. Diagn. Investig.* **2012**, *24*, 1172–1176. [CrossRef] [PubMed]
9. Angen, Ø.; Thomsen, J.; Larsen, L.E.; Larsen, J.; Kokotovic, B.; Heegaard, P.M.H.; Enemark, J.M.D. Respiratory disease in calves: Microbiological investigations on trans-tracheally aspirated bronchoalveolar fluid and acute phase protein response. *Vet. Microbiol.* **2009**, *137*, 165–171. [CrossRef] [PubMed]
10. Bell, C.J.; Blackburn, P.; Elliott, M.; Patterson, T.I.A.P.; Ellison, S.; Lahuerta-Marin, A.; Ball, H.J. Investigation of polymerase chain reaction assays to improve detection of bacterial involvement in bovine respiratory disease. *J. Vet. Diagn. Investig.* **2014**, *26*, 631–634. [CrossRef] [PubMed]
11. Booker, C.W.; Abutarbush, S.M.; Morley, P.S.; Jim, G.K.; Pittman, T.J.; Schunicht, O.C.; Perrett, T.; Wildman, B.K.; Fenton, R.K.; Guichon, P.T.; et al. Microbiological and histopathological findings in cases of fatal bovine respiratory disease of feedlot cattle in western Canada. *Can. Vet. J.* **2008**, *49*, 473. [PubMed]
12. O'Neill, R.; Mooney, J.; Connaghan, E.; Furphy, C.; Graham, D.A. Patterns of detection of respiratory viruses in nasal swabs from calves in Ireland: A retrospective study. *Vet. Rec.* **2014**, *175*, 35. [CrossRef] [PubMed]

13. Stein, R.A.; Katz, D.E. Escherichia coli, cattle and the propagation of disease. *FEMS Microbiol. Lett.* **2017**, *364*, 1–11. [CrossRef]
14. Abdelhay Kaoud, H. Introductory Chapter: Bacterial Cattle Diseases—Economic Impact and Their Control. In *Bacterial Cattle Diseases*; IntechOpen: London, UK, 2019.
15. Catania, S.; Gobbo, F.; Bilato, D.; Gagliazzo, L.; Moronato, M.L.; Terregino, C.; Bradbury, J.M.; Ramírez, A.S. Two strains of Mycoplasma synoviae from chicken flocks on the same layer farm differ in their ability to produce eggshell apex abnormality. *Vet. Microbiol.* **2016**, *193*, 60–66. [CrossRef] [PubMed]
16. Catania, S.; Bilato, D.; Gobbo, F.; Granato, A.; Terregino, C.; Iob, L.; Nicholas, R.A.J. Treatment of Eggshell Abnormalities and Reduced Egg Production Caused by Mycoplasma synoviae Infection. *Avian Dis.* **2010**, *54*, 961–964. [CrossRef] [PubMed]
17. McAuliffe, L.; Ellis, R.J.; Lawes, J.R.; Ayling, R.D.; Nicholas, R.A.J. 16S rDNA PCR and denaturing gradient gel electrophoresis; a single generic test for detecting and differentiating Mycoplasma species. *J. Med. Microbiol.* **2005**, *54*, 731–739. [CrossRef] [PubMed]
18. Butler, J.A.; Pinnow, C.C.; Thomson, J.U.; Levisohn, S.; Rosenbusch, R.F. Use of arbitrarily primed polymerase chain reaction to investigate Mycoplasma bovis outbreaks. *Vet. Microbiol.* **2001**, *78*, 175–181. [CrossRef]
19. R Core Team. *R: A Language and Environment for Statistical Computing 2019*; R Foundation for Statistical Computing: Vienna, Austria; Available online: https://www.R-project.org/ (accessed on 1 July 2020).
20. Bates, D.; Mächler, M.; Bolker, B.; Walker, S. Fitting Linear Mixed-Effects Models Using {lme4}. *J. Stat. Softw.* **2015**, *67*, 1–48. [CrossRef]
21. Chung, Y.; Rabe-Hesketh, S.; Dorie, V.; Gelman, A.; Liu, J. A nondegenerate penalized likelihood estimator for variance parameters in multilevel models. *Psychometrika* **2013**, *78*, 685–709. [CrossRef] [PubMed]
22. Lenth, R. Emmeans: Estimated Marginal Means, Aka Least-Squares Means. R Package Version 1.4.6. 2019. Available online: https://CRAN.R-project.org/package=emmean (accessed on 1 July 2020).

13

Epidemiology and Management of BVDV in Rangeland Beef Breeding Herds in Northern Australia

Michael McGowan [1,*], Kieren McCosker [2], Geoff Fordyce [3] and Peter Kirkland [4]

1 School of Veterinary Science, The University of Queensland, Gatton, QLD 4343, Australia
2 Department of Primary Industry and Resources, Katherine, NT 0851, Australia; kieren.mccosker@nt.gov.au
3 Queensland Alliance for Agriculture and Food Innovation, Centre for Animal Science, The University of Queensland, St Lucia, QLD 4072, Australia; g.fordyce@uq.edu.au
4 Elizabeth Macarthur Agricultural Institute, PMB 4008, Narellan, NSW 2567, Australia; peter.kirkland@dpi.nsw.gov.au
* Correspondence: m.mcgowan@uq.edu.au

Abstract: Approximately 60% of Australia's beef cattle are located in the vast rangelands of northern Australia. Despite the often low stocking densities and extensive management practices of the observed herd, animal prevalence of BVDV infection and typical rates of transmission are similar to those observed in intensively managed herds in southern Australia and elsewhere in the world. A recent large three- to four-year study of factors affecting the reproductive performance of breeding herds in this region found that where there was evidence of widespread and/or recent BVDV infection, the percentage of lactating cows that became pregnant within four months of calving was reduced by 23%, and calf wastage was increased by 9%. BVDV is now considered the second most important endemic disease affecting beef cattle in northern Australia, costing the industry an estimated AUD 50.9 million annually. Although an effective killed vaccine was released in Australia in 2003, the adoption of routine whole herd vaccination by commercial beef farmers has been slow. However, routine testing to identify persistently infected replacement breeding bulls and heifers has been more widely adopted.

Keywords: epidemiology; BVDV; rangeland beef herds; northern Australia

---

1. Introduction

Approximately 60% of Australia's beef cattle are located in northern Australia, which includes the state of Queensland, the Northern Territory, and the northern part of the state of Western Australia [1]. This is a subtropical-tropical region with a characteristic wet and dry season dominated by a summer rainfall pattern. Cattle predominantly graze either native rangeland pastures or those containing introduced tropical grasses and legumes, which all vary considerably in dry matter digestibility and crude protein content according to the season. Approximately 85% of beef cattle in this region contain at least some *Bos indicus* genetics, enabling them to better cope with high environmental temperatures, low quality grazing pastures, and internal and external parasitism, in particular cattle tick (*Rhipicephalus microplus*) and buffalo fly (*Haematobia irritans exigua*) infestations. Median property and paddock size [1] vary considerably across this region (60 to 1250 km^2 and 419 to 2611 ha, respectively) and stocking rates are typically moderate to low; one adult equivalent (AE) in 5–30 ha, but in some areas, this is as low as 1 AE to 150 ha. Cattle are extensively managed, typically only being mustered (brought in from the paddock and handled through the cattle yards and crush or chute) twice a year, between April to June and August to October, when a number of husbandry and management practices are performed, such as branding and weaning, pregnancy diagnosis, drafting cattle into new management groups, and identification and removal of cull cows and bulls. Notably, this is generally the only time when disease control measures, such as the vaccination of cattle, are conducted. Approximately two-thirds of cow herds in the northern dry tropical rangelands are continuously mated [1], whereas in the more intensively managed southern areas of this region, herds are control mated, typically for periods of four to seven months. Peak calving occurs from October through to January. A consequence of the long mating periods in this region is that at any time there are always some cattle being mated through to six months of gestation, and thus at risk of bovine viral diarrhoea virus (BVDV) induced disease.

In Australia, BVDV was first reported to have been isolated from cases of acute and chronic mucosal disease of cattle in 1964 [2]. Several years later, the findings of the first serological survey of Australian cattle were published [3], and reported a 91% crude prevalence of seropositive cattle sampled from herds located north of the Tropic of Capricorn compared to a prevalence of 54% for those located south of the Tropic. The proportion of seropositive herds was similar, 96% and 84%, respectively. Overall, the estimated prevalence of seropositive herds was 89%, confirming that the national herd was already endemically infected. In 2007 [4], phylogenetic analysis of Australian isolates of BVDV, primarily from persistently infected (PI) cattle collected over a 25-year study, found that 96.3% were BVDV-1c strains, with the remainder being either BVDV-1a (3.1%) or 1b strains (0.3%). No type-2 isolates or Hobi-like (type 3) were identified. Notably, subgenotype 1c has only been reported in Japan, Chile, Argentina, Spain, and South Africa [4]; the first cattle imported into Australia came from South Africa.

It has been estimated [5] that approximately 1% of cattle in the Australian national herd are PI. This is supported by the results of antigen capture ELISA testing of young cattle (9–24 months of age) for export (n = 24,035) and health certification (n = 13,800) conducted at the Elizabeth MacArthur Agricultural Institute between approximately 2004 and 2010; 1.1% and 1.53% of cattle were confirmed PI, respectively (P. Kirkland pers. comm.). The prevalence of PI cattle amongst breeding-age bulls and heifers in Queensland, where approximately half of Australia's cattle reside, was 0.35%. This review focuses on updating the knowledge and understanding of the epidemiology and management of BVDV in northern Australia.

2. Prevalence

In the mid-1990s, as part of a structured animal health surveillance programme conducted by the Queensland government, a sample of heifers and cows from 213 Queensland beef herds was bled, and the BVDV seroprevalence was determined using a virus neutralisation test [6]. The overall individual animal seroprevalence was 45%. Despite significant differences between regions with respect to environment and herd management, there was no significant difference between two consecutive years in the percentage of heifer groups and herds, which were estimated to be entirely seronegative (28–41% and 9–13%, respectively). However, herds with 500 or more cattle had a significantly higher likelihood of containing one or more seropositive cattle. In small herds, spontaneous elimination of infection is likely more common because following an outbreak of infection, most cattle become naturally immune and PI cattle have a significantly shortened life expectancy. In larger herds with multiple management groups, typically there are some groups with a high proportion of naïve cattle, with the mixing of cattle from different groups resulting in the ongoing birth of PI cattle. For example, the seroprevalence of seven breeding groups of heifers and cows on a farm in south-east Queensland ranged from 0–80%, with four groups having a very low seroprevalence and one group having a high seroprevalence (Marbach pers. comm.).

In a four-year (2007–2011) longitudinal study [1] of factors affecting the reproductive performance of 73 commercial beef herds across northern Australia, sera from a cross-sectional sample of cattle in each enrolled breeding group were tested using a BVDV Agar Gel Immunodiffusion test (AGID) [7]. The advantage of using this serological test is that both the prevalence of seropositive cattle and the prevalence of recently infected cattle (those with an AGID test result of three or greater) can be estimated, and test results are not affected by vaccination.

The overall seroprevalence was similar for heifers and cows and between years, varying between 50% and 55%. The median management group seroprevalence was also similar across regions and years. Approximately one in four and one in five heifer and cow groups, respectively, were mostly naïve (<20% seroprevalence), and 3 in 10 and 4 in 10 heifer and cow groups, respectively, were mostly naturally immune (>80% seroprevalence; Table 1). Although the stocking rate is generally low, the typical behaviour of cattle in this hot region of Australia, including the daily close congregation of animals around watering points and nutritional supplementation sites, is likely to encourage the transmission of BVDV.

Table 1. Distribution of cow and heifer mobs by observed BVDV seroprevalence category [1].

Animal Class	Year	No. of Management Groups	Group Seroprevalence Category *		
			Low	Moderate	High
Heifers	2009	42	31.0%	35.7%	33.3%
	2011	25	24.0%	48.0%	28.0%
Cows #	2009	62	21.0%	38.7%	40.3%
	2011	60	15.0%	50.0%	35.0%

Some cow groups contained both heifers and cows; * Seroprevalence category defined as: Low, <20%; Moderate, 20–80%; and High, >80% seropositive.

The frequency of management groups likely to have experienced an outbreak of BVDV infection (i.e., >30% of AGID test results were ≥3; Table 2) varied between years. In 2009, approximately 3 in 10 and 2 in 10 heifer and cow groups, respectively (Table 2), were likely to have experienced an outbreak of BVDV infection. However, in 2011 only 1 in 10 and 1 in 20 heifer and cow groups, respectively (Table 2), were likely to have experienced an outbreak of BVDV infection. Outbreaks of BVDV infection in groups of heifers are relatively common due to the recognised generally lower age-specific seroprevalence [6]. A serological study of groups of mating age heifers and first-lactation cows in 12 herds in the Northern Territory found that in nearly half of the herds most of the cattle were likely to be susceptible to infection [8]. Further, these estimates of the prevalence of outbreaks of BVDV infection are similar to those derived from collation of laboratory investigations conducted in Queensland and the Northern Territory [9]. Differences between years in the prevalence of outbreaks of infection are likely to reflect the cyclical changes in proportion of naïve and PI cattle in management groups, strongly influenced by herd culling and heifer replacement practices.

Overall, there is no evidence that the prevalence of infection in beef cattle in northern Australia, either at the herd or animal level, has changed significantly between 1967 and 2009 to 2011.

Table 2. Distribution of management groups of unvaccinated heifers and cows by prevalence of recent BVDV infection [1].

Animal Class	Year	No. of Management Groups	Frequency of Recent Infection *		
			Low	Moderate	High
Heifers	2009	36	41.7%	30.6%	27.8%
	2011	22	63.6%	27.3%	9.1%
Cows #	2009	57	42.1%	42.1%	15.8%
	2011	54	68.5%	27.8%	3.7%

Some cow mobs contained both heifers and cows; * Mob prevalence of recent BVDV infection defined as Low: <10%; Moderate: 10–30% and High: >30% AGID test result ≥3.

3. Transmission

Reported rates of transmission of BVDV vary considerably depending particularly on the opportunities for close contact between susceptible and PI cattle. When susceptible cattle were placed in close proximity to a PI animal (e.g., kept in a small yard with common water and hay feeder),

60% became infected [10,11] within 24 hours. Under stocking rates of approximately one animal per hectare, transmission rates of 30–60% per month (1–2% per day) are often observed from the temperate beef grazing regions of Australia [10]. However, the birth of a cluster of PI calves can result in approximately 1–4% of susceptible cows becoming infected per day [10].

There have been few reports on transmission of BVDV in the extensively managed beef herds of northern Australia. A study of BVDV transmission on two commercial beef properties in central Queensland [12] found that between two days prior to artificial insemination (AI) through to day 51 after AI, 70% and 32% of the seronegative cows and heifers, respectively, seroconverted, but between day 51 and 210, only 17% and 3% of the seronegative cows and heifers, respectively, seroconverted. Thus, during the period in which there was frequent handling to synchronise oestrous and conduct AI and later pregnancy diagnosis (up to day 51), 1% and 0.6% of susceptible cows and heifers became infected per day, respectively; though after this, when cattle were not handled, only 0.1% and 0.02% of susceptible cows and heifers became infected per day, respectively. However, the marked decrease in the rate of transmission after the period of frequent handling cannot be simply explained by the lack of handling alone, but is more likely to have been due to the removal (at the time of pregnancy diagnosis), relocation (planned or inadvertent) or death of some or all of the PI cattle in these herds.

In a north Queensland study [9] of rates of transmission over a two- to six-month period during the dry season in groups (n = 199 to 506) of recently weaned calves (3 to 7 months of age), managed in large paddocks (~4000 ha) at stocking rates of one AE per 2–8 ha, 0.5% to 1% of susceptible cattle became infected per day. These rates of transmission are similar to those observed in intensively managed beef herds. Typically in these rangeland herds, calves weaned from different breeding groups are accumulated in large holding yards over one or more weeks, and after processing (castration, dehorning, etc.) graze together in a single paddock, all of which increases the likelihood of transmission of BVDV. A serological study of heifers in herds in the Northern Territory [8] found that although only approximately half the cattle had seroconverted by the time of weaning, by the age of first mating (two to three years of age), virtually all had seroconverted. However, in one herd, there was no evidence of seroconversion at the time of weaning, and by the time of mating, only about 20% had seroconverted. Therefore, although the typical management of young cattle in these herds is likely to encourage the transmission of BVDV, by chance alone in a given year, PI animal(s) may not be present in a paddock of weaned calves, or the PI may associate with only some of the group (particularly in very large paddocks with multiple watering points). This results in a high proportion of cattle being susceptible to infection at the time of their first mating at around two years of age.

In a serological study [13] of BVDV infection in central Queensland, beef herds showed no significant difference between heifers and young cows in the estimated annual incidence of infection (22% to 29%). A larger study of beef herds across Queensland conducted in 1994–1995 [7] reported similar, albeit lower, estimates of annual incidence of seroconversion (12% to 24%), with again no observed age-related effect.

4. Clinical Presentation

In the first 20 years after its initial detection in Australia, BVDV was considered to primarily cause acute or chronic mucosal disease, with the latter being a much more common presentation. However, fundamental research conducted at the Central Veterinary Laboratory, Glenfield, in the mid-1980s [11] demonstrated that infection of immunologically naïve female cattle around the time of mating resulted in a significantly lower conception rate and an increased rate of late embryonic and early fetal loss without any evidence of clinical disease in the females. Further work by this research group [14] demonstrated that infection of females between 25 to 40 days of gestation resulted in almost all surviving fetuses being born persistently infected.

Although in northern Australia most mixing of cattle from different paddocks and properties typically occurs around the bi-annual mustering events, problems with maintaining fence security (floods, bushfires, wildlife, and bulls) means that introductions of new cattle to a breeding group can occur at any time. Based on the findings [1] presented in Table 2, about 2 in 10 and 1 in 10 management groups of unvaccinated heifers and cows, respectively, are at risk of experiencing an outbreak of BVDV infection during mating across northern Australia. The most common clinical presentations observed as a consequence of outbreaks of infection in this region are lower than expected pregnancy rates and/or weaning rates, and a higher than expected incidence of weak non-viable calves born and/or ill-thrifty calves at time of weaning. Cases of chronic mucosal disease in yearling and older cattle presenting primarily as marked loss of body condition, and cases of BVDV-induced neurological disease in calves, are only sporadically observed due to paddocks being large and the terrain and vegetation markedly hinder observation of individual cattle.

In these extensively managed herds, the recommended approach to determining whether BVDV infection is likely to have contributed to the observed lower than expected reproductive performance requires, firstly, accounting for the likely impact of the major factors known to affect performance [1], and, secondly, cross-sectional blood sampling of cattle from affected management groups for AGID serology [15]. Multivariable modelling [1] of the impact of the magnitude of BVDV seroprevalence predicted that in management groups with a high seroprevalence (>80% seropositive) at the time of pregnancy diagnosis, the mean percentage of lactating cows that became pregnant within four months of calving was 23% lower ($p < 0.05$; Table 3) than in management groups with a low seroprevalence (<20% seropositive) [1]. In the majority of high seroprevalence management groups, there was evidence from AGID serology of some (>10% of samples tested) recent BVDV infection. Modelling also showed that in management groups that showed evidence of widespread recent BVDV infection (>30% of samples had an AGID test result of ≥3) either at the time of pregnancy diagnosis or weaning, the predicted calf wastage (losses between confirmed pregnancy and weaning) was approximately twice as great (Table 4) as that in groups with evidence of only a low-to-moderate prevalence of recent infection.

Table 3. Predicted percentage of lactating cows that became pregnant within four months of calving (P4M) by BVDV seroprevalence category [1].

BVDV Seroprevalence *	Mean % P4M	95% Confidence Interval	
		Lower	Upper
Low	57.3 ^{A}	43.8	70.9
Moderate	43.2 ^{AB}	26.2	60.1
High	34.3 ^{B}	17.0	51.6

* Seroprevalence category defined as Low: <20%; Moderate: 20–80% and High: >80% seropositive. Means not sharing a common superscript are significantly different ($p < 0.05$).

Table 4. Predicted mean percentage of calf wastage by category of recent BVDV infection [1].

Prevalence * of Recent BVDV	Mean % Calf Wastage	95% Confidence Interval	
		Lower	Upper
Low	11.45 ^{A}	6.51	16.39
Moderate	12.08 ^{A}	7.00	17.16%
High	20.84 ^{B}	12.49	29.19

* Mob prevalence of recent BVDV infection defined as Low: <10%; Moderate: 10–30% and High: >30% AGID test result ≥3. Means not sharing a common superscript are significantly different ($p < 0.05$).

5. Economic Impact

In Meat Livestock Australia's most recent (2015) assessment of the economic cost of endemic disease in the cattle and sheep industries [16], BVDV was considered the second most important disease problem in both southern and northern Australia. Using Australian findings from both experimental and field studies [11,12,14,17,18] of the impact of BVDV infection during mating and gestation, the estimated prevalence of PI cattle [9] and the distribution of prevalence of susceptible cattle in herds in northern Australia [1], it was estimated that a population-level weaning rate would be conservatively reduced by 1–4.5% as a result of between 3% to 7% of heifers/cows being infected each year. Overall the estimated annual economic cost of BVDV infection in the beef industry in northern Australia was AUD 50.9 million.

6. Management Strategies

Australian cattle veterinarians and farmers only began to recognise the potential impact of BVDV infection on beef herd performance in the late 1980s, with those involved in the artificial breeding industry being most interested in strategies to prevent outbreaks of infection in groups of cattle undergoing artificial insemination or embryo collection and transfer. However, in contrast to other countries, Australia has only had access to a BVDV vaccine since 2003. Therefore, initial strategies such as blood sample testing of cattle suspected of being PI (e.g., ill-thrifty cattle) and then deliberately exposing selected unmated/non-pregnant females to confirmed PI cattle, or inoculation of these cattle with the live virus either derived from a PI animal [19] or from laboratory culture were used.

Due to recognised differences in strains of BVDV found in Australian cattle and national biosecurity concerns, an Australian killed vaccine was developed by Pfizer Animal Health (Zoetis) using isolates provided by Dr. Peter Kirkland's laboratory (EMAI). A field evaluation [20] conducted in 2007–2009 demonstrated that in groups of heifers experiencing significant outbreaks of BVDV during mating, the efficacy of the Pestigard®vaccine in preventing infection in progeny of vaccinates was 80% (95% CI, 71–86). Despite the demonstrated efficacy of the vaccine, adoption of routine vaccination of breeding cattle has been relatively slow. A survey [1] of 73 commercial breeding herds located across northern Australia found that in only 6% of herds all breeding cattle were vaccinated, and in 3% of herds, only heifers were vaccinated. Cost of vaccinations and requirement to initially vaccinate cattle twice have been cited as reasons for lack of adoption. The latter issue has been greatly assisted by research, which demonstrated that the interval between the first and second vaccination could be extended to six months, which more readily enables vaccination to be incorporated into routine herd management. Further, with the greater recognition of the impact on beef breeding businesses of an outbreak of BVDV in bull-breeding herds, those using artificial breeding and those using short mating periods are increasingly adopting either vaccination of their heifers only or whole herd vaccination. In some cases, the decision on whether to vaccinate is based on the findings of AGID testing of a cross-section of cattle in each breeding group.

Perhaps the most common BVDV control measure being used by cattle producers in northern Australia is requiring that all purchased replacement bulls be certified as being not PI. Seedstock producers increasingly test to assess the PI status of their bulls at the time of conducting breeding soundness examinations prior to sale. The availability of a reliable antigen capture by ELISA with high sensitivity and specificity, combined with the convenience of testing either hair or ear-notch samples, has encouraged the adoption of testing to confirm that replacement breeding animals are not PI.

To support the ongoing efforts of veterinarians and cattle producers to control BVDV in Australia, a technical advisory group has developed comprehensive guidelines defining the approach to investigating and managing BVDV in beef and dairy herds [15]. Further, although there has been some discussion about the possibility of eradicating BVDV from Australian cattle, due to the high prevalence of infection at a herd and animal level, strategic prevention of infection via testing and quarantining of introduced cattle, and vaccination of groups/herds of cattle at risk of an outbreak of infection will be the main approach to BVDV control in Australia for the foreseeable future.

Acknowledgments: Funding for major research projects cited in this review was provided by Meat Livestock Australia. The authors wish to thank the collaborating beef cattle producers and their veterinarians across Northern Australia for their wonderful co-operation in completing these projects.

References

1. McGowan, M.R.; McCosker, K.; Fordyce, G.; Smith, D.; O'Rourke, P.K.; Perkins, N.; Barnes, T.; Marquet, L.; Morton, J.; Newsome, T.; et al. *North Australian Beef Fertility Project: Cash Cow*; Final Report, Project B.NBP.0382; Meat and Livestock Australia: Sydney, Australia, 2014.
2. French, E.L.; Snowdon, W.A. Mucosal Disease in Australian Cattle. *Aust. Vet. J.* **1964**, *40*, 99–105. [CrossRef]
3. St George, T.D.; Snowdon, W.A.; Parsonson, I.M.; French, E.L. A serological survey of mucosal disease and infectious bovine rhinotracheitis in cattle in Australia and New Guinea. *Aust. Vet. J.* **1967**, *43*, 549–556. [CrossRef] [PubMed]
4. Ridpath, J.F.; Fulton, R.W.; Kirkland, P.D.; Neill, J.D. Prevalence and antigenic differences observed between Bovine viral diarrhea virus subgenotypes isolated from cattle in Australia and feedlots in the southwestern United States. *J. Vet. Diagn. Investig.* **2010**, *22*, 84–191. [CrossRef] [PubMed]
5. Littlejohns, I.R.; Horner, G.W. Incidence, Epidemiology and control of bovine pestivirus infections and disease in Australia and New Zealand. *Rev. Sci. Tech.* **1990**, *9*, 195–205. [CrossRef] [PubMed]
6. Taylor, L.F.; Black, P.F.; Pitt, D.J.; MacKenzie, A.R.; Johnson, S.J.; Rodwell, B.J. A seroepidemiological study of bovine pestivirus in Queensland beef and dairy herds conducted in 1994/95. *Aust. Vet. J.* **2006**, *84*, 163–168. [CrossRef] [PubMed]
7. Kirkland, P.D.; MacKintosh, S.G. *Ruminant Pestivirus Infections*; Australia and New Zealand Standard Diagnostic Procedures: Camden, Australia, 2006.
8. Schatz, T.J.; Melville, L.F.; Davis, S.S. Pestivirus (BVDV) prevalence on Northern Territory cattle properties. *Proc. Aust. Soc. Anim. Prod.* **2008**, *27*, 38.
9. Kirkland, P.D.; Fordyce, G.; Holroyd Taylor, J.; McGowan, M.R. *Impact of Infectious Diseases on Beef Cattle Reproduction: Investigations of Pestivirus and Neospora in Beef Herds in Eastern Australia*; Final Report, Project AHW.042; Meat and Livestock Australia: Sydney, Australia, 2009.
10. Littlejohns, I.R. Complications to the study of the relationship between bovine lymphocyte antigens and mucosal disease. In *Characterization of the Bovine Immune System and the Genes Regulating Expression of Immunity with Particular Reference to their Role in Disease Resistance*; Davis, W.C., Shelton, J.N., Weems, C.W., Eds.; Washington State University: Pullman, DC, USA, 1985; pp. 179–190.
11. McGowan, M.R.; Kirkland, P.D.; Richards, S.G.; Littlejohns, I.R. Increased reproductive losses in cattle infected with bovine pestivirus around the time of insemination. *Vet. Rec.* **1993**, *133*, 39–43. [CrossRef]
12. McGowan, M.R.; Kirkland, P.D.; Rodwell, B.J.; Kerr, D.R.; Carroll, C.L. A field investigation of the effects on reproductive performance of Bovine Viral Diarrhoea (BVD) virus infection around the time of insemination. *Theriogenology* **1993**, *39*, 443–449. [PubMed]
13. McGowan, M.R.; Baldock, F.C.; Kirkland, P.D.; Ward, M.P.; Holroyd, R.G. A Preliminary Estimate of the Economic Impact of Bovine Pestivirus Infection in Beef Cattle Herds in Central Queensland. In Proceedings of the Annual Conference of Australian Association of Cattle Veterinarians, Townsville, Australia, 14–18 May 1992; pp. 129–132.
14. Kirkland, P.D.; McGowan, M.R.; MacKintosh, S.G. Factors influencing the development of persistent infection of cattle with pestivirus. In *Proceedings of the 2nd Symposium on Pestiviruses*; Edwards, S., Ed.; Foundation Marcel Merieux: Lyon, France, 1993; pp. 117–121.
15. McGowan, M.; Kirkland, P.; Howard, R.; Morton, J.; Younis, P.; Bergman, E.; Cusack, P. *Guidelines for the Investigation and Control of BVDV in Beef and Dairy Herds and Feedlots*, 3rd ed.; Pfizer Animal Health: Sydney, Australia, 2011.
16. Lane, J.; Jubb, T.; Shepherd, R.; Webb-Ware, J.; Fordyce, G. *Priority List of Endemic Diseases for the Red Meat Industries*; Final Report, Project B.AHE.0010; Meat and Livestock Australia: Sydney, Australia, 2015.
17. Kirkland, P.D.; Hart, K.G.; Moyle, A.M.; Rogan, E. The Impact of pestivirus on an artificial breeding program for cattle. *Aust. Vet. J.* **1990**, *67*, 261–263. [CrossRef] [PubMed]
18. Kirkland, P.D.; MacKintosh, S.G.; Moyle, A.M. The outcome of widespread use of semen from a bull persistently infected with pestivirus. *Vet. Rec.* **1994**, *135*, 527–529. [CrossRef] [PubMed]
19. Cook, L.G.; Littlejohns, I.R.; Jessep, T. Induced sero-conversion in heifers with a field strain of bovine pestivirus—A comparison of methods and doses. *Aust. Vet. J.* **1990**, *67*, 393–395. [CrossRef] [PubMed]
20. Morton, J.M.; Phillips, N.J.; Taylor, L.F.; McGowan, M.R. Bovine viral diarrhea virus in beef heifers in commercial herds in Australia: Mob-level seroprevalences and incidences of seroconversion, and vaccine efficacy. *Aust. Vet. J.* **2013**, *91*, 517–524. [CrossRef] [PubMed]

14

The Outcome of Porcine Foetal Infection with Bungowannah Virus is Dependent on the Stage of Gestation at which Infection Occurs: Serology and Virology

Deborah S. Finlaison * and Peter D. Kirkland

Virology Laboratory, Elizabeth Macarthur Agricultural Institute, New South Wales Department of Primary Industries, Menangle, NSW 2568, Australia; peter.kirkland@dpi.nsw.gov.au
* Correspondence: deborah.finlaison@dpi.nsw.gov.au

Abstract: Bungowannah virus is a novel porcine pestivirus identified in a disease outbreak in Australia in 2003. The aim of this study was to determine the outcome of infection of the pregnant pig with this virus. Twenty-four pregnant pigs were infected at days 35, 55, 75 or 90 of gestation. Blood, tonsillar and rectal swabs were collected from each pig at birth and then weekly until euthanasia or death. Tissues were sampled at necropsy. Viral load was measured by real-time reverse-transcription polymerase chain reaction (qRT-PCR) and antibody levels in serum by peroxidase-linked immunoassay. Bungowannah virus was detected in the serum and excretions of all infected pigs at birth regardless of the stage of gestation at which infection occurred. Persistent infections occurred following infection prior to the development of foetal immunocompetence. Unexpectedly some animals infected at day 55 of gestation later cleared the virus and seroconverted. Viraemia and viral shedding resolved quickest following infection in late gestation.

Keywords: Bungowannah virus; foetus; pestivirus; porcine; real-time PCR; serology; virology

---

1. Introduction

Bungowannah virus is a novel pestivirus identified from an outbreak of disease in a piggery in New South Wales, Australia, in June 2003 [1]. It is genetically distinct from the other recognised pestiviruses of pigs, classical swine fever virus (CSFV) and atypical porcine pestivirus (APPV) [2,3] with its closest genetic relationship to the recently identified Linda virus [4]. The disease was referred to as the porcine myocarditis syndrome, or PMC, because histological changes in affected animals consist almost exclusively of a multifocal non-suppurative myocarditis, with myonecrosis in some cases. The outbreak initially presented as sudden death in 2- to 3-week-old weaning age pigs, but soon after the onset there was a marked increase in the birth of stillborn foetuses and a slight increase in the occurrence of mummified pigs. Cumulative losses in some weeks exceeded 50% of pigs born, and it is estimated that as many as 50,000 pigs died in the initial outbreak. Due to the reproductive effects and disease occurring almost exclusively in the first 2–3 weeks of life it was presumed to be predominantly the consequence of in utero infection. This hypothesis was supported by the detection of elevated serum IgG levels in up to 50% of stillborn pigs and by the absence of disease in pigs soon after weaning or in sows farrowing affected litters [1].

The pestiviruses are well recognised reproductive pathogens where the outcome of infection is dependent on a number of factors including the pathogenicity of the infecting strain, the stage of gestation that infection occurs in relation to organogenesis and development of immune competence, where infection prior to foetal immunocompetence may result in a persistent infection due to immunotolerance [5–14]. Persistently infected (PI) animals remain serologically negative and demonstrate cell-mediated unresponsiveness to the infecting strain, shed virus throughout their lives, and are usually epidemiologically more important in ongoing virus transmission than acute, transiently infected animals [5,13–22]. It has been shown experimentally that pigs infected post-natally with Bungowannah virus develop transient infections that resolve over a 10-day period and transmit the virus inefficiently [23]. PI animals are usually the reservoirs of pestiviruses in nature but no PI pigs surviving past 6–8 weeks old have been identified in the affected piggery. Therefore, to better understand how virus transmission is maintained in an infected population it is important to know if long-term infections can occur and to clarify the significance and sources of viral shedding following in utero infections.

This study examined the virological and serological characteristics of in utero infection of the porcine foetus with Bungowannah virus at different stages of gestation. The primary objectives were to determine:

1. If the porcine foetus becomes infected in utero following intra-nasal exposure of the sow;
2. The concentrations of Bungowannah virus RNA in serum, and shed in oropharyngeal secretions and faeces, and whether this is affected by the stage of pregnancy at which the sow is infected;
3. If the pig foetus mounts a humoral immune response following in utero infection;
4. If persistent infections with Bungowannah virus occur and whether there is a critical stage of gestation at which infection results in this outcome;
5. The optimal tissue samples for the detection of Bungowannah virus;
6. If PI pigs can readily transmit infection to naïve pigs.

Infection of the porcine foetus with Bungowannah virus was successful, and the virological and serological characteristics following in utero infection at different stages of gestation are reported. The clinical signs and gross pathology are described in an accompanying manuscript [24].

2. Materials and Methods

2.1. Londitudinal Study Design

Twenty-four pregnant pigs (22 gilts and two parity-1 sows) with known joining dates were obtained from a piggery known to be free of Bungowannah virus, and sampled and shown to be seronegative on the day of inoculation. Pregnancy was confirmed by ultrasound examination prior to selection for the study. Gilts from this piggery were routinely vaccinated against parvovirus, leptospirosis, erysipelas and *E. coli* with commercial vaccines at selection and again 4 weeks later. Both gilts and sows were also vaccinated against leptospirosis, erysipelas and E. coli at 13 weeks of pregnancy. The animals were moved to facilities at the Elizabeth Macarthur Agricultural Institute 3–5 days before they were due to be infected.

The pigs were challenged intranasally at approximately day 35 (34–36), 55 (55–58), 75 (72–76) or 90 (90–92) of gestation (n = 6 per group referred to as D35, D55, D75 and D90) [24]. These time-points were selected as they were similar to those used in a previous study where foetuses were directly inoculated [25] and they span the gestational age at which the pig foetus is considered to become immunocompetent (70 days). Due to animal accommodation availability and the logistics of undertaking a study of this size, the four treatment groups were challenged and managed separately. The four batch farrowings occurred over a 5-month period. To facilitate intranasal challenge, the pregnant pigs were sedated approximately 30 minutes prior with Azaperone (40 mg/mL—up to 2 mL/20 kg).

All pregnancies were allowed to proceed to 113 days of gestation when all pigs were induced to farrow on day 114 to optimise collection of blood from pigs prior to suckling. Farrowing was induced with 500 μg cloprostenol given intramuscularly on the morning of day 113 and, if required, followed 24 h later with Oxytocin (10 i.u.) intramuscularly.

Pigs from infected litters were weaned when 21–25 days old. As the presence of Bungowannah virus could still be detected at weaning in several challenge groups, as many pigs as the secure containment facilities could hold were weaned and retained until at least 5 to 8 weeks of age (D35, n = 11; D55, n = 22; D75, n = 23; D90, n = 20). Selected pigs from D35 and D55 were kept in the study for a longer period of time to allow ongoing monitoring of virological and serological parameters and clinical signs [24]. Throughout the study, pigs that were moribund, not feeding or did not appear to be viable were euthanased by an intravenous overdose of pentobarbitone sodium.

Pigs from the three litters that did not become infected with Bungowannah virus (on the basis that the virus could not be detected in serum or body fluid for any of the pigs in the litter in a real-time reverse-transcription polymerase chain reaction (qRT-PCR) assay and negative precolostral serology results) were kept as control pigs until they were 14 to 21 days old, at which time they were euthanased.

Individual pig identifications (IDs) have been retained in the text where relevant to facilitate comparison between virological, serological, clinical signs, gross [24] and histopathology findings described in related manuscripts. The first number relates to the litter ID and the second the animal ID within the litter (generally in order of birth) e.g., 8-01 indicates the first piglet to be born in litter 8.

The animal studies were approved by the Animal Ethics Committee of the Elizabeth Macarthur Agricultural Institute, AEC Reference No. M09/02 (6 March 2009).

2.2. Inoculum

The pregnant pigs were challenged with approximately 5.3–5.8 $\log_{10}$ $TCID_{50}$ of Bungowannah virus in 5 mL of phosphate buffered gelatin saline (PBGS; pH 7.3, 2.5 mL per nostril), with the exception of Litter 11 where the sow only received approximately 3.8 $\log_{10}$ $TCID_{50}$ of virus. This inoculum was prepared as previously described [23] and confirmed to be free of porcine parvovirus, porcine circovirus type 2 and other pestiviruses by PCR [26,27]. Testing for porcine reproductive and respiratory syndrome virus was not performed because Australia is free of this virus.

2.3. Sample Collection—Pregnant Animals

A vaginal swab was collected from each sow on the day of farrowing. In addition, a piece of placenta was collected and swabbed. Vaginal swabs were then collected every 2–3 days until 14 days post-farrowing and then once to twice weekly until 21–28 days.

All swabs collected during the course of the study were placed in 2 mL of PBGS and stored at 4 °C prior to testing.

2.4. Sample Collection—Piglets

A clotted blood sample, and oropharyngeal and rectal swabs were collected from pigs shortly after birth and where possible before they suckled. While this was achieved in most instances, some animals farrowed earlier than 114 days or commenced farrowing earlier than 24 h after receiving the cloprostenol injection and had suckled. For pigs that were stillborn, body cavity fluid (in preferential order of pericardial>pleural>abdominal fluid) was collected rather than serum.

Thereafter, oropharyngeal and rectal swabs and clotted blood samples were collected weekly up to 8 weeks of age. After this time-point, any remaining pigs were sampled every 10–14 days up to 3 months of age. Three animals from the D55 group that were seronegative at birth were followed for an extended period (10-1 to 189 days, and 8-01 and 8-05 to 329 days of age). Urine was collected opportunistically from weaned pigs.

All pigs were subjected to a detailed necropsy and a wide range of samples were collected for virology, serology and histopathology. Samples for qRT-PCR were collected by firmly rubbing a swab across the freshly cut surface of a section of heart, lung, thymus, spleen, small intestine, inguinal lymph node and brain, and from the surface of the tonsil from pigs of infected litters; from pigs of uninfected litters, swabs were collected directly from the surface of the tonsil and from a cut section of lung and spleen.

2.5. Transmission Study Design

Two 5-and-a-half week-old pigs were obtained from the same piggery as the pregnant animals. After an acclimatisation period of 2 days in isolation, the two naïve pigs were housed for 28 days in the same room and pen with two pigs from D55 (8-01 and 10-01) considered PI with Bungowannah virus. The PI pigs were selected for the study based on low pre-suckle IgG levels (448 and 135 μg/mL), and high quantities of Bungowannah virus RNA in serum (6.9 and 5.5 $\log_{10}$ copies/mL serum) and on oropharyngeal swabs (6.1 and 6.8 $\log_{10}$ copies/swab) at 6 weeks of age compared with cohorts. Retrospective testing demonstrated both were seronegative for Bungowannah virus antibodies at birth, when tested in the peroxidase-linked immunoassay.

2.6. Sample Collection—Transmission Study

Serum, oropharyngeal and rectal swabs were collected from the introduced pigs on day 0, and then from the introduced and PI pigs on days 1, 8 (serum) or 9 (oropharyngeal and rectal swabs), 15, 22 and 28 days post-introduction.

2.7. RNA Extraction and Real-Time Reverse-Transcription Polymerase Chain Reaction (qRT-PCR)

Total nucleic acid was extracted from 50 uL of sera and PBGS containing swabs using the MagMax™-96 Viral RNA Isolation Kit (Ambion, Austin, Texas Cat. No. 1836). A Kingfisher®96 magnetic particle handling system (Thermo Fisher Scientific, Waltham, MA, USA) was used for the extraction process and the purified nucleic acid was eluted in 50 μL of buffer.

qRT-PCR was used for the detection and quantification of Bungowannah virus RNA. Five microlitres of nucleic acid was amplified using the AgPath-ID™ One-Step RT-PCR kit (Applied Biosystems, Foster City, CA, USA, Cat No. 4387424) with primers and probe as previously published [28]. The reaction was run in an Applied Biosystems 7500 Fast or 7900HT Real-Time PCR System (Foster City, CA, USA) both run in standard mode. A 10-fold dilution series of Bungowannah virus RNA standards ranging from 10^7–10^2 RNA copies/5 μL [25] was included in each assay and the quantity of Bungowannah virus RNA in a sample determined from the standard curve. For quantification purposes 2.3 and 2.6 $\log_{10}$ copies/mL were considered the sensitivity of the assay for serum and swabs/tissues respectively although the accuracy of quantification was considered likely to be variable below 4.3 or 4.6 $\log_{10}$ copies/mL. Additionally, means were calculated against a baseline of 2.3 or 2.6 $\log_{10}$ copies/mL for negative samples depending on the sample type.

2.8. Serology

A peroxidase-linked immunoassay was used for the detection of Bungowannah virus antibodies [28]. Where an animal recorded an antibody titre ≥5120, a titre of 5120 (12.3 $\log_2$) was used for calculation of means; where no antibody was detected, a titre of 8 (3 $\log_2$) was assigned for calculation of means.

2.9. Analysis of Results

To facilitate analysis of data, Bungowannah qRT-PCR results for serum, oropharyngeal and rectal swabs for each challenge time-point were grouped into time intervals based on the age of the pigs (0–1, 2–9, 10–17, 18–24, 25–31, 32–38, 39–45, 46–52, 53–60, 61–70 and 71–80 days). The same process was applied for serology results although the first time intervals were 0 and 1–9 days. Pigs that where known to have suckled prior to Day 0 sampling were classified as having been sampled on day 1 for the purpose of this study. Where an animal had been sampled twice within one of these intervals, the mean result for that animal was used when calculating the time-point mean. In addition, the results for animals in the D35 and D55 challenge groups were subdivided based on the presence or absence of antibodies to Bungowannah virus in samples collected prior to suckling.

3. Results

3.1. Longitudinal Study

3.1.1. Pregnant Pigs

All pregnant pigs became infected with Bungowannah virus (as confirmed by seroconversion), with transplacental infection detected for 20 of the 23 (87%) litters. Transplacental infection did not occur for one pregnant pig in each of the D35, D55 and D75 challenge groups [24]. One pig from D55 was found to be not pregnant. For each sow that produced an infected litter, virus was detected in high quantities on vaginal swabs (mean 7.2 $\log_{10}$ copies/swab; range 5.8–8.2 $\log_{10}$ copies/swab) on the day of farrowing, decreasing rapidly by 5–7 days post-farrowing (mean 3.3 $\log_{10}$ copies/swab; range <2.6–5.4 $\log_{10}$ copies/swab) (Figure 1). By day 12–14 post-farrowing the mean amount of virus detected was 2.9 $\log_{10}$ copies/swab (range <2.6–4.3 $\log_{10}$ copies/swab). Viral RNA was not detected on any vaginal swabs collected after 23 days post-farrowing (n = 15). The mean quantity of Bungowannah virus RNA detected on placental swabs at day 0 (7.0 $\log_{10}$ copies/swab; range 5.7–8.1 $\log_{10}$ copies/swab) from the infected litters was comparable to that detected on vaginal swabs. Bungowannah virus RNA was not detected on vaginal or placental swabs collected from sows farrowing uninfected litters.

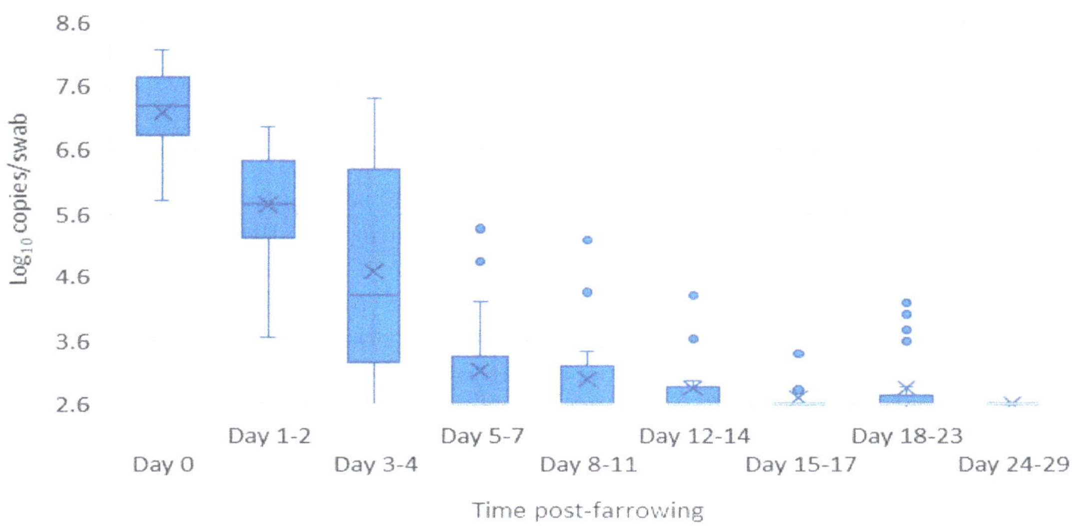

Figure 1. Box and whisker plot summarising the quantity of Bungowannah virus detected in vaginal swabs between 0–29 days post-farrowing following in utero infection (x = mean; — = median; the whiskers extend up from the top of the box to the largest data element that is less than or equal to 1.5 times the interquartile range (IQR) and down from the bottom of the box to the smallest data element that is larger than 1.5 times the IQR. Values outside this range are considered outliers and are represented by dots).

3.1.2. Piglets—qRT-PCR

Bungowannah virus RNA was detected in the serum, body cavity fluid or internal tissues of 225/226 pigs in the 20 infected litters at birth regardless of the stage of gestation that the dam had been infected. It was concluded that one pig (11-15) had not become infected in utero based on the absence of viraemia at birth and because it became seronegative at 9 weeks old indicating the absence of a humoral immune response to infection. This pig was born after it was believed farrowing had concluded and had an antibody titre of ≥10,240 when sampled the next day, presumably due to ingestion of colostrum. No viraemia was detected during the 10 weeks it was followed in the study.

All pigs from three litters (n = 42) were uninfected at birth (based on the absence of viraemia and seronegative serology at birth). The pigs in these three litters all developed high antibody titres after ingestion of colostrum. They did not become infected with Bungowannah virus (based on the absence of a viraemia) despite being in the same room as pigs from infected litters where no direct contact was possible. Occasionally low quantities of Bungowannah virus were detected on oropharyngeal (n = 4; mean 3.5 $\log_{10}$ copies/swab; range 3.3–3.9 $\log_{10}$ copies/swab) and rectal swabs (n = 7; mean 3.2 $\log_{10}$ copies/swab; range 2.7–4.9 $\log_{10}$ copies/swab), presumably due to environmental contamination as a result of sharing a room with an infected litter. Viral RNA was never detected on oropharyngeal swabs from the animal in which 4.9 $\log_{10}$ copies were detected on the rectal swab, or on tissue samples at necropsy. Additionally, all tissue samples collected from these pigs were negative for Bungowannah virus RNA.

Results for the D35 and D55 groups have been subdivided based on whether Bungowannah virus antibodies were detected at birth (Ab +ve) or not (Ab −ve). Samples were collected from all weaned/surviving pigs in the D35, D75 and D90 groups until 75, 56 and 35 days of age respectively. In some cases on the day of euthanasia a direct tonsillar swab was collected rather than an oropharyngeal swab. This result is captured under the results for tissues. In the D55 group, samples were collected through until 120 days in the Ab +ve group (n = 4) and to 329 days in the Ab −ve group (n = 2; 8-01 and 8-05). The number of animals from which serum or body fluid was collected at each time-point for Bungowannah virus PCR is summarised in Table S1.

- Serum: the mean quantity of Bungowannah virus RNA detected in serum at birth exceeded 6.4 $\log_{10}$ copies/mL for all groups of pigs, with the highest levels recorded in those animals where no antibody was detected at birth and where the sow had been infected prior to foetal immunocompetence (D35 (Ab −ve) 7.8 $\log_{10}$ copies/mL; D55 (Ab −ve) 8.4 $\log_{10}$ copies/mL) (Figure 2). For those animals seropositive at birth, the infection gradually cleared over time, although low-level viraemias were still detected at 75 days of age in some animals. At around 28 days of age when maternal antibodies started to wane (Figure 3) the viral load in serum started to rise for the pigs born seronegative in the D35 and D55 groups (Figure 2). By day 120 viral RNA could no longer be detected in the serum of the four remaining D55 (Ab +ve) pigs (data not shown).
- Oropharyngeal swabs: the mean quantity of viral RNA detected on oropharyngeal swabs at birth ranged from 6.5 (D90) to 7.2 $\log_{10}$ copies/swab (D55 Ab −ve & Ab +ve) (Figure 4). Through to 75 days of age the amount of RNA detected on oropharyngeal swabs remained elevated for the D35 (Ab −ve) and D55 (Ab −ve) groups (Figure 4). In contrast, for all other groups, the amount of RNA decreased over time, reducing most rapidly for the D75 and D90 animals. By day 120 viral RNA could no longer be detected on oropharyngeal swabs of the three D55 (Ab +ve) pigs sampled (data not shown).
- Rectal swabs: the mean level of viral RNA detected on rectal swabs at birth ranged from 6.3 (D90) to 7.1 $\log_{10}$ copies/swab (D55 Ab −ve) (Figure 5). As observed for oropharyngeal swabs, the amount of RNA detected on rectal swabs remained elevated for the D35 (Ab −ve) and D55 (Ab −ve) animals through to day 75. In contrast, for all other groups where the pigs were seropositive at birth, the amount of RNA decreased over time, reducing most rapidly for the D75 and D90 animals. By day 120 viral RNA could not be detected on rectal swabs from the four remaining D55 (Ab +ve) pigs (data not shown). Three animals from the D55 (Ab −ve) group were followed for >6 months (8-01, 8-05 and 10-01). Pig 10-01 appeared to seroconvert between 42 to 49 days old, with a marked reduction in viral load in serum and on rectal swabs from around 84 days of age, and oropharyngeal swabs on day 98 (Figure 6A). Virus was not detected in the serum of 10-01 at time of euthanasia on day 189, but low levels of viral RNA were still detected on oropharyngeal and rectal swabs. Pigs 8-01 and 8-05 seroconverted between 127 and 190 days of age (Figure 6B,C) after which the viraemia was cleared. The amount of virus detected on oropharyngeal and rectal swabs decreased more rapidly after seroconversion for 8-01 compared with 8-05 (Figure 6B,C).

- Mummified foetuses: the mean quantity of viral RNA detected on swabs of the internal organs of mummified foetuses was 5.6 $\log_{10}$ copies/swab for D35 (n = 13; range 4.9–6.9 $\log_{10}$ copies/swab), 5.6 $\log_{10}$ copies/swab for D75 (n = 2; range 5.5–5.7 $\log_{10}$ copies/swab) and 3.0 $\log_{10}$ copies/swab for D90 (n = 1).
- Tissues: at birth and in the first 10 days of life, virus was readily detected in all tissues collected from infected pigs in groups D35, D55 and D75 (Table 1). For group D90, virus was not always detected in tissues sampled at birth but was most likely to be detected in tonsillar swabs and from lymph nodes and heart. For all groups, in the first 10 days of life, the greatest quantity of viral RNA was detected from the tonsils (range of means 5.8 to 7.2 $\log_{10}$ copies/swab) and the brain (range of means 4.8 to 7.0 $\log_{10}$ copies/swab). Subsequently, the amount of Bungowannah viral RNA detected in tissues decreased over time and the proportion of tissues in which viral RNA was detected decreased in those groups where the pigs were seropositive at birth. This decrease occurred most rapidly for the D75 and D90 animals (Table 1). There were only two D35 (Ab +ve) animals identified and by the end of the study (day 75) Bungowannah viral RNA was either no longer detected in tissues or was at low levels, with the highest levels in lymph nodes followed by tonsil (Table 1). In contrast, for D35 (Ab −ve) virus was detected at all time-points for all animals and remained elevated in all tissues with highest quantities detected from tonsil, and in lymph nodes and brain. For the D55 (Ab −ve) group the amount of RNA detected in tissues was generally higher for the first two time-points compared with D55 (Ab +ve) although the number of animals sampled was low. An extensive range of tissues was collected from the presumptively PI pigs (8-01 and 8-05) that were followed until 11 months of age (Table 2). The quantity of Bungowannah virus RNA detected in epididymal semen (9.8 $\log_{10}$ copies/mL) is the highest amount of viral RNA detected in any sample collected throughout the course of the study.
- Urine: urine was collected directly from the bladder of six D35 (Ab −ve) animals at necropsy at between 57–77 days of age in with a mean 6.2 $\log_{10}$ copies/mL (range 5.1–6.9) of viral RNA detected. Virus was also detected in the urine of four D55 (Ab +ve) pigs between 80–90 days of age (mean 4.4 $\log_{10}$ copies/mL) but by day 117 viral RNA was no longer detectable in three. In contrast, Bungowannah virus RNA was only detected in the urine of 2/12 animals from D90 in low quantities when euthanased between 19 and 22 days of age (2.7 $\log_{10}$ copies/mL).

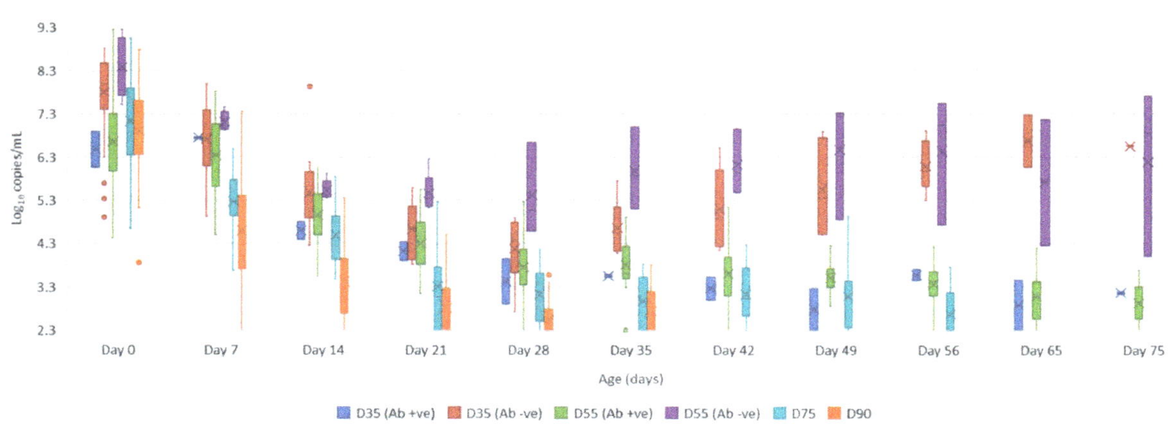

Figure 2. Box and whisker plot summarising the quantity of Bungowannah virus detected in serum between 0 to 75 days of age following in utero infection at one of four stages of gestation (x = mean; — = median; the whiskers extend up from the top of the box to the largest data element that is less than or equal to 1.5 times the interquartile range (IQR) and down from the bottom of the box to the smallest data element that is larger than 1.5 times the IQR. Values outside this range are considered outliers and are represented by dots).

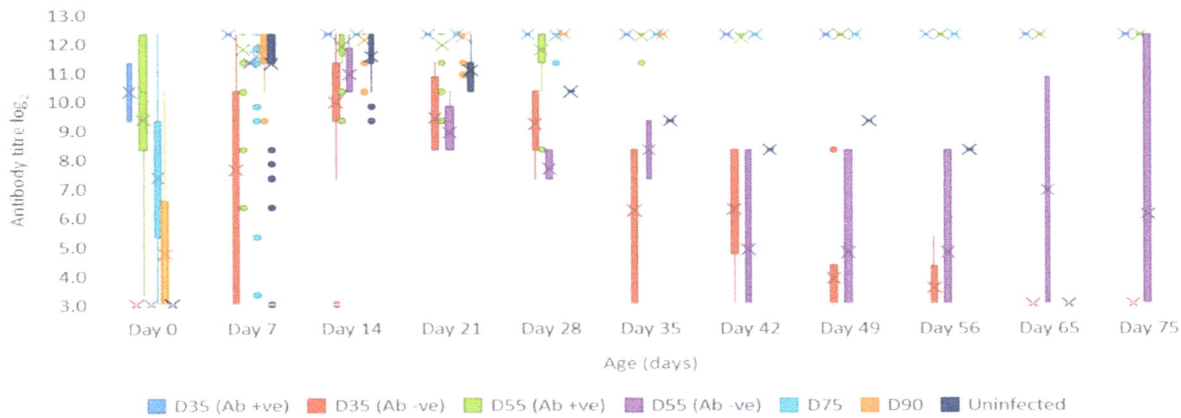

Figure 3. Box and whisker plot summarising the antibody titre against Bungowannah virus in serum as measured by peroxidase-linked immune assay between 0 to 75 days of age following in utero infection at one of four stages of gestation (x = mean; — = median; the whiskers extend up from the top of the box to the largest data element that is less than or equal to 1.5 times the interquartile range (IQR) and down from the bottom of the box to the smallest data element that is larger than 1.5 times the IQR. Values outside this range are considered outliers and are represented by dots).

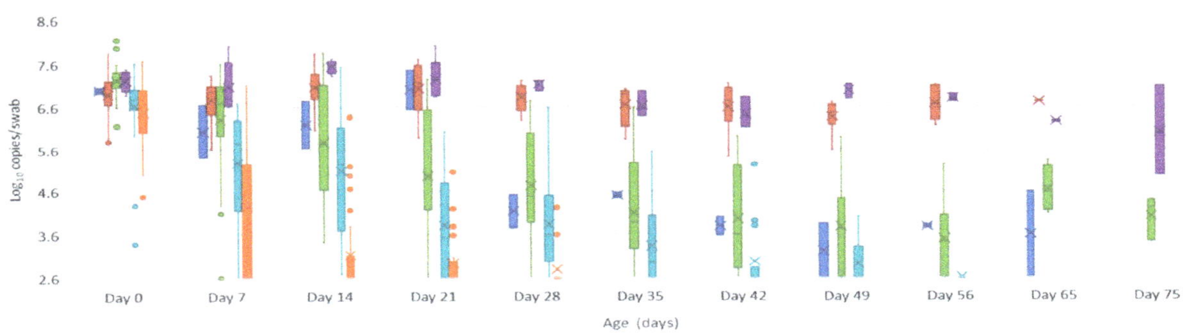

Figure 4. Box and whisker plot summarising the quantity of Bungowannah virus detected on oropharyngeal swabs between 0 to 75 days of age following in utero infection at one of four stages of gestation (x = mean; — = median; the whiskers extend up from the top of the box to the largest data element that is less than or equal to 1.5 times the interquartile range (IQR) and down from the bottom of the box to the smallest data element that is larger than 1.5 times the IQR. Values outside this range are considered outliers and are represented by dots).

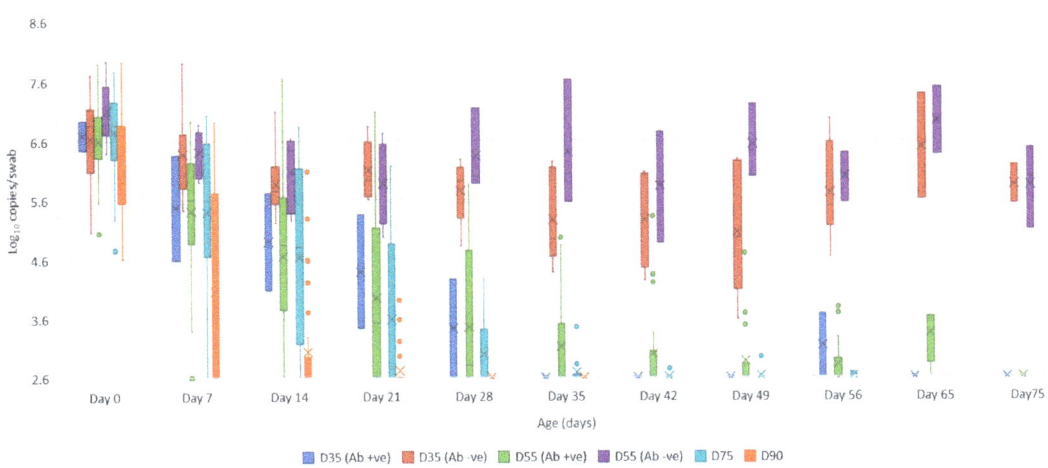

Figure 5. Box and whisker plot summarising the quantity of Bungowannah virus detected on rectal

swabs between 0 to 75 days of age following in utero infection at one of four stages of gestation (x = mean; — = median; the whiskers extend up from the top of the box to the largest data element that is less than or equal to 1.5 times the interquartile range (IQR) and down from the bottom of the box to the smallest data element that is larger than 1.5 times the IQR. Values outside this range are considered outliers and are represented by dots).

3.1.3. Piglets—Serology

The antibody titres of surviving pigs in each of the challenge groups between age 0 to 75 days are presented in Figure 3. Pigs that were known to have fed and were seropositive were excluded from the day 0 antibody titre calculations. The results can be broadly divided into four groups:

- Animals are detected with antibody prior to suckling (or are presumably in the process of seroconverting – D90). The percentage of seropositive (titres ≥10) pigs for each challenge group seropositive was 4% (D35), 82% (D55), 98% (D75) and 50% (D90). The highest antibody titres were detected in those litters infected earliest in gestation: D35 (mean = 1280; n = 2), D55 (mean = 654; n = 32), D75 (mean = 164; n = 45) and D90 (mean = 27; n = 50). After ingestion of maternal antibodies, the antibody titre rises and stays elevated for the remainder of the study (D35 (Ab +ve); D55 (Ab +ve); D75; D90).

- Animals are seronegative at birth; antibody levels increase with ingestion of maternal antibody and then gradually wane with the animal becoming seronegative again at around 40–60 days of age (D35 (Ab −ve)).

- Animals are seronegative at birth (D55 (Ab −ve); n = 7). These animals have the same serological profile as the D35 group after the ingestion of colostrum. At a variable time after losing maternal antibody these animals seroconvert (10-01 at between 42–49 days of age; 8-01 and 8-05 between 127 and 190 days of age; Figure 6). Note that the seroconversion of 10-01 has resulted in the large box plot for D55 (Ab −ve) from day 42 onwards, as the other two animals in the group (8-01 and 8-05) were seronegative at these time-points.

- Uninfected (seronegative) pigs born to an infected dam; antibody levels increase with ingestion of maternal antibody and then gradually wane with the animal becoming seronegative again at around 60–70 days of age.

3.2. Transmission Study

Bungowannah viral RNA was detected on oropharyngeal swabs collected from the introduced pigs at 24 h after their entry to the room/pen containing the presumptively PI animals. Peak viraemia and viral shedding were detected at 8 (serum) or 9 (oropharyngeal and rectal swabs) days post-introduction. Both introduced pigs seroconverted between days 8 and 15 with a titre of 5120 recorded at day 15. Figure 7 illustrates the differences in levels of viraemia and shedding observed between the PI and transiently infected pigs in this study. The differences in viral load detected on oropharyngeal swabs were >2 $\log_{10}$ copies per swab higher for the PI pigs compared to the transiently infected in-contact pigs at peak shedding on day 9. This difference was more than 10-fold higher for the rectal swabs. At the time of peak viraemia in the transiently infected pigs the viral load was equal to that of pig 10-01 but still >2 $\log_{10}$ copies/mL less than that detected in 8-01.

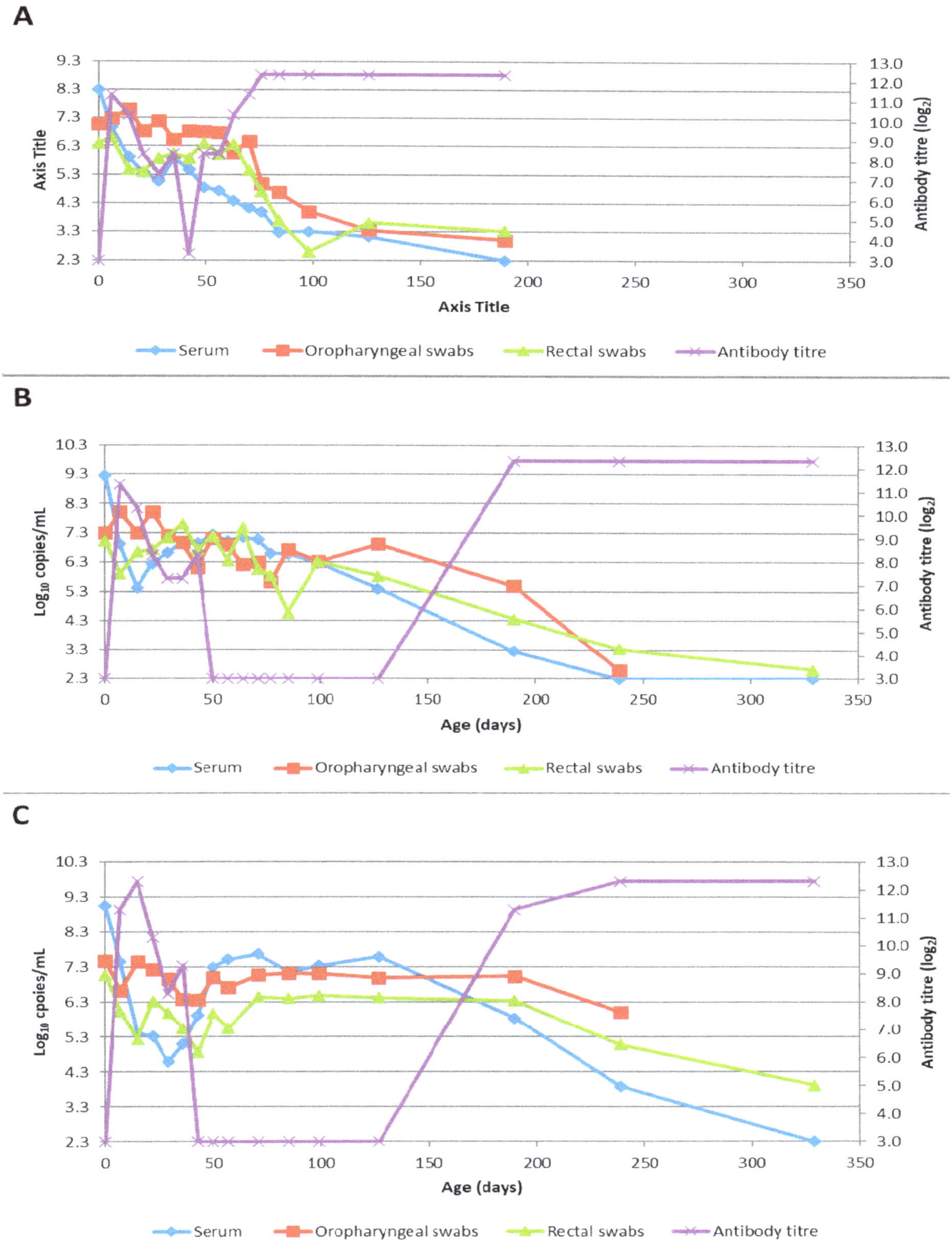

Figure 6. Quantity of Bungowannah virus detected in serum, oropharyngeal and rectal swabs, and antibody titre against Bungowannah virus detected in: (**A**) 10-01 from birth to 189 days of age; (**B**) 8-01 (D55 Ab −ve) from birth to 329 days of age; (**C**) 8-05 (D55 Ab −ve) from birth to 329 days of age.

Table 1. Quantity of Bungowannah virus RNA detected in selected tissues at four time periods after birth in challenge groups D35, D55, D75 and D90.

		D35 (Ab +ve)			D35 (Ab −ve)			D55 (Ab +ve)			D55 (Ab −ve)			D75			D90		
Tissue	Age	No. +ve (%) [a]	Mean [b]	Range [b]	No. +ve (%)	Mean	Range	No. +ve (%)	Mean	Range	No. +ve (%)	Mean	Range	No. +ve (%)	Mean	Range	No. +ve (%)	Mean	Range
Tonsil	0–10				28 (100%)	7.1	6.2–8.3	10 (100%)	7.2	6.3–7.8	2 (100%)	7.2	7.0–7.5	30 (100%)	6.7	5.0–7.8	24 (96%)	5.8	ND–7.7
	11–30				4 (100%)	6.7	5.2–7.6	5 (71%)	4.4	ND–7.1	2 (100%)	6.5	6.4–6.6	3 (75%)	4.0	ND–6.4	1 (5%)	2.6	ND–2.8
	31–60				5 (100%)	6.9	6.4–7.4							8 (44%)	2.9	ND–4.3	1 (8%)	2.6	ND–2.8
	>60	1 (50%)	3.3	ND–4.0	3 (100%)	7.0	6.5–7.4	10 (48%)	3.2	ND–6.8	0 (0%)	<2.6	NA						
Lymph Node	0–10				31 (100%)	5.3	4.4–6.3	10 (100%)	5.4	4.5–6.4	2 (100%)	4.5	3.9–5.2	34 (100%)	5.3	3.9–6.5	26 (100%)	4.7	3.2–6.4
	11–30				4 (100%)	4.5	3.4–5.7	7 (100%)	5.1	2.8–6.0	2 (100%)	5.5	5.0–6.1	4 (100%)	4.8	3.7–5.4	12 (55%)	3.6	ND–5.6
	31–60				5 (100%)	5.3	4.5–6.6							12 (71%)	3.9	ND–6.3	10 (77%)	3.9	ND–5.4
	>60	2 (100%)	4.2	4.0–4.5	3 (100%)	6.0	5.7–6.2	17 (77%)	4.5	ND–6.5	1 (100%)	6.5	NA						
Spleen	0–10				30 (100%)	5.9	4.5–7.3	10 (100%)	5.2	4.7–5.8	2 (100%)	4.9	4.7–5.0	34 (100%)	5.4	3.6–6.9	18 (69%)	3.6	ND–5.2
	11–30				4 (100%)	4.5	3.4–5.9	7 (100%)	3.8	2.9–4.7	2 (100%)	4.3	3.8–4.8	4 (100%)	3.5	2.8–4.6	1 (5%)	2.6	ND–2.8
	31–60				5 (100%)	4.6	3.8–5.8							9 (50%)	3.1	ND–4.4	0 (0%)	<2.6	NA
	>60	1 (50%)	2.8	ND–3.1	3 (100%)	5.8	5.3–6.4	14 (67%)	3.3	ND–4.9	1 (100%)	3.9	NA						
Thymus	0–10				29 (100%)	5.6	4.1–6.4	10 (100%)	5.2	4.3–5.8	2 (100%)	4.9	4.8–5.1	32 (100%)	5.4	3.3–6.8	19 (79%)	4.1	ND–5.7
	11–30				4 (100%)	4.3	3.0–5.1	7 (100%)	3.8	2.9–4.9	2 (100%)	4.5	4.5–4.6	1 (25%)	2.9	ND–3.7	2 (10%)	2.6	ND–3.2
	31–60				5 (100%)	4.6	4.0–5.4							7 (39%)	2.8	ND–3.9	1 (8%)	2.6	ND–3.0
	>60	0 (0%)	<2.6	ND	3 (100%)	5.2	4.7–5.5	9 (41%)	3.0	ND–4.5	1 (100%)	3.0	NA						
Lung	0–10				31 (100%)	6.4	5.1–7.6	10 (100%)	6.0	5.2–6.8	2 (100%)	6.2	6.2–6.2	33 (100%)	6.5	4.4–8.2	21 (81%)	4.2	ND–6.2
	11–30				4 (100%)	4.8	4.2–5.6	7 (100%)	3.8	2.7–5.5	2 (100%)	4.7	4.5–4.9	4 (100%)	3.9	3.6–4.2	1 (5%)	2.6	ND–2.9
	31–60				5 (100%)	4.8	4.3–5.5							11 (61%)	3.4	ND–6.8	2 (15%)	2.7	ND–3.1
	>60	0 (0%)	<2.6	ND	3 (100%)	5.0	4.4–6.1	12 (57%)	3.2	ND–5.5	1 (100%)	4.1	NA						
Heart	0–10				31 (100%)	6.1	4.3–7.2	10 (100%)	6.0	4.9–7.0	2 (100%)	5.6	5.5–5.8	34 (100%)	6.0	4.2–7.9	26 (100%)	5.4	3.9–6.9
	11–30				4 (100%)	4.3	3.7–5.2	7 (100%)	3.7	2.6–4.8	2 (100%)	4.2	4.2–4.2	4 (100%)	3.4	2.9–4.2	8 (36%)	2.9	ND–4.1
	31–60				5 (100%)	4.2	3.4–5.2							4 (22%)	2.8	ND–4.3	4 (31%)	2.7	ND–3.1
	>60	0 (0%)	<2.6	ND	3 (100%)	4.3	3.8–5.1	7 (32%)	2.9	ND–4.9	0 (0%)	<2.6	NA						
Intestine	0–10				31 (100%)	5.4	3.4–7.4	10 (100%)	4.3	3.3–5.7	2 (100%)	4.6	4.4–4.8	34 (100%)	5.0	2.6–6.8	17 (68%)	3.7	ND–5.5
	11–30				4 (80%)	4.4	ND–5.4	3 (43%)	3.0	ND–4.5	1 (50%)	3.8	2.6–5.1	3 (75%)	3.5	ND–4.3	2 (10%)	2.7	ND–3.8
	31–60				5 (100%)	6.2	4.2–7.1							3 (17%)	2.7	ND–3.7	4 (31%)	2.8	ND–3.3
	>60	0 (0%)	<2.6	ND	3 (100%)	5.7	5.2–6.1	10 (45%)	3.1	ND–6.2	1 (100%)	4.5	NA						
Brain	0–10				32 (100%)	7.0	6.1–7.8	10 (100%)	6.5	5.4–7.7	2 (100%)	6.8	6.5–7.2	30 (100%)	6.3	5.2–7.4	23 (92%)	4.8	ND–6.2
	11–30				4 (100%)	6.1	5.8–6.5	7 (100%)	5.3	4.4–6.1	2 (100%)	5.9	5.8–6.0	4 (100%)	4.3	3.8–5.0	4 (18%)	2.9	ND–4.8
	31–60				5 (100%)	6.0	5.5–6.5							14 (78%)	3.5	ND–4.5	8 (62%)	3.1	ND–3.9
	>60	1 (50%)	3.1	ND–3.7	3 (100%)	6.4	5.8–7.2	17 (77%)	4.0	ND–5.9	1 (100%)	3.3	NA						

[a] Percentage positive of total animals sampled at that time–point; [b] Log_{10} copies/swab; ND = Not detected.

Table 2. Quantity of Bungowannah virus RNA detected in selected tissues and fluids from pigs 8-01 and 8-05 (D55 Ab −ve) at 11 months of age.

Animal ID	Sample	Viral Load [a]	Animal ID	Sample	Viral Load [a]
08-01	Tonsil	4.74	08-05	Tonsil	7.46
	Lymph node	4.82		Lymph node	7.31
	Spleen	4.36		Spleen	4.93
	Thymus	ND		Thymus	ND
	Brain	ND		Brain	4.18
	Heart	4.25		Heart	3.78
	Lung	ND		Lung	ND
	Intestine	4.78		Intestine	6.34
	Urine	6.9		Urine	5.8
	Kidney	ND		Kidney	3.7
	Epididymal semen	9.8		Ovarian follicular fluid	ND
	Seminal fluid	3.4		Cervix	ND
	Bulbourethral gland	5.8		Ovary	2.8
	Epididymis (head)	6.2		Uterus	4.3
	Epididymis (tail)	8.0		Vagina	5.2
	Prostate	4.1			
	Seminal vesicle	ND			
	Testis	6.3			

[a] Log_{10} copies/mL or swab; ND = Not detected.

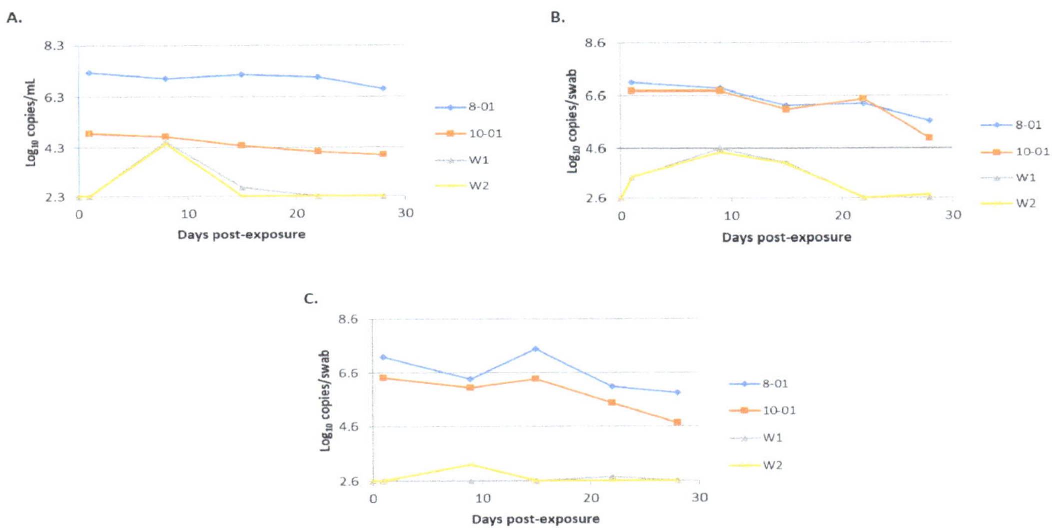

Figure 7. Comparison of the quantity of virus detected in serum (**A**), oropharyngeal swabs (**B**) and rectal swabs (**C**) for persistently infected (PI) animals (8-01 and 10-01) and transiently infected in-contact animals (W1 and W2).

4. Discussion

This study demonstrates that the porcine foetus can become infected with Bungowannah virus following intranasal challenge of the dam and characterises the virological and serological responses following in utero infection of the porcine foetus at different stages of gestation. Persistent infections, as described for other pestiviruses, were observed, as was a chronic infection state where animals that had been presumed to be PI animals later seroconverted and cleared the viral infection. Transmission of Bungowannah virus infection from chronically infected pigs to naïve pigs was readily achieved, with evidence of virus transfer within 24 h.

Preliminary investigations to identify the causative agent of the porcine myocarditis syndrome utilised a direct foetal inoculation route [25]. In the current study, the goal was to determine the outcomes using a natural route of infection at different stages of gestation. Transplacental infection was successfully achieved following intra-nasal exposure of the dam in 87% (20/23) of the litters. In addition, this outcome was not affected by the stage of gestation of the sow at the time of challenge.

Regardless of the stage of gestation that infection occurred, Bungowannah virus was detected in the serum, body fluid and excretions of infected pigs at birth and this was unrelated to the presence of precolostral Bungowannah virus-specific antibody in these animals. Generally, there was minimal difference in virus shedding between the pigs in the different challenge groups at birth, although the mean and median were lowest for the D90 group. The highest viral loads in serum or body fluid were recorded in the D35 (Ab −ve) and D55 (Ab −ve) groups. Over the course of the study it was noted that viral shedding reduced more quickly the later in gestation that the dam was challenged for those pigs which were seropositive at birth or in the D90 group. For those pigs seronegative at birth (D35 and D55 groups), viral shedding remained elevated throughout the course of the study. The exception was those animals that seroconverted after 6–7 weeks (10-01) and between 18 and 28 weeks (8-01 and 8-05) after which viral shedding gradually decreased, although the reduction varied between pigs. In contrast, the viral load in serum declined for all challenge groups after the ingestion of colostrum, but, as maternal antibodies waned in those animals that were seronegative at birth (D35 and D55), the viral load in serum increased as has been described for CSFV [13–15]. Despite animals 8-01, 8-05 and 10-01 seroconverting, it still took approximately 3 months for the viraemia to clear after this event.

It is interesting to compare our results with experimental studies of classical swine fever virus in the porcine foetus which were conducted 40–50 years ago with the less sensitive technologies of virus isolation and antigen detection by immunofluorescence [13,14,21,29]. While test sensitivity may affect the direct comparison of the proportion of animals infected with CSFV at birth compared to Bungowannah virus, the findings are similar. Virus could be detected in a proportion of all pigs born following infection with CSFV both pre- and post-immunocompetence as we have observed. Van Oirschot [13] also described congenitally infected pigs that cleared their CSFV infection by 2 weeks of age. The proportion of pigs that recovered increased the later in gestation that infection took place and was also associated with a low viral load in serum at birth. While precolostral CSFV neutralising antibodies were only detected in one animal (sow infected at 90 days of gestation), these virology findings are similar to those observed for congenital Bungowannah virus infections.

The pig foetus is able to mount a humoral immune response to Bungowannah virus following in utero infection. The highest antibody titres at birth were observed in those pigs that seroconverted and were the progeny of sows challenged at D35 and D55. Only one pig at D70 had no detectable antibody and it was stillborn. Antibody titres in the D90 group were generally low at birth presumably due to the short interval between infection and birth. However, the detection of viraemia indicates that all pigs in the D90 litters were infected prior to birth. Pigs infected post-natally generally seroconvert from 12–14 days post-infection [23]. Therefore, based on the D90 data, it is considered that transplacental and subsequent foetal infection had occurred within 8–10 days of intra-nasal exposure of the sow.

Unfortunately, farrowings were not monitored throughout the night and in some cases pigs were able to feed prior to precolostral blood samples being collected. While not optimal, we were still able to identify pigs in the D35 and D55 groups that did and did not mount a humoral immune response in utero and demonstrate that the time of gestation at which infection occurs has an influence on the ability of the porcine foetus to mount a humoral immune response to Bungowannah virus. The porcine foetus becomes competent to respond to infection with CSFV between days 70–90 of gestation and the serological findings of this study would suggest that the timing is similar, although likely closer to 70 days for Bungowannah virus [13,14,21]. The failure of some pigs in the D35 and D55 litters to seroconvert is indicative of immunotolerance, which occurs following infection prior to foetal immunocompetence and is recognised with other in utero pestivirus infections [5,13,14,21]. In the D55 group it was in Litters 8 and 10, that were challenged at 56 and 55 days of gestation, respectively, that the birth of litters with a mix of both seronegative and seropositive pigs resulted. A previous study [25], suggested that direct in utero transmission of Bungowannah virus to adjacent foetuses is probable and this has also been suggested for CSFV [22]. We speculate that the mixed outcomes of seronegative and seropositive pigs at birth in the D55 and to a lesser extent the D35 group are a consequence of the timing of foetal infection following transplacental transmission, and timing of any subsequent infections that result from direct in utero transmission.

While the current study did not measure neutralising antibody, the findings have similarities to those of Frey et al. [21] who did not detect neutralising antibody against CSFV in progeny at term when pregnant gilts were infected with CFSV at 65–67 days of gestation. In contrast, 3/4 (75%) of foetuses from gilts infected at 85 days of gestation had neutralising antibodies at term; additionally, antibodies were only detected in 2/6 (33%) of infected pigs when infection occurred after 94 days of gestation. As these foetuses were collected via hysterectomy at term it is not possible to determine if the failure to detect a neutralising antibody response is due to insufficient time between infection and sampling or the result of immunotolerance. Interestingly, Van Oirschot [13] with one exception did not detect precolostral antibodies in any pigs following challenge of the dam with CSFV at 40, 65 or 90 days gestation although the ability of some pigs (highest percentage at 90 days) to clear their infection by 2 weeks of age indicates they were not immunotolerant. Further comparison of antibody titres as measured by PLA and the virus neutralisation test may clarify the nature of the humoral immune response that develops in the period immediately following the development of immunocompetence compared with later in gestation.

The results also suggest that the cell-mediated immune response to Bungowannah virus may be suppressed if the foetus is infected before 90 days gestation or that the antibody response at this time is non-neutralising. In those foetuses from dams infected at 75 days of gestation or earlier that mounted an antibody response, even after ingestion of colostrum, the time taken for these animals to clear the infection was generally delayed compared to those from dams infected at 90 days gestation.

The identification of viraemic pigs that were seronegative following infection of the sow with Bungowannah virus at 35 or 55 days of gestation suggests that persistent infections may result. Persistent pestivirus infections occur following in utero infection of the foetus prior to it becoming immunocompetent and have been described following infection prior to day 70 to 90 of gestation for CSFV, bovine viral diarrhoea virus (BVDV) and Border disease-like viruses in the pig [13,14,30,31]. Despite two pigs in D35 not becoming PI, infection at this stage of gestation results in a high probability of occurrence. By day 55 of gestation the likelihood of maternal infection resulting in persistent infections is declining and may result in a mixed outcome for foetuses within that litter. Based on the results of this study and direct foetal inoculation [25], infection of the pregnant pig after approximately day 60 of gestation (approximately day 70 for foetal infection) seems unlikely to result in persistent infections.

At birth, PI animals could only be differentiated in the laboratory by their seronegative status. While the mean viral load in serum at birth was higher than for those animals born seropositive, individual animal variation was sufficient to prevent the titre of viraemia being a distinguishing feature. Furthermore, it was not until maternal antibodies began to wane from approximately 4–5 weeks of age in the PI pigs that the viral load in serum was higher than the non-PI animals. In contrast, the viral load on oropharyngeal and rectal swabs from PI animals remained elevated throughout the study period but the viral load on swabs for those animals seropositive at birth declined from 3 weeks of age. PI pigs from the D35 group grew poorly and died or were euthanased by 75 days of age [24]. While those from the D55 group were stunted [24], they had survived longer.

Three pigs, from the D55 group (8-01, 8-05 and 10-01) were monitored over a 6 to 11 month period to assess their virological and serological status over time and for any abnormal clinical signs [24]. Unexpectedly, these animals that appeared to be PI seroconverted at varying times during this observation period. This phenomenon has been described rarely in pigs infected with BVDV or border disease virus (BDV) [30,31]. Like these previous studies with BVDV and BDV, the Bungowannah virus viraemia ceased after seroconversion but virus could still be detected in many tissues for a further 5–6 months and at high levels for the female (8-05). For the male (8-01), the highest viral load was 9.8 log_{10} copies/mL in epididymal semen and was generally above 6.0 log_{10} copies/mL for other testicular samples (Table 2). Such high virus levels have also been observed in a PI bull [32] and in the pig 8-01 presumably remained high following seroconversion due to the immunologically privileged status of the testes. In contrast, for the female (8-05) the highest viral loads were detected in lymphoid tissues (tonsil and lymph node) (Table 2). It is also of interest to note the high quantity of Bungowannah virus detected in the seminal fluid of the male in the absence of spermatozoa [24]. This has also been described in a boar PI with BVDV [32]. The mechanism for the failure of virus to be cleared from tissues at the same time as the resolution of the viraemia is not clear but may be related to clearance from infected cells being dependent on cell-mediated immunity rather than just the presence of antibody and its inability to access immunologically privileged sites.

Chronic infections resulting from in utero infections with pestivirus have not been reported in ruminants with one exception of BDV in a sheep [17]. It seems probable that the mechanism for development of the chronic infections observed in pigs are related to differences in the time required for maturation of the immune system of ruminants and pigs given that the porcine foetus becomes immunocompetent at a proportionately later stage of gestation compared to ruminants.

While the two chronically infected pigs followed to 11 months of age were quite stunted and would not have been selected as breeding animals [24], they have the potential to be more important in the ongoing transmission of Bungowannah virus than the PI pigs that die early in life. To this end, we were able to show that Bungowannah virus is readily transmitted by these animals to naïve pigs in close proximity.

At least 100–1000 times more Bungowannah virus RNA was detected on oropharyngeal and faecal swabs from pigs at birth in this study compared with peak viral shedding of transiently infected animals [23]. The difference in quantity of virus shed by persistently/chronically infected animals in oropharyngeal swabs compared with peak shedding by transiently infected animals remained approximately 100 times higher until seroconversion was detected in the chronically infected animals. In addition, while the virus load in faeces is negligible in the transiently infected pig, faeces along with urine appear to be an important route of shedding in the PI pig (100–1000 times greater quantity), emphasising the role of PI animals in the epidemiology of pestivirus infections. Placental and vaginal secretions also appear to be an important source of virus for environmental contamination and ongoing transmission and has previously been recognised for BVDV [33]. High quantities of viral RNA could be detected in the placental and vaginal secretions of recently farrowed animals that carried infected foetuses. Although the quantity detected decreased rapidly over the first 5–7 days after farrowing, these reproductive materials could provide a significant source of virus in a population of pregnant animals to sustain transmission cycles even in the absence of a PI animal. This study indicates that all recently farrowed Bungowannah virus infected litters are also potentially adding large quantities of virus into the environment. Further studies are required to determine if these animals are shedding an infectious virus and, therefore, a source of virus for ongoing transmission, although given the quantities of Bungowannah virus RNA detected on oropharyngeal swabs we believe this is highly likely to be the case.

Finally, examination of the virus loads in tissue samples indicates that Bungowannah virus is widely disseminated in the porcine foetus at birth and provides an insight into sample selection for diagnostic purposes from live and dead animals. While the virus could usually be detected in a wide range of samples collected at birth, the optimal tissues to sample for virus detection were serum/body fluid, oropharyngeal swabs, tonsils and lungs. In older animals, virus can also be readily detected in a wide range of samples from PI animals, although serum, oropharyngeal swabs and lymph nodes are preferred for the greatest chance of detection of infection in animals greater than 10 days of age that may not be PI. The high quantity of virus detected in tonsillar samples suggests that the tonsils are the primary source of Bungowannah virus found in oropharyngeal secretions.

5. Conclusions

The results of this study provide a unique insight into the biology of Bungowannah virus infections in the porcine foetus and the subsequent pre- and post-weaning period following infection at different stages of gestation. While the birth of PI animals was expected based on our knowledge of pestivirus infections in other species, the birth of chronically infected pigs that later went on to seroconvert was unexpected. This study provides further information about how the porcine foetus responds to in utero pestivirus infections.

Author Contributions: Conceptualization, D.S.F. and P.D.K.; methodology, D.S.F. and P.D.K.; investigation, D.S.F.; resources, D.S.F. and P.D.K.; data curation, D.S.F.; writing—original draft preparation, D.S.F.; writing—review and editing, D.S.F. and P.D.K.; visualization, D.S.F. and P.D.K.; supervision, P.D.K.; project administration, D.S.F. and P.D.K.; funding acquisition, P.D.K. All authors have read and agreed to the published version of the manuscript.

Acknowledgments: We gratefully acknowledge the staff of the Virology Laboratory at the Elizabeth Macarthur Agricultural Institute (EMAI) for technical assistance (particularly Katherine King), veterinary assistance (Andrew Read), and assistance with sample collection, and both farm and laboratory staff, especially Glenda Macnamara, for their care of the animals used in this study.

References

1. McOrist, S.; Thornton, E.; Peake, A.; Walker, R.; Robson, S.; Finlaison, D.; Kirkland, P.; Reece, R.; Ross, A.; Walker, K.; et al. An infectious myocarditis syndrome affecting late-term and neonatal piglets. *Aust. Vet. J.* **2004**, *82*, 509–511. [CrossRef]
2. Kirkland, P.D.; Frost, M.J.; Finlaison, D.S.; King, K.R.; Ridpath, J.F.; Gu, X. Identification of a novel virus in pigs-Bungowannah virus: A possible new species of pestivirus. *Virus Res.* **2007**, *129*, 26–34. [CrossRef]
3. Hause, B.M.; Collin, E.A.; Peddireddi, L.; Yuan, F.; Chen, Z.; Hesse, R.A.; Gauger, P.C.; Clement, T.; Fang, Y.; Anderson, G. Discovery of a novel putative atypical porcine pestivirus in pigs in the USA. *J. Gen. Virol.* **2015**, *96*, 2994–2998. [CrossRef]
4. Lamp, B.; Schwarz, L.; Hogler, S.; Riedel, C.; Sinn, L.; Rebel-Bauder, B.; Weissenbock, H.; Ladinig, A.; Rumenapf, T. Novel pestivirus species in pigs, Austria, 2015. *Emerg. Infect. Dis.* **2017**, *23*, 1176–1179. [CrossRef]
5. Moennig, V.; Liess, B. Pathogenesis of intrauterine infections with bovine viral diarrhea virus. *Vet. Clin. North Am. Food Anim. Pract.* **1995**, *11*, 477–487. [CrossRef]
6. Roeder, P.L.; Jeffrey, M.; Cranwell, M.P. Pestivirus fetopathogenicity in cattle: Changing sequelae with fetal maturation. *Vet. Rec.* **1986**, *118*, 44–48. [CrossRef]
7. Baker, J.C. The Clinical Manifestations of Bovine Viral Diarrhea Infection. *Vet. Clin. N. Am.-Food A.* **1995**, *11*, 425–445. [CrossRef]
8. McGowan, M.R.; Kirkland, P.D. Early reproductive loss due to bovine pestivirus infection. *Br. Vet. J.* **1995**, *151*, 263–270. [CrossRef]
9. Garcia-Perez, A.L.; Minguijon, E.; Estevez, L.; Barandika, J.F.; Aduriz, G.; Juste, R.A.; Hurtado, A. Clinical and laboratorial findings in pregnant ewes and their progeny infected with Border disease virus (BDV-4 genotype). *Res. Vet. Sci.* **2009**, *86*, 345–352. [CrossRef] [PubMed]
10. Arruda, B.L.; Arruda, P.H.; Magstadt, D.R.; Schwartz, K.J.; Dohlman, T.; Schleining, J.A.; Patterson, A.R.; Visek, C.A.; Victoria, J.G. Identification of a divergent lineage porcine pestivirus in nursing piglets with congenital tremors and reproduction of disease following experimental inoculation. *PLoS ONE* **2016**, *11*, e0150104. [CrossRef]
11. Nettleton, P.F. Border disease. In *Infectious Diseases of Livestock*, 2nd ed.; Coetzer, J.A.W., Tustin, R.C., Eds.; Oxford University Press Southern Africa: Cape Town, South Africa, 2004; Volume 2, pp. 970–974.
12. Trautwein, G.; Hewicker, M.; Liess, B.; Orban, S.; Grunert, E. Studies on transplacental transmissibility of a bovine virus diarrhoea (BVD) vaccine virus in cattle III. Occurrence of central nervous system malformations in calves born from vaccinated cows. *J. Vet. Med. B.* **1986**, *33*, 260–268. [CrossRef] [PubMed]
13. Van Oirschot, J.T. Experimental production of congenital persistent swine fever infections: I. Clinical, pathological and virological observations. *Vet. Microbiol.* **1979**, *4*, 117–132. [CrossRef]
14. Meyer, H.; Liess, B.; Frey, H.R.; Hermanns, W.; Trautwein, G. Experimental transplacental transmission of hog cholera virus in pigs. IV. Virological and serological studies in newborn piglets. *Zentralbl Veterinarmed B* **1981**, *28*, 659–668. [CrossRef]
15. Van Oirschot, J.T.; Terpstra, C. A congenital persistent swine fever infection. I. Clinical and virological observations. *Vet. Microbiol.* **1977**, *2*, 121–132. [CrossRef]
16. Van Oirschot, J.T. A congenital persistent swine fever infection. II. Immune response to swine fever virus and unrelated antigens. *Vet. Microbiol.* **1977**, *2*, 133–142. [CrossRef]

17. Nettleton, P.F.; Gilmour, J.S.; Herring, J.A.; Sinclair, J.A. The production and survival of lambs persistently infected with border disease virus. *Comp. Immunol. Microbiol. Infect. Dis.* **1992**, *15*, 179–188. [CrossRef]
18. Barlow, R.M.; Vantsis, J.T.; Gardiner, A.C.; Rennie, J.C.; Herring, J.A.; Scott, F.M.M. Mechanisms of natural transmission of Border disease. *J. Comp. Pathol.* **1980**, *90*, 57–65. [CrossRef]
19. Plateau, E.; Vannier, P.; Tillon, J.P. Atypical hog cholera infection: Viral isolation and clinical study of in utero transmission. *Am. J. Vet. Res.* **1980**, *41*, 2012–2015.
20. Moennig, V.; Floegel-Niesmann, G.; Greiser-Wilke, I. Clinical signs and epidemiology of classical swine fever: A review of new knowledge. *Vet. J.* **2003**, *165*, 11–20. [CrossRef]
21. Frey, H.R.; Liess, B.; Richter-Reichhelm, H.B.; von Benten, K.; Trautwein, G. Experimental transplacental transmission of hog cholera virus in pigs. I. Virological and serological studies. *Zentralbl Veterinarmed B* **1980**, *27*, 154–164. [CrossRef] [PubMed]
22. Van Oirschot, J.T. Congenital infections with nonarbo togaviruses. *Vet. Microbiol.* **1983**, *8*, 321–361. [CrossRef]
23. Finlaison, D.S.; King, K.R.; Gabor, M.; Kirkland, P.D. An experimental study of Bungowannah virus infection in weaner aged pigs. *Vet. Microbiol.* **2012**, *160*, 245–250. [CrossRef]
24. Finlaison, D.S.; Kirkland, P.D. The outcome of porcine foetal infection with Bungowannah virus is dependent on the stage of gestation at which infection occurs. Part 2: Clinical signs and gross pathology. *Viruses* **2020**. submitted for publication.
25. Finlaison, D.S.; Cook, R.W.; Srivastava, M.; Frost, M.J.; King, K.R.; Kirkland, P.D. Experimental infections of the porcine foetus with Bungowannah virus, a novel pestivirus. *Vet Microbiol* **2010**, *144*, 32–40. [CrossRef] [PubMed]
26. Kim, J.; Choi, C.; Han, D.U.; Chae, C. Simultaneous detection of porcine circovirus type 2 and porcine parvovirus in pigs with PMWS by multiplex PCR. *Vet. Rec.* **2001**, *149*, 304–305. [CrossRef]
27. Hoffmann, B.; Depner, K.; Schirrmeier, H.; Beer, M. A universal heterologous internal control system for duplex real-time RT-PCR assays used in a detection system for pestiviruses. *J. Virol. Methods* **2006**, *136*, 200–209. [CrossRef]
28. Finlaison, D.S.; King, K.R.; Frost, M.J.; Kirkland, P.D. Field and laboratory evidence that Bungowannah virus, a recently recognised pestivirus, is the causative agent of the porcine myocarditis syndrome (PMC). *Vet. Microbiol.* **2009**, *136*, 259–265. [CrossRef]
29. Cowart, W.O.; Morehouse, L. Effects of attenuated hog cholera virus in pregnant swine at various stages of gestation. *J. Am. Vet. Med. Assoc.* **1967**, *151*, 1788–1794.
30. Paton, D.J.; Done, S.H. Congenital infection of pigs with ruminant-type pestiviruses. *J. Comp. Pathol.* **1994**, *111*, 151–163. [CrossRef]
31. Terpstra, C.; Wensvoort, G. A congenital persistent infection of bovine virus diarrhoea virus in pigs: Clinical, virological and immunological observations. *Vet. Q.* **1997**, *19*, 97–101. [CrossRef]
32. Kirkland, P.D.; Richards, S.G.; Rothwell, J.T.; Stanley, D.F. Replication of bovine viral diarrhoea virus in the bovine reproductive tract and excretion of virus in semen during acute and chronic infections. *Vet. Rec.* **1991**, *128*, 587–590. [CrossRef] [PubMed]
33. Kirkland, P.D.; McGowan, M.R.; Mackintosh, S.G.; Moyle, A. Insemination of cattle with semen from a bull transiently infected with pestivirus. *Vet. Rec.* **1997**, *140*, 124–127. [CrossRef] [PubMed]

Bovine Pestivirus Heterogeneity and its Potential Impact on Vaccination and Diagnosis

Victor Riitho [1,†], Rebecca Strong [1], Magdalena Larska [2], Simon P. Graham [3,4] and Falko Steinbach [1,4,*]

1 Virology Department, Animal and Plant Health Agency, APHA-Weybridge, Woodham Lane, New Haw, Addlestone KT15 3NB, UK; vriitho@gmail.com (V.R.); Rebecca.Strong@apha.gov.uk (R.S.)
2 Department of Virology, National Veterinary Research Institute, Al. Partyzantów 57, 24-100 Puławy, Poland; maglar7@wp.pl
3 The Pirbright Institute, Ash Road, Pirbright GU24 0NF, UK; simon.graham@pirbright.ac.uk
4 School of Veterinary Medicine, University of Surrey, Guilford GU2 7XH, UK
* Correspondence: falko.steinbach@apha.gov.uk
† Current Address: Centre of Genomics and Child Health, The Blizard Institute, Queen Mary University of London, London E1 2AT, UK.

Abstract: Bovine Pestiviruses A and B, formerly known as bovine viral diarrhoea viruses (BVDV)-1 and 2, respectively, are important pathogens of cattle worldwide, responsible for significant economic losses. Bovine viral diarrhoea control programmes are in effect in several high-income countries but less so in low- and middle-income countries where bovine pestiviruses are not considered in disease control programmes. However, bovine pestiviruses are genetically and antigenically diverse, which affects the efficiency of the control programmes. The emergence of atypical ruminant pestiviruses (Pestivirus H or BVDV-3) from various parts of the world and the detection of Pestivirus D (border disease virus) in cattle highlights the challenge that pestiviruses continue to pose to control measures including the development of vaccines with improved cross-protective potential and enhanced diagnostics. This review examines the effect of bovine pestivirus diversity and emergence of atypical pestiviruses in disease control by vaccination and diagnosis.

Keywords: bovine pestiviruses; bovine viral diarrhoea; vaccination; control; diagnosis; antigenic cross-reactivity

---

1. Bovine Pestiviruses

The Pestivirus genus within the family Flaviviridae of single stranded positive sense RNA viruses comprises eleven recognized species, Pestivirus A-K [1]. The previously recognised species included bovine viral diarrhoea virus 1 (BVDV-1, now known as Pestivirus A), BVDV-2 (Pestivirus B), classical swine fever virus (CSFV, Pestivirus C) and border disease virus (BDV, Pestivirus D). In addition, a further 7 other species were designated as Pestivirus E-K: Pestivirus E (pronghorn antelope virus), Pestivirus F (porcine Pestivirus), Pestivirus G (giraffe Pestivirus), Pestivirus H (Hobi-like Pestivirus, atypical ruminant Pestivirus, also known as BVDV-3), Pestivirus I (Aydin-like Pestivirus, sheep Pestivirus), Pestivirus J (rat Pestivirus) and Pestivirus K (atypical porcine Pestivirus). The reclassification of species names is relatively new, and still not widely used, and thus for ease of comparing the literature, both nomenclatures will be used here throughout.

The classification of pestiviruses is based on genetic and antigenic relatedness as well as the host of origin [2]. Genetic likeness of pestiviruses has been shown to be consistent with antigenic relatedness as defined by binding assays with monoclonal antibodies (mAbs) or serum cross-neutralisation relative to the type virus of a particular species [3]. Pestiviruses differ in their host tropism with Pestivirus A,

B and H mainly found in Bovidae or material thereof, hence the original naming as BVDV-1, -2 and -3. Phylogenetic analysis has identified 21 Pestivirus A subtypes (BVDV-1a-u) and 4 Pestivirus B subtypes (BVDV-2a-d) [4]. Pestiviruses H (BVDV-3), formerly referred to as atypical bovine pestiviruses, are a species with similar variability, but no defined subtypes as of yet [5]. Bovine pestiviruses can also infect other domestic livestock species such as sheep, goats and pigs [6]. Conversely, publications have demonstrated the infection of cattle with Pestivirus D (border disease virus) normally associated with the infection of small ruminants, including the ability to establish a persistent infection in bulls [7–9]. There is a need to understand the role of heterologous hosts in the transmission, spill over and emergence of bovine pestiviruses [10].

Pestivirus H (BVDV-3) represents a group of atypical ruminant pestiviruses that were first detected in commercial foetal bovine serum (FBS), originating from South America [11], Southeast Asia [12] or with unknown origin [13]. Other viruses have also been isolated from aborted bovine foetuses [14] and from buffalo in Brazil [15]. It is not clear whether cattle or other bovids are the natural reservoir/host of atypical ruminant pestiviruses. More recently, a Pestivirus H strain has been associated with a severe respiratory disease outbreak and abortions in multiparous cows in Italy [16]. Accordingly, there is evidence suggesting that Pestivirus H is spreading in cattle in South America [14], Southeast Asia [17] and Europe [16]. The extent to which they are present in the cattle population worldwide needs to be further assessed since the genetic and antigenic diversity between bovine pestiviruses poses a significant challenge in BVD diagnosis and vaccination [18].

2. Impact and Control of Bovine Pestiviruses

Bovine pestiviruses are an important group of pathogens that cause significant economic losses to the cattle industry worldwide [19]. BVD is well recognised as an economic factor of cattle production in the western world but less so in the developing world including emerging economies, such as Brazil, where it is not yet considered in disease control programmes. A meta-analysis of bovine pestivirus prevalence in 325 studies across 73 countries showed global prevalence with significantly higher prevalence in countries without BVDV control programmes [20]. The prevalence and impact of Pestivirus H is yet to be fully considered in such studies.

As a result of their economic impact, significant efforts are being made to prevent and control bovine pestiviruses in many developed countries, particularly in Europe. BVD control programmes have been classified as either systematic, involving a monitored, goal-oriented reduction in incidence and prevalence across a regional or national cattle industry, non-systematic, where measures are implemented on a herd basis as a bottom-up approach without wider systematic monitoring [21]. Three key elements for the systematic control of bovine pestiviruses have been described: the identification and elimination of congenitally persistently infected (PI) immunotolerant animals [22]; increased surveillance to monitor the progress of interventions and detect new infections [23] and measures to prevent the infection of pestivirus naïve animals and (re-) introduction of the virus into BVD-free herds. All of this might be achieved by strict biosecurity protocols, including quarantine for incoming animals, but in most cases will require the assistance of vaccines to make the control measures more sustainable, particularly in farms where biosecurity is difficult to maintain [24].

3. Immunity to Bovine Pestiviruses

Antibodies against pestiviruses are acquired from maternal colostrum or following an active immune response due to infection or vaccination and the importance of neutralising antibodies has been well documented [25,26]. Neutralising antibody responses have been described to target envelope glycoproteins E1 and E2, with E2 being immunodominant, playing a major role in the attachment of the virus on to a target/host cell that the neutralising antibodies inhibit [27,28]. Studies of the immune response to Pestivirus A (BVDV-1) have suggested a role for both antibody and T cell responses in protection [29–32]. The further characterisation of antibody and T cell targets that elicit protective immune responses to pestiviruses therefore remains an important prerequisite in the design of next-generation vaccines.

There is good evidence for the role of T cell responses in BVD immunity. Calves vaccinated in the presence of maternal antibodies, whilst unable to mount an effective antibody response, do generate memory T cells sufficient to protect against subsequent viral challenge [33]. Both $CD4^+$ and $CD8^+$ T cell responses have been shown to be evoked by Pestivirus A (BVDV-1) [34], although the antibody depletion of $CD4^+$ T cells, but not $CD8^+$ or γ/δ T cells, has been shown to increase the duration of virus shedding [35]. These $CD4^+$ T cell responses have been shown to be directed principally against E2 and NS3 but also to other proteins such as the N^{pro}, C and E^{rns} proteins [36–38]. An assessment of longitudinal responses to all the different BVDV proteins in the course of natural infection has not been conducted. However, E2 and NS3 have been shown to be the immunodominant proteins by assessment of ex vivo T cell responses to peptide pools representing the whole Pestivirus A (BVDV-1) proteome following experimental infection [39].

4. Cross-Protection between Bovine Pestiviruses

Given the range of Pestivirus species that may infect cattle and cause BVD, it is evident that broadly cross-protective vaccines are required for the control of pestiviruses in cattle, buffalo and other bovid species. While good cross-protection has been observed within the wide range of Pestivirus A (BVDV-1) genotypes, the need to adapt vaccines to include atypical bovine pestiviruses (Pestiviruses H/BVDV-3) has been considered in the development of vaccines [40,41].

Clinical cross-protection against Pestivirus B (BVDV-2) challenge has been reported using Pestivirus A based MLV vaccines [42]. However, the inability to fully prevent foetal infection, postnatal infection and virus shedding has, in part at least, been attributed to antigenic diversity [18,43]. Accordingly, Pestivirus B has been included in some newer vaccine preparations [44,45]. The comparison of T cell and antibody responses observed after infection with a Pestivirus A and/or a Pestivirus H (BVDV-3) virus showed limited immune reactivity to Pestivirus H in Pestivirus A infected animals but good reactivity to Pestivirus A in Pestivirus H inoculated animals [46]. Highly conserved targets such as non-structural protein NS3 generated recall T cell responses in both groups, while viral glycoprotein E2 responses were virus species specific.

Considering the proteomes of bovine pestiviruses these results are not surprising, but they allow for the rationale design of future vaccines that should convey a broad cross-protection. It has been well described that Pestivirus A can be separated into genotypes a-u [4,47], but all of these belong to the same serotype with antibodies widely cross-reacting. Indeed, the amino acid (aa) identity of Pestivirus A genotypes is >85% for the polyprotein, compared to the identity between Pestiviruses A, B and H of 71–76% (data not shown).

The differences within and between pestiviruses are the highest in the E2 glycoprotein that mediates the viral attachment and is under selective pressure from neutralising antibodies. Here, the identity among Pestivirus A E2 proteins is 68–78% and between Pestivirus A to B is 61–66%, while between Pestivirus A and H it is only 57–63%. Accordingly, the aforementioned lack of T-cell cross-reaction between E2 of different pestiviruses and a limited ability to cross-neutralise is not surprising. More so, when we focus on the E2 aa 1-271 that are known to contain the host-cell interaction mediating domains DA, DB, and DC [48], the aa identity among Pestivirus A is further reduced to 66–76% and between the three pestivirus species A, B and H to 50–62% (Table 1). These figures give an approximation of the challenge for vaccine design, without taking discontinuous, conformational epitopes into account while conversely some of the changes might not affect the neutralising epitopes. More research is needed to precisely identify the molecular events and binding partners involved in virus attachment and fusion, as well as defining neutralising epitopes on the pestivirus envelope E2 protein.

Table 1. E2 amino acid homology of selected Pestivirus A, B and H strains. Full genome sequences of selected strains were downloaded from GenBank; the respective accession numbers are provided. Additional information as per strain name and/or country of origin are provided in the left column. Sequences were translated into proteins where necessary and aligned with Clustal W and the sequences trimmed to contain the aa 1-271 of the E2 protein using the MacVector software package. The matrix depicts identities of amino acids (aa) above and homologies below the diagonal. The identities between the same virus species: Pestivirus A (BVDV-1), B (BVDV-2) or H (BVDV-3) are highlighted in green. The identities of Pestivirus B or H compared to Pestivirus A are highlighted in yellow.

	MH379638.1	M96687	KX987157	KR866116	LC089876	JN400273	JQ799141	AF502399	KJ000672	MH231148	KY683847	FJ040215	JQ612704
MH379638.1 BVDV-1a GB Ho916	100	75.6	73.3	73.7	71.9	69.6	66.3	58.5	56.7	60.4	54.1	52.6	53
M96687 BVDV-1b OSLOSS	84.5	100	69	72.3	72.3	69.7	64.9	57.2	56.1	59.4	52.8	52.4	52.4
KX987157 BVDV-1f SLO	82.6	79.3	100	72.2	75.2	73.7	71.1	59.6	58.1	61.5	56.7	54.4	56.7
KR866116 BVDV-1m CN	84.1	81.2	85.2	100	70.7	74.4	66.7	55.9	57.4	59.6	57.4	56.3	58.1
LC089876 BVDV-1n JP	79.6	81.2	83	81.5	100	67.4	68.5	58.5	57	58.5	55.9	55.2	54.4
JN400273 BVDV-1q SD0803 pig	82.2	81.9	84.1	83.7	78.9	100	65.9	58.1	59.3	60.7	55.2	53.3	55.9
JQ799141 BVDV-1u Yak CN	78.5	77.1	81.1	80.4	79.6	81.9	100	58.1	60.4	63	52.6	52.2	52.6
AF502399 BVDV-2a NY-93	71.9	70.5	73.3	72.2	68.1	74.4	75.2	100	80.6	80.6	52.2	54.1	51.1
KJ000672 BVDV-2b SD1301	70.4	67.5	71.1	71.5	66.3	73.7	74.1	88.4	100	81	50.7	53	50.4
MH231148 BVDV-2c 12-149150	72.2	70.5	73.3	73.3	68.1	73.7	77	90.7	87.7	100	53.7	54.4	53
KY683847 BVDV-3 BRA Bos Ind	67	67.2	71.9	71.9	71.1	70.4	67.8	65.9	65.2	66.3	100	90	94.1
FJ040215 BVDV-3 Thai KK	68.5	67.9	71.9	70.7	73	70	68.5	67.8	67	67.4	94.8	100	86.2
JQ612704 BVDV-3 IT	66.3	66.4	71.1	72.2	69.6	71.1	68.1	65.6	65.9	65.6	97	92.6	100

Conversely, NS3, the other main immunogenic protein identified, is highly conserved among Pestivirus A (>94%) and between Pestiviruses A, B and H (>89%, Table 2). Accordingly, broad cross-reactivity for the T-cells directed against NS3 can be assumed. This cross-reactivity would support both cytotoxic $CD8^+$ T cell and $CD4^+$ helper T cell responses and thus indirectly support B cell responses. Accordingly, it is tempting to speculate that the observed clinical cross-protection at least observed by Pestivirus A vaccines, or after infection of cattle with other pestiviruses is indeed T cell driven.

Table 2. NS3 amino acid homology of selected Pestivirus A, B and H strains. Approach and methods used are similar to Table 1. For this analysis, the full length NS3 protein sequences were used.

	MH379638.1	M96687	KX987157	KR866116	LC089876	JN400273	JQ799141	AF502399	KJ000672	MH231148	KY683847	FJ040215	JQ612704
MH379638.1 BVDV-1a GB Ho916	100	97.5	97.4	97.4	97.4	97.4	94	91.9	91.1	92.1	92.4	91.8	92.2
M96687 BVDV-1b OSLOSS	99.4	100	97.4	97.8	97.8	97.8	94.3	92.1	90.6	91.9	92.5	91.9	92.4
KX987157 BVDV-1f SLO	99.4	99.4	100	98.1	97.4	98	94.4	92.1	90.8	91.9	92.5	91.9	92.4
KR866116 BVDV-1m CN	99.4	99.4	99.4	100	97.8	98.2	94	92.7	91.4	92.5	92.4	91.5	92.2
LC089876 BVDV-1n JP	99.4	99.4	99.4	99.4	100	97.7	94	91.8	90.3	91.7	92.4	91.9	91.9
JN400273 BVDV-1q SD0803 pig	99.1	99.4	99	99.1	99.1	100	94.6	91.7	90.5	91.5	92.4	91.7	92.2
JQ799141 BVDV-1u Yak CN	98.2	98.2	98.1	98	98	98	100	90.6	89.5	89.9	91.5	91.4	91.5
AF502399 BVDV-2a NY-93	98.2	98	98.4	98.2	98	97.7	97.1	100	97.5	98.1	91.7	90.9	91.5
KJ000672 BVDV-2b SD1301	97.5	97.5	98	97.8	97.5	97.2	96.3	99	100	97.7	90.3	89.9	90.8
MH231148 BVDV-2c 12-149150	98.1	97.8	98.2	98.1	97.8	97.5	96.9	99.6	99.1	100	91.1	90.3	91.2
KY683847 BVDV-3 BRA Bos Ind	97.2	97.2	96.9	97.4	97.2	97.2	96.6	96.6	95.9	96.5	100	98.5	99.6
FJ040215 BVDV-3 Thai KK	97.2	97.2	96.9	97.2	97.2	96.9	96.6	96.3	95.9	96.2	99.3	100	98.4
JQ612704 BVDV-3 IT	97.2	97.2	96.9	97.4	96.9	97.2	96.6	96.6	96.2	96.5	99.7	99.3	100

It seems feasible to consider a vaccine design that takes only a limited amount of conserved T cell reactive antigens such as NS3 and a mix of E2 (possibly only domains DA-DC) to induce neutralising antibodies into account. This, however, highlights crucial limitations of both the immune system and some of the current state-of-the-art approaches to design modern vaccines: the immune system cannot make a rational decision; it will induce B (antibody) and T cell responses to all antigens presented in a vaccine. Accordingly, traditional inactivated vaccines would likely distract the immune response into too many unnecessary and unhelpful directions. Conversely, some of the promising modern platforms that can mimic MLV will struggle with this design too. Both replication deficient and recombinant pestiviruses use the exchange of one protein (or parts of it). Such a vaccine cannot be designed carrying multiple E2 variants. Similarly, the delivery of multiple proteins is a challenge for viral vector vaccines—unless variants of these are combined in one product. DNA, RNA or subunit vaccines would have an advantage here but are not (yet) ready in their design and proof of concept for production that they can be used with same efficacy as MLV or surrogates thereof.

5. Vaccination against Bovine Pestiviruses

According to VeVax, an online licensed veterinary vaccines database [49], there are more than 120 registered BVD vaccine products currently in use around the world, mostly in North and South America. These are conventional modified live virus (MLV) or inactivated/killed virus vaccines, formulated as either Pestivirus A and/or B (BVDV-1 and/or -2) preparations or multivalent vaccines including other pathogens implicated in the bovine respiratory disease complex, such as members of the Pasteurellaceae family (including *Mannheimia haemolytica*, *Pasturella multicoda* and *Haemophilus somni*), bovine herpesvirus-1, parainfluenza type 3 virus and bovine respiratory syncytial virus [50].

Vaccination against bovine pestiviruses is an additional control measure aimed at the protection of post-natal calves against infection after maternally-derived antibody wanes and of heifers to prevent foetal infections which may result in reproductive failure, foetal losses and birth of PI calves, which continuously spread the virus [51]. The adoption of BVD vaccination in Europe is voluntary with uptake ranging from 20–75% [52]. BVD eradication without vaccination has been successfully carried out by large-scale eradication schemes in Scandinavian countries where 90–99% of herds are considered free of Pestiviruses A and B (BVDV-1 and -2) [53]. These schemes are, however, expensive and intensive and take a long time to implement. The addition of vaccination remains a cost-effective measure for disease control [54]. Furthermore, in regions with high cattle densities and BVDV prevalence, and therefore an increased probability of virus reintroduction into naïve herds, vaccination can easily be incorporated into systematic control strategies [55].

5.1. *Modified Live Virus Vaccines*

MLV vaccines are more efficacious since they induce high titres of virus neutralising antibodies and provide a longer duration of protection from clinical disease than inactivated vaccines that often require booster immunizations to achieve sustained protection [56]. However, there is a risk that MLVs may revert to a virulent form or recombine with field viruses and cause disease and vaccinated animals have been reported to develop transient viremia and to shed vaccine virus [57,58]. MLV vaccines have also been shown to confer foetal protection after Pestivirus A (BVDV-1) and, in a few instances, Pestivirus B (BVDV-2) challenge following vaccination with Pestivirus A based MLV vaccines [59–61]. In pregnant animals, however, live vaccines pose the risk of the vertical transmission of vaccine virus that can occasionally result in foetal complications or birth of PI calves [62]. MLV vaccination has also been implicated in post-vaccination mucosal disease, when PI animals do not mount an immune response to BVDV, due to their intra-uterine infection, and a fatal condition develops, characterised by severe lesions of the oral and intestinal mucosa [63]. As a result of these safety concerns, MLVs are not licensed in all countries.

5.2. *Inactivated Vaccines*

Whilst inactivated vaccines are generally safer and therefore preferred for the vaccination of breeding cattle, bovine neonatal pancytopenia (BNP) has highlighted that there too problems may arise. BNP was a syndrome associated with an inactivated BVD vaccine that affected calves in their first month of life, characterised by pancytopenia, severe bleeding and high lethality that had originally been described in Europe. The vaccine design was rational: prepare the virus in a bovine cell line to reduce allergic or other reactions [64]. What had not been considered sufficiently was the ability of such a preparation to induce some form of auto-immune reaction as it seems to have occurred. The vaccine in question contained a significant amount of bovine (cell line derived) non-viral antigens [65] and the transfer (ingestion) of colostrum from vaccinated affected dams (i.e., those that had given birth to BNP calves) was sufficient to induce disease in several (albeit not all) calves [66]. The underlying pathogenesis of BNP is far from being fully resolved as blood transfusion to affected calves was not sufficient to overcome this problem. The nature of alloreactive antibodies associated with BNP [67] remains debatable, with bovine MHC class I molecules suggested to be the alloantigens responsible [10,68,69]. It is worth noting that BNP affected only some dams in some herds, thus an unresolved genetic component also seems to have played a role. The disease was a highly unusual event that could have been avoided through improved vaccine preparations. In principle, however, this highlights the potential for a safety problem in the use of crude inactivated BVDV preparations that contain significant amounts of host cell derived material.

5.3. *Differentiation of Infection from Vaccination (DIVA)*

Importantly, neither MLV nor inactivated vaccines allow for DIVA [70], which reduces their suitability for use in BVD eradication efforts when vaccination and control could be monitored by Ab ELISA tests. Inactivated vaccines were previously thought to facilitate DIVA because of a lack of production of non-structural proteins such as NS3 and hence the diminished responses to these target antigens [71]. This has, however, in a number of studies proved not be the case [72,73], due to the presence of non-structural proteins in the crude virus preparations used in inactivated vaccines.

5.4. *Sub-Unit and Next-Generation Vaccines*

Recent BVD vaccine developments aim to address the shortcomings of the existing vaccines. An ideal vaccine should prevent disease, prevent vertical and horizontal virus transmission, be safe in pregnant animals, unable to revert to virulence, have broad efficacy to account for virus diversity and permit DIVA [40]. Various approaches towards the development of the next generation of BVD vaccines have been made and some already evaluated in cattle, but most still face challenges [74–77]. One such approach, DNA vaccination, has been trialled with mixed success and is generally deemed to be effective but comes with challenges such as the optimal route of delivery. The use of recombinant subunit proteins had earlier been deemed insufficient to provide effective protection, not least when focusing on E2 [39,78–81]. The combination of antigens (e.g., E2 and NS3) in formulations with molecular adjuvants to stimulate antigen-presenting cells [58,59] has been more successful, but requires further refinement. The combination of approaches such as a DNA prime, protein boost regimes [82–84] is overall more promising than either of the two alone, but comes with the inherent drawback of requiring at least two vaccinations. Accordingly, these types of vaccines are a challenge to the manufacturer, the veterinarian and the farmer. Vaccinations of animals in remote areas of under-developed countries are a challenge already, but additionally, farmers in developed countries and industrialised settings prefer single, possibly multivalent, or fewer multiple vaccines that require minimal inoculations. Defective viral vectored replicons [85–89], synthetic attenuated infectious cDNA clones [90,91], as well as chimeric pestivirus marker vaccines [92], all aim to build upon the success of MLV vaccines, but face regulatory challenges in some countries as they are genetically engineered microorganisms and those built on recombinant pestiviruses might (with regards to recombination) come with similar limitations as MLVs.

In summary, BVD vaccine development efforts are the subject of ongoing research, following the trends of modern vaccine innovation, and have contributed to pave the way for such, including the use of RNA vaccination [70]. To further improve the design of safe and efficacious vaccines that cross-protect against several related pestiviruses and are sufficiently cheap to manufacture and apply, an improved understanding of the immunology in bovine pestivirus infections is required.

6. Diagnosis of Bovine Pestiviruses

Virus isolation has historically been considered the gold standard for the detection of pestiviruses in blood and milk samples. Antigen detection by immunohistochemistry, antigen-capture ELISA and nucleic acid detection by polymerase chain reaction (PCR) based tests are now broadly applied [93,94]. The detection of bovine pestivirus-specific antibody in milk or blood samples by ELISA or by virus neutralisation test is also possible, although these tests are not able to differentiate infected from vaccinated animals (DIVA), which is a significant limitation for BVD control programmes [70]. Antibody and antigen tests, when used together, help to distinguish acutely infected from persistently infected (PI) animals. The diagnoses of both virus and immune responses can be hampered by the genetic and antigenic variability of pestiviruses. More robust approaches are required to assess antigenic relationships between the various Pestivirus species and subtypes [95]. Most tests were established against Pestiviruses A and B (BVDV-1 and -2) and have not been fully validated to detect Pestivirus H (BVDV-3) or Pestivirus D (BDV). Whilst the comparative performance of different Pestivirus A and B assays to detect antibodies against atypical Pestiviruses has been assessed [96], the existing tests are not sensitive enough and no specific tests are available. This makes the comprehensive detection of all potential bovine pestiviruses a diagnostic challenge that can be addressed by focusing on conserved parts of the genome/proteome [11,17,97].

7. Conclusions

Bovine pestivirus diversity, heterologous hosts and the emergence of novel ruminant pestiviruses all pose a significant challenge to control and vaccination [10]. Vaccine efficacy studies should include challenges with heterotypic bovine pestivirus species and vaccines will have to be designed with at least Pestivirus A, B and H (BVDV-1, -2 and -3) in mind. A better understanding of this diversity and consideration of vaccine correlates of protection, cross-protective potential and efficacy against various bovine Pestivirus species will improve vaccine design and thus support global BVD control to reduce the disease burden and economic impact.

Author Contributions: Conceptualization: V.R. and S.P.G.; writing—original draft preparation: V.R.; writing—review and editing: R.S., M.L., S.P.G. and F.S.; supervision: S.P.G. and F.S. All authors have read and agreed to the published version of the manuscript.

References

1. King, A.M.Q.; Lefkowitz, E.J.; Mushegian, A.R.; Adams, M.J.; Dutilh, B.E.; Gorbalenya, A.E.; Harrach, B.; Harrison, R.L.; Junglen, S.; Knowles, N.J.; et al. Changes to taxonomy and the International Code of Virus Classification and Nomenclature ratified by the International Committee on Taxonomy of Viruses (2018). *Arch. Virol.* **2018**, *163*, 2601–2631. [CrossRef]
2. Simmonds, P.; Becher, P.; Bukh, J.; Gould, E.A.; Meyers, G.; Monath, T.; Muerhoff, S.; Pletnev, A.; Rico-Hesse, R.; Smith, D.B.; et al. ICTV Virus Taxonomy Profile: Flaviviridae. *J. Gen. Virol.* **2017**, *98*, 2–3. [CrossRef]
3. Becher, P.; Ramirez, R.A.; Orlich, M.; Cedillo-Rosales, S.; König, M.; Schweizer, M.; Stalder, H.; Schirrmeier, H.; Thiel, H.-J. Genetic and antigenic characterization of novel pestivirus genotypes: Implications for classification. *Virology* **2003**, *311*, 96–104. [CrossRef]
4. Yeşilbağ, K.; Alpay, G.; Becher, P. Variability and Global Distribution of Subgenotypes of Bovine Viral Diarrhea Virus. *Viruses* **2017**, *9*, 128. [CrossRef]
5. Bauermann, F.V.; Ridpath, J.F.; Weiblen, R.; Flores, E.F. HoBi-like viruses: An emerging group of pestiviruses. *J. Veter. Diagn. Investig.* **2013**, *25*, 6–15. [CrossRef]
6. Tao, J.; Liao, J.; Wang, Y.; Zhang, X.; Wang, J.; Zhu, G. Bovine viral diarrhea virus (BVDV) infections in pigs. *Veter. Microbiol.* **2013**, *165*, 185–189. [CrossRef]
7. Braun, U.; Hilbe, M.; Peterhans, E.; Schweizer, M. Border disease in cattle. *Veter. J.* **2019**, *246*, 12–20. [CrossRef]
8. Strong, R.; La Rocca, S.A.; Ibata, G.; Sandvik, T. Antigenic and genetic characterisation of border disease viruses isolated from UK cattle. *Veter. Microbiol.* **2010**, *141*, 208–215. [CrossRef]

9. McFadden, A.M.; Tisdall, D.J.; Hill, F.I.; Otterson, P.; Pulford, D.J.; Peake, J.; Finnegan, C.J.; La Rocca, S.A.; Kok-Mun, T.; Weir, A.M. The first case of a bull persistently infected with Border disease virus in N. Z. *N. Z. Veter. J.* **2012**, *60*, 290–296. [CrossRef]
10. Walz, P.H.; Chamorro, M.F.; Falkenberg, S.M.; Passler, T.; Van Der Meer, F.; Woolums, A.R. Bovine viral diarrhea virus: An updated American College of Veterinary Internal Medicine consensus statement with focus on virus biology, hosts, immunosuppression, and vaccination. *J. Veter. Intern. Med.* **2020**. [CrossRef]
11. Schirrmeier, H.; Strebelow, G.; Depner, K.; Hoffmann, B.; Beer, M. Genetic and antigenic characterization of an atypical pestivirus isolate, a putative member of a novel pestivirus species. *J. Gen. Virol.* **2004**, *85*, 3647–3652. [CrossRef]
12. Liu, L.; Xia, H.; Baule, C.; Belák, S. Maximum likelihood and Bayesian analyses of a combined nucleotide sequence dataset for genetic characterization of a novel pestivirus, SVA/cont-08. *Arch. Virol.* **2009**, *154*, 1111–1116. [CrossRef]
13. Peletto, S.; Zuccon, F.; Pitti, M.; Gobbi, E.; De Marco, L.; Caramelli, M.; Masoero, L.; Acutis, P.L. Detection and phylogenetic analysis of an atypical pestivirus, strain IZSPLV_To. *Res. Veter. Sci.* **2012**, *92*, 147–150. [CrossRef]
14. Cortez, A.; Heinemann, M.B.; De Castro, A.M.M.G.; Soares, R.M.; Pinto, A.M.V.; Alfieri, A.F.; Flores, E.F.; Leite, R.C.; Richtzenhain, L.J. Genetic characterization of Brazilian bovine viral diarrhea virus isolates by partial nucleotide sequencing of the 5′-UTR region. *Pesqui. Veterinária Bras.* **2006**, *26*, 211–216. [CrossRef]
15. Stalder, H.; Meier, P.; Pfaffen, G.; Canal, C.W.; Rufenacht, J.; Schaller, P.; Bachofen, C.; Marti, S.; Vogt, H.; Peterhans, E. Genetic heterogeneity of pestiviruses of ruminants in Switzerland. *Prev. Veter. Med.* **2005**, *72*, 37–41. [CrossRef]
16. DeCaro, N.; Lucente, M.S.; Mari, V.; Cirone, F.; Cordioli, P.; Camero, M.; Sciarretta, R.; Losurdo, M.; Lorusso, E.; Buonavoglia, C. Atypical Pestivirus and Severe Respiratory Disease in Calves, Europe. *Emerg. Infect. Dis.* **2011**, *17*, 1549–1552. [CrossRef]
17. Ståhl, K.; Kampa, J.; Alenius, S.; Wadman, A.P.; Baule, C.; Aiumlamai, S.; Belák, S. Natural infection of cattle with an atypical 'HoBi'-like pestivirus – Implications for BVD control and for the safety of biological products. *Veter. Res.* **2007**, *38*, 517–523. [CrossRef]
18. Bolin, S.R.; Grooms, D.L. Origination and consequences of bovine viral diarrhea virus diversity. *Veter. Clin. N. Am. Food Anim. Pract.* **2004**, *20*, 51–68. [CrossRef]
19. Pinior, B.; Garcia, S.; Minviel, J.J.; Raboisson, D. Epidemiological factors and mitigation measures influencing production losses in cattle due to bovine viral diarrhoea virus infection: A meta-analysis. *Transbound. Emerg. Dis.* **2019**, *66*, 2426–2439. [CrossRef]
20. Scharnböck, B.; Roch, F.-F.; Richter, V.; Funke, C.; Firth, C.L.; Obritzhauser, W.; Baumgartner, W.; Käsbohrer, A.; Pinior, B. A meta-analysis of bovine viral diarrhoea virus (BVDV) prevalences in the global cattle population. *Sci. Rep.* **2018**, *8*, 1–15. [CrossRef]
21. Lindberg, A.; Houe, H. Characteristics in the epidemiology of bovine viral diarrhea virus (BVDV) of relevance to control. *Prev. Veter. Med.* **2005**, *72*, 55–73. [CrossRef] [PubMed]
22. Schweizer, M.; Peterhans, E. Pestiviruses. *Annu. Rev. Anim. Biosci.* **2014**, *2*, 141–163. [CrossRef] [PubMed]
23. Lindberg, A.; Brownlie, J.; Gunn, G.J.; Houe, H.; Moennig, V.; Saatkamp, H.W.; Sandvik, T.; Valle, P. The control of bovine viral diarrhoea virus in Europe: Today and in the future. *Rev. Sci. Tech.* **2006**, *25*, 961–979. [CrossRef] [PubMed]
24. Negron, M.; Raizman, E.A.; Pogranichniy, R.; Hilton, W.M.; Levy, M. Survey on management practices related to the prevention and control of bovine viral diarrhea virus on dairy farms in Indiana, United States. *Prev. Veter. Med.* **2011**, *99*, 130–135. [CrossRef] [PubMed]
25. Bolin, S.R.; Ridpath, J.F. Assessment of protection from systemic infection or disease afforded by low to intermediate titers of passively acquired neutralizing antibody against bovine viral diarrhea virus in calves. *Am. J. Veter. Res.* **1995**, *56*, 755–759.
26. Howard, C.J.; Clarke, M.C.; Brownlie, J. Protection against respiratory infection with bovine virus diarrhoea virus by passively acquired antibody. *Veter. Microbiol.* **1989**, *19*, 195–203. [CrossRef]
27. Bolin, S.R. Immunogens of bovine viral diarrhea virus. *Veter. Microbiol.* **1993**, *37*, 263–271. [CrossRef]
28. Mignon, B.; Waxweiler, S.; Thiry, E.; Boulanger, D.; Dubuisson, J.; Pastoret, P.-P. Epidemiological evaluation of a monoclonal ELISA detecting bovine viral diarrhoea pestivirus antigens in field blood samples of persistently infected cattle. *J. Virol. Methods* **1992**, *40*, 85–93. [CrossRef]

29. Chase, C.C.; Elmowalid, G.; Yousif, A.A. The immune response to bovine viral diarrhea virus: A constantlychanging picture. *Veter. Clin. N. Am. Food Anim. Pract.* **2004**, *20*, 95–114. [CrossRef]
30. Kapil, S.; Walz, P.; Wilkerson, M.; Minocha, H. Immunity and Immunosuppression. In *Bovine Viral Diarrhea Virus*; Blackwell Publishing Ltd.: Hoboken, NJ, USA, 2008; pp. 157–170. [CrossRef]
31. Howard, C.J. Immunological responses to bovine virus diarrhoea virus infections. *Rev. Sci. Tech.* **1990**, *9*, 95–103. [CrossRef]
32. Potgieter, L.N. Immunology of Bovine Viral Diarrhea Virus. *Veter. Clin. N. Am. Food Anim. Pract.* **1995**, *11*, 501–520. [CrossRef]
33. Endsley, J.J.; Roth, J.A.; Ridpath, J.; Neill, J. Maternal antibody blocks humoral but not T cell responses to BVDV. *Boiologicals* **2003**, *31*, 123–125. [CrossRef]
34. Rhodes, S.G.; Cocksedge, J.M.; A Collins, R.; I Morrison, W. Differential cytokine responses of CD4+ and CD8+ T cells in response to bovine viral diarrhoea virus in cattle. *J. Gen. Virol.* **1999**, *80*, 1673–1679. [CrossRef] [PubMed]
35. Howard, C.; Clarke, M.; Sopp, P.; Brownlie, J. Immunity to bovine virus diarrhoea virus in calves: The role of different T-cell subpopulations analysed by specific depletion in vivo with monoclonal antibodies. *Veter. Immunol. Immunopathol.* **1992**, *32*, 303–314. [CrossRef]
36. Lambot, M.; Letesson, J.-J.; Douart, A.; Pastoret, P.P.; Joris, E. Characterization of the immune response of cattle against non-cytopathic and cytopathic biotypes of bovine viral diarrhoea virus. *J. Gen. Virol.* **1997**, *78 Pt 5*, 1041–1047. [CrossRef]
37. Collen, T.; Morrison, W.I. CD4+ T-cell responses to bovine viral diarrhoea virus in cattle. *Virus Res.* **2000**, *67*, 67–80. [CrossRef]
38. Collen, T.; Carr, V.; Parsons, K.; Charleston, B.; Morrison, W.I. Analysis of the repertoire of cattle CD4(+) T cells reactive with bovine viral diarrhoea virus. *Veter. Immunol. Immunopathol.* **2002**, *87*, 235–238. [CrossRef]
39. Riitho, V.; Walters, A.A.; Somavarapu, S.; Lamp, B.; Rümenapf, T.; Krey, T.; Rey, F.A.; Oviedo-Orta, E.; Stewart, G.R.; Locker, N.; et al. Design and evaluation of the immunogenicity and efficacy of a biomimetic particulate formulation of viral antigens. *Sci. Rep.* **2017**, *7*, 13743. [CrossRef]
40. Fulton, R.W. Vaccines. In *Bovine Viral Diarrhea Virus*; Blackwell Publishing Ltd.: Hoboken, NJ, USA, 2008; pp. 209–222. [CrossRef]
41. Fulton, R.W. Impact of species and subgenotypes of bovine viral diarrhea virus on control by vaccination. *Anim. Health Res. Rev.* **2015**, *16*, 40–54. [CrossRef]
42. Kelling, C.L.; Hunsaker, B.D.; Steffen, D.J.; Topliff, C.L.; Eskridge, K.M. Characterization of protection against systemic infection and disease from experimental bovine viral diarrhea virus type 2 infection by use of a modified-live noncytopathic type 1 vaccine in calves. *Am. J. Veter. Res.* **2007**, *68*, 788–796. [CrossRef]
43. Newcomer, B.W.; Chamorro, M.F.; Walz, P.H. Vaccination of cattle against bovine viral diarrhea virus. *Veter. Microbiol.* **2017**, *206*, 78–83. [CrossRef] [PubMed]
44. Ridpath, J.F. Practical significance of heterogeneity among BVDV strains: Impact of biotype and genotype on U.S. control programs. *Prev. Veter. Med.* **2005**, *72*, 17–30. [CrossRef] [PubMed]
45. Fulton, R.W.; Cook, B.J.; Payton, M.E.; Burge, L.J.; Step, D.L. Immune response to bovine viral diarrhea virus (BVDV) vaccines detecting antibodies to BVDV subtypes 1a, 1b, 2a, and 2c. *Vaccine* **2020**, *38*, 4032–4037. [CrossRef] [PubMed]
46. Riitho, V.; Larska, M.; Strong, R.; La Rocca, S.A.; Locker, N.; Alenius, S.; Steinbach, F.; Liu, L.; Uttenthal, A.; Graham, S.P. Comparative analysis of adaptive immune responses following experimental infections of cattle with bovine viral diarrhoea virus-1 and an Asiatic atypical ruminant pestivirus. *Vaccine* **2018**, *36*, 4494–4500. [CrossRef]
47. Mirosław, P.; Polak, M. Increased genetic variation of bovine viral diarrhea virus in dairy cattle in Poland. *BMC Veter. Res.* **2019**, *15*, 1–12. [CrossRef]
48. El Omari, K.; Iourin, O.; Harlos, K.; Grimes, J.M.; Stuart, D.I. Structure of a Pestivirus Envelope Glycoprotein E2 Clarifies Its Role in Cell Entry. *Cell Rep.* **2013**, *3*, 30–35. [CrossRef]
49. He, Y.; Racz, R.; Sayers, S.; Lin, Y.; Todd, T.; Hur, J.; Li, X.; Patel, M.; Zhao, B.; Chung, M.; et al. Updates on the web-based VIOLIN vaccine database and analysis system. *Nucleic Acids Res.* **2014**, *42*, D1124–D1132. [CrossRef]
50. Allen, J.W.; Viel, L.; Bateman, K.G.; Nagy, E.; Røsendal, S.; Shewen, P.E. Serological titers to bovine herpesvirus 1, bovine viral diarrhea virus, parainfluenza 3 virus, bovine respiratory syncytial virus and Pasteurella

haemolytica in feedlot calves with respiratory disease: Associations with bacteriological and pulmonary cytological variables. *Can. J. Veter. Res.* **1992** *56*, 281–288.

51. Fulton, R.W.; Ridpath, J.; Confer, A.W.; Saliki, J.T.; Burge, L.J.; Payton, M.E. Bovine viral diarrhoea virus antigenic diversity: Impact on disease and vaccination programmes. *Boiologicals* **2003**, *31*, 89–95. [CrossRef]
52. Moennig, V.; Brownlie, J. Position paper: Vaccines and vaccination strategies. *EU Themat. Netw. BVDV Control* **2006**.
53. Bitsch, V.; Rønsholt, L. Control of Bovine Viral Diarrhea Virus Infection Without Vaccines. *Veter. Clin. N. Am. Food Anim. Pract.* **1995**, *11*, 627–640. [CrossRef]
54. Van Oirschot, J.T.; Bruschke, C.J.; Van Rijn, P.A. Vaccination of cattle against bovine viral diarrhoea. *Veter. Microbiol.* **1999**, *64*, 169–183. [CrossRef]
55. Moennig, V.; Eicken, K.; Flebbe, U.; Frey, H.-R.; Grummer, B.; Haas, L.; Greiser-Wilke, I.; Liess, B. Implementation of two-step vaccination in the control of bovine viral diarrhoea (BVD). *Prev. Veter. Med.* **2005**, *72*, 109–114. [CrossRef] [PubMed]
56. Theurer, M.E.; Larson, R.L.; White, B.J. Systematic review and meta-analysis of the effectiveness of commercially available vaccines against bovine herpesvirus, bovine viral diarrhea virus, bovine respiratory syncytial virus, and parainfluenza type 3 virus for mitigation of bovine respiratory disease complex in cattle. *J. Am. Veter. Med. Assoc.* **2015**, *246*, 126–142. [CrossRef]
57. Fulton, R.W.; Saliki, J.T.; Burge, L.J.; Payton, M.E. Humoral Immune Response and Assessment of Vaccine Virus Shedding in Calves Receiving Modified Live Virus Vaccines Containing Bovine Herpesvirus-1 and Bovine Viral Diarrhoea Virus 1a. *J. Veter. Med. Ser. B* **2003**, *50*, 31–37. [CrossRef] [PubMed]
58. Grooms, D.L.; Brock, K.V.; Ward, L.A. Detection of cytopathic bovine viral diarrhea virus in the ovaries of cattle following immunization with a modified live bovine viral diarrhea virus vaccine. *J. Veter. Diagn. Investig.* **1998**, *10*, 130–134. [CrossRef]
59. Xue, W.; Mattick, D.; Smith, L.; Maxwell, J. Fetal protection against bovine viral diarrhea virus types 1 and 2 after the use of a modified-live virus vaccine. *Can. J. Veter. Res.* **2009**, *73*, 292–297.
60. Fairbanks, K.K.; Rinehart, C.L.; Ohnesorge, W.C.; Loughin, M.M.; Chase, C.C. Evaluation of fetal protection against experimental infection with type 1 and type 2 bovine viral diarrhea virus after vaccination of the dam with a bivalent modified-live virus vaccine. *J. Am. Veter. Med. Assoc.* **2004**, *225*, 1898–1904. [CrossRef]
61. Kovács, F.; Magyar, T.; Rinehart, C.; Elbers, K.; Schlesinger, K.; Ohnesorge, W.C. The live attenuated bovine viral diarrhea virus components of a multi-valent vaccine confer protection against fetal infection. *Veter. Microbiol.* **2003**, *96*, 117–131. [CrossRef]
62. Ficken, M.D.; Ellsworth, M.A.; Tucker, C.M.; Cortese, V.S. Effects of modified-live bovine viral diarrhea virus vaccines containing either type 1 or types 1 and 2 BVDV on heifers and their offspring after challenge with noncytopathic type 2 BVDV during gestation. *J. Am. Veter. Med. Assoc.* **2006**, *228*, 1559–1564. [CrossRef]
63. Becher, P.; Orlich, M.; Thiel, H.-J. RNA Recombination between Persisting Pestivirus and a Vaccine Strain: Generation of Cytopathogenic Virus and Induction of Lethal Disease. *J. Virol.* **2001**, *75*, 6256–6264. [CrossRef] [PubMed]
64. Benedictus, L.; Bell, C.R. The risks of using allogeneic cell lines for vaccine production: The example of Bovine Neonatal Pancytopenia. *Expert Rev. Vaccines* **2016**, *16*, 65–71. [CrossRef] [PubMed]
65. Euler, K.N.; Hauck, S.M.; Ueffing, M.; Deeg, C.A. Bovine neonatal pancytopenia—Comparative proteomic characterization of two BVD vaccines and the producer cell surface proteome (MDBK). *BMC Veter. Res.* **2013**, *9*, 18. [CrossRef] [PubMed]
66. Friedrich, A.; Büttner, M.; Rademacher, G.; Klee, W.; Weber, B.K.; Müller, M.; Carlin, A.; Assad, A.; Hafner-Marx, A.; Sauter-Louis, C.M. Ingestion of colostrum from specific cows induces Bovine Neonatal Pancytopenia (BNP) in some calves. *BMC Veter. Res.* **2011**, *7*, 10. [CrossRef]
67. Pardon, B.; Stuyven, E.; Stuyvaert, S.; Hostens, M.; Dewulf, J.; Goddeeris, B.M.; Cox, E.; Deprez, P. Sera from dams of calves with bovine neonatal pancytopenia contain alloimmune antibodies directed against calf leukocytes. *Veter. Immunol. Immunopathol.* **2011**, *141*, 293–300. [CrossRef]
68. Bastian, M.; Holsteg, M.; Hanke-Robinson, H.; Duchow, K.; Cussler, K. Bovine Neonatal Pancytopenia: Is this alloimmune syndrome caused by vaccine-induced alloreactive antibodies? *Vaccine* **2011**, *29*, 5267–5275. [CrossRef]
69. Foucras, G.; Corbière, F.; Tasca, C.; Pichereaux, C.; Caubet, C.; Trumel, C.; Lacroux, C.; Franchi, C.; Burlet-Schiltz, O.; Schelcher, F.; et al. Alloantibodies against MHC Class I: A Novel Mechanism of Neonatal

Pancytopenia Linked to Vaccination. *J. Immunol.* **2011**, *187*, 6564–6570. [CrossRef]
70. Van Oirschot, J.T. Diva vaccines that reduce virus transmission. *J. Biotechnol.* **1999**, *73*, 195–205. [CrossRef]
71. Makoschey, B.; Sonnemans, D.; Bielsa, J.M.; Franken, P.; Mars, M.; Santos, L.; Alvarez, M. Evaluation of the induction of NS3 specific BVDV antibodies using a commercial inactivated BVDV vaccine in immunization and challenge trials. *Vaccine* **2007**, *25*, 6140–6145. [CrossRef]
72. Álvarez, M.; Donate, J.; Makoschey, B. Antibody responses against non-structural protein 3 of bovine viral diarrhoea virus in milk and serum samples from animals immunised with an inactivated vaccine. *Veter. J.* **2012**, *191*, 371–376. [CrossRef]
73. Raue, R.; Harmeyer, S.S.; Nanjiani, I.A. Antibody responses to inactivated vaccines and natural infection in cattle using bovine viral diarrhoea virus ELISA kits: Assessment of potential to differentiate infected and vaccinated animals. *Veter. J.* **2011**, *187*, 330–334. [CrossRef] [PubMed]
74. Nobiron, I.; Thompson, I.; Brownlie, J.; Collins, M.E. DNA vaccination against bovine viral diarrhoea virus induces humoral and cellular responses in cattle with evidence for protection against viral challenge. *Vaccine* **2003**, *21*, 2082–2092. [CrossRef]
75. Young, N.J.; Thomas, C.J.; Thompson, I.; Collins, M.E.; Brownlie, J. Immune responses to non-structural protein 3 (NS3) of bovine viral diarrhoea virus (BVDV) in NS3 DNA vaccinated and naturally infected cattle. *Prev. Veter. Med.* **2005**, *72*, 115–120. [CrossRef] [PubMed]
76. Liang, R.; van den Hurk, J.V.; Zheng, C.; Yu, H.; Pontarollo, R.A.; Babiuk, L.A.; van Drunen Littel-van den Hurk, S. Immunization with plasmid DNA encoding a truncated, secreted form of the bovine viral diarrhea virus E2 protein elicits strong humoral and cellular immune responses. *Vaccine* **2005**, *23*, 5252–5262. [CrossRef] [PubMed]
77. Harpin, S.; Hurley, D.J.; Mbikay, M.; Talbot, B.; Elazhary, Y. Vaccination of cattle with a DNA plasmid encoding the bovine viral diarrhoea virus major glycoprotein E2. *J. Gen. Virol.* **1999**, *80 Pt 12*, 3137–3144. [CrossRef]
78. Thomas, C.J.; Young, N.J.; Heaney, J.; Collins, M.E.; Brownlie, J. Evaluation of efficacy of mammalian and baculovirus expressed E2 subunit vaccine candidates to bovine viral diarrhoea virus. *Vaccine* **2009**, *27*, 2387–2393. [CrossRef]
79. Bolin, S.R.; Ridpath, J.F. Glycoprotein E2 of bovine viral diarrhea virus expressed in insect cells provides calves limited protection from systemic infection and disease. *Arch. Virol.* **1996**, *141*, 1463–1477. [CrossRef]
80. Zoth, S.C.; Leunda, M.R.; Odeón, A.; Taboga, O. Recombinant E2 glycoprotein of bovine viral diarrhea virus induces a solid humoral neutralizing immune response but fails to confer total protection in cattle. *Braz. J. Med. Biol. Res.* **2007**, *40*, 813–818. [CrossRef]
81. Wang, S.; Yang, G.; Nie, J.; Yang, R.; Du, M.; Su, J.; Wang, J.; Wang, J.; Zhu, Y. Recombinant Erns-E2 protein vaccine formulated with MF59 and CPG-ODN promotes T cell immunity against bovine viral diarrhea virus infection. *Vaccine* **2020**, *38*, 3881–3891. [CrossRef]
82. Liang, R.; van den Hurk, J.V.; Landi, A.; Lawman, Z.; Deregt, D.; Townsend, H.; Babiuk, L.A.; van Drunen Littel-van den Hurk, S. DNA prime–protein boost strategies protect cattle from bovine viral diarrhea virus type 2 challenge. *J. Gen. Virol.* **2008**, *89*, 453–466. [CrossRef]
83. Liang, R.; van den Hurk, J.V.; Babiuk, L.A.; van Drunen Littel-van den Hurk, S. Priming with DNA encoding E2 and boosting with E2 protein formulated with CpG oligodeoxynucleotides induces strong immune responses and protection from Bovine viral diarrhea virus in cattle. *J. Gen. Virol.* **2006**, *87*, 2971–2982. [CrossRef] [PubMed]
84. Cai, D.; Song, Q.; Duan, C.; Wang, S.; Wang, J.; Zhu, Y. Enhanced immune responses to E2 protein and DNA formulated with ISA 61 VG administered as a DNA prime-protein boost regimen against bovine viral diarrhea virus. *Vaccine* **2018**, *36*, 5591–5599. [CrossRef] [PubMed]
85. Elahi, S.M.; Shen, S.H.; Talbot, B.G.; Massie, B.; Harpin, S.; Elazhary, Y. Recombinant adenoviruses expressing the E2 protein of bovine viral diarrhea virus induce humoral and cellular immune responses. *FEMS Microbiol. Lett.* **1999**, *177*, 159–166. [CrossRef] [PubMed]
86. Elahi, S.M.; Bergeron, J.; Nagy, E.; Talbot, B.G.; Harpin, S.; Shen, S.H.; Elazhary, Y. Induction of humoral and cellular immune responses in mice by a recombinant fowlpox virus expressing the E2 protein of bovine viral diarrhea virus. *FEMS Microbiol. Lett.* **1999**, *171*, 107–114. [CrossRef]
87. Toth, R.L.; Nettleton, P.F.; McCrae, M.A. Expression of the E2 envelope glycoprotein of bovine viral diarrhoea virus (BVDV) elicits virus-type specific neutralising antibodies. *Veter. Microbiol.* **1999** *65*, 87–101. [CrossRef]

88. Baxi, M.K.; Deregt, D.; Robertson, J.; Babiuk, L.A.; Schlapp, T.; Tikoo, S.K. Recombinant Bovine Adenovirus Type 3 Expressing Bovine Viral Diarrhea Virus Glycoprotein E2 Induces an Immune Response in Cotton Rats. *Virology* **2000**, *278*, 234–243. [CrossRef]
89. Elahi, S.M.; Shen, S.-H.; Talbot, B.G.; Massie, B.; Harpin, S.; Elazhary, Y. Induction of Humoral and Cellular Immune Responses against the Nucleocapsid of Bovine Viral Diarrhea Virus by an Adenovirus Vector with an Inducible Promoter. *Virology* **1999**, *261*, 1–7. [CrossRef]
90. Meyer, C.; Von Freyburg, M.; Elbers, K.; Meyers, G. Recovery of Virulent and RNase-Negative Attenuated Type 2 Bovine Viral Diarrhea Viruses from Infectious cDNA Clones. *J. Virol.* **2002**, *76*, 8494–8503. [CrossRef]
91. Meyers, G.; Tautz, N.; Becher, P.; Thiel, H.J.; Kümmerer, B.M. Recovery of cytopathogenic and noncytopathogenic bovine viral diarrhea viruses from cDNA constructs. *J. Virol.* **1996**, *70*, 8606–8613. [CrossRef]
92. Luo, Y.; Yuan, Y.; Ankenbauer, R.G.; Nelson, L.D.; Witte, S.B.; Jackson, J.A.; Welch, S.-K.W. Construction of chimeric bovine viral diarrhea viruses containing glycoprotein Erns of heterologous pestiviruses and evaluation of the chimeras as potential marker vaccines against BVDV. *Vaccine* **2012**, *30*, 3843–3848. [CrossRef]
93. Saliki, J.T.; Dubovi, E.J. Laboratory diagnosis of bovine viral diarrhea virus infections. *Veter. Clin. N. Am. Food Anim. Pract.* **2004**, *20*, 69–83. [CrossRef] [PubMed]
94. Sandvik, T. Selection and use of laboratory diagnostic assays in BVD control programmes. *Prev. Veter. Med.* **2005**, *72*, 3–16. [CrossRef] [PubMed]
95. Mosena, A.C.S.; Falkenberg, S.M.; Ma, H.; Casas, E.; Dassanayake, R.P.; Walz, P.H.; Canal, C.W.; Neill, J.D. Multivariate analysis as a method to evaluate antigenic relationships between BVDV vaccine and field strains. *Vaccine* **2020**, *38*, 5764–5772. [CrossRef] [PubMed]
96. Larska, M.; Polak, M.P.; Liu, L.; Alenius, S.; Uttenthal, A. Comparison of the performance of five different immunoassays to detect specific antibodies against emerging atypical bovine pestivirus. *J. Virol. Methods* **2013**, *187*, 103–109. [CrossRef]
97. Bauermann, F.V.; Flores, E.F.; Ridpath, J.F. Antigenic relationships between Bovine viral diarrhea virus 1 and 2 and HoBi virus: Possible impacts on diagnosis and control. *J. Veter. Diagn. Investig.* **2012**, *24*, 253–261. [CrossRef]

16

Identification of Antimicrobial Resistance-Associated Genes through Whole Genome Sequencing of *Mycoplasma bovis* Isolates with Different Antimicrobial Resistances

Lisa Ledger, Jason Eidt and Hugh Y. Cai *

Animal Health Lab, University of Guelph, 419 Gordon St., Guelph, ON N1H 6R8, Canada; lledger@uoguelph.ca (L.L.); jeidt@uoguelph.ca (J.E.)

* Correspondence: hcai@uoguelph.ca

Abstract: Antimicrobial resistance (AMR) in *Mycoplasma bovis* has been previously associated with topoisomerase and ribosomal gene mutations rather than specific resistance-conferring genes. Using whole genome sequencing (WGS) to identify potential new AMR mechanisms for *M. bovis*, it was found that a 2019 clinical isolate with high MIC (2019-043682) for fluoroquinolones, macrolides, lincosamides, pleuromutilins and tetracyclines had a new core genome multilocus sequencing (cgMLST) type (ST10-like) and 91% sequence similarity to the published genome of *M. bovis* PG45. Closely related to PG45, a 1982 isolate (1982-M6152) shared the same cgMLST type (ST17), 97.2% sequence similarity and low MIC results. Known and potential AMR- associated genetic events were identified through multiple sequence alignment of the three genomes. Isolate 2019-043682 had 507 genes with non-synonymous mutations (NSMs) and 67 genes disrupted. Isolate 1982-M6152 had 81 NSMs and 20 disruptions. Using functional roles and known mechanisms of antimicrobials, a 55 gene subset was assessed for AMR potential. Seventeen were previously identified from other bacteria as sites of AMR mutation, 38 shared similar functions to them, and 11 contained gene-disrupting mutations. This study indicated that *M. bovis* may obtain high AMR characteristics by mutating or disrupting other functional genes, in addition to topoisomerases and ribosomal genes.

Keywords: *Mycoplasma bovis*; antimicrobial resistance; whole genome sequencing; MIC; cgMLST

---

1. Introduction

Mycoplasma bovis is a member of the Mollicutes; membrane-bound bacteria which lack a cell wall, precluding the use of many common antimicrobial agents such as the β-lactams [1]. In cattle, *M. bovis* is a causative agent of pneumonia, arthritis, otitis media, and reproductive disease and is a contributor to the bovine respiratory disease (BRD) complex, also known as 'shipping fever', which is a major source of morbidity, mortality and financial loss in calf and feedlot operations. Additionally, *M. bovis* is capable of persisting for the life of a colonized animal, which may remain asymptomatic while acting as a source of infection for herdmates or offspring [1,2].

Of note, many of the antibiotics to which *M. bovis* shows resistance are not licensed for usage in treating *M. bovis* infections [3] but may be used in the treatment of other bovine bacterial pathogens. Given the asymptomatic nature of many *M. bovis* infections, and the high rates of colonization when animals are co-mingled (potentially over 90%) [4,5], conditions are favourable for the development of multi-drug resistant strains. With global rates of antimicrobial resistance increasing, understanding the molecular mechanisms underlying antimicrobial resistance, particularly for multi-drug resistant (MDR) strains, is critical for determining effective treatment [6], or potentially to design treatment protocols that use evolutionary approaches to counter or reverse antimicrobial resistance [7].

Unlike other members of the BRD complex such as *Mannheimia haemolytica*, *Histophilus somni* or *Pasteurella multocida*, *M. bovis* is not known to possess defined antimicrobial resistance genes [8] but appears to have the molecular mechanisms of its resistance rooted in point mutations within several ribosomal and topoisomerase genes. Previous studies have used whole-genome sequencing (WGS) paired with minimum inhibitory concentration (MIC) testing to establish that mutations within *gyrA* and *parC* are linked to increased resistance to fluoroquinolones, that increased resistance to spectinomycin and the tetracyclines is linked to *rrs1-rrs2* (16S rRNA gene) mutations, and that *rrl1-rrl2* (23S rRNA gene) mutations are linked to increased resistance to florfenicol, lincosamides, macrolides and pleuromutilins [9], with *rrl3* (23S rRNA gene) also implicated in macrolide resistance [10].

In a large-scale MIC study of *M. bovis* strains isolated between 1978 to 2009, fluctuations in antimicrobial susceptibility over time were observed [3] with the MIC50 values, and thus resistance, increasing for several tetracycline and macrolide-class antimicrobial drugs over the span of the study. Additionally, associations between MIC50 values were observed for different antimicrobials; although sequencing these isolates fell beyond the scope of the study, the association between lincosamides, pleuromutilins and florfenicol in terms of *rrl1-rrl2* mutations was mirrored by a similar observed association in MIC50 values with these historical samples.

A high MIC *M. bovis* was isolated from lung tissues of a two-week old male Holstein calf submitted to the Animal Health Lab in July of 2019 for post-mortem examination. In the interest of determining possible genetic factors for this high level of resistance, whole-genome sequencing using the Illumina MiSeq platform was conducted, in tandem with WGS of a historical isolate of *M. bovis* (1982-M6152) previously categorized as low MIC for most antimicrobials [3]. The MICs and sequence data for both isolates were compared to *M. bovis* strain PG45, a reference strain with a fully sequenced and circularized genome, in order to identify any gaps in sequencing coverage, to determine if any new genes were present in the isolates as opposed to a reference strain, and to better elucidate which mutations in the high MIC isolate were potentially significant for AMR by ruling out any shared mutations with the low MIC isolate.

2. Results

2.1. MIC Testing

Cultures of two isolates of *M. bovis* (1982-M6152 and 2019-043682) and *M. bovis* strain PG45 (used as a reference strain) were tested in triplicate for minimum inhibitory concentration of 16 antimicrobials (Table 1), with the results of MIC testing identical within each triplicate. Relative to *M. bovis* PG45, isolate 1982-M6152 shows a two-fold increase in MIC for oxytetracycline but is otherwise identical in response to other antimicrobial compounds. Isolate 2019-043682 shows increased MICs for multiple fluoroquinolones, macrolides and tetracyclines, as well as a lincosamide, a pleuromutilin and two inhibitors of protein synthesis (gentamicin and florfenicol). For aminoglycosides the results are mixed, with increased MIC observed for spectinomycin, but no change in MIC for neomycin. All three strains have high MICs for sulfonamides, although they retain a low MIC for combination trimethoprim/sulfa.

2.2. Whole-Genome Sequencing

Raw sequencing yield for the two sequenced isolates was 167.8 Mb for 1982-M6152 (GenBank accession: CP058969), and 54.02 Mb for 2019-043682 (GenBank accession: CP058968). Given the sequencing yields and the documented genome size of 1.003 Mb for *M. bovis* PG45 (GenBank accession NC_014760.1), raw sequencing coverage (where C = yield/genome size) was 167× for 1982-M6152 and 54× for 2019-043682, which is sufficient for analysis of mutations and SNPs. Assembled using SPAdes 3.9.0 [11] in Illumina's BaseSpace hub (Illumina, Inc., San Diego, CA, USA) genome sizes were 978,895 bp for 1982-M6152 and 941,076 bp for 2019-043682. Also within BaseSpace, core genome multilocus squence typing (cgMLST) was conducted for both isolates sequenced, using Bacterial

Analysis Pipeline v1.0.4 [12]. Isolate 2019-043682 had an undescribed cgMLST type (ST10-like) while isolate 1982-M6152 had the same cgMLST type (ST17) as PG45.

Table 1. Average results of MIC testing for two isolates of Mycoplasma bovis, compared to reference strain PG45, by μg of antimicrobial compound required to inhibit growth. Isolates and the reference strain were tested in triplicate with identical results within each triplicate for all antimicrobials tested.

Antimicrobial	PG45	2019-043682	1982-M6152
Neomycin	>32	>32	>32
Spectinomycin	<8	16	<8
Trimethoprim/Sulfa	>2/38	>2/38	>2/38
Danofloxacin	0.5	>1	0.5
Enrofloxacin	0.5	2	0.5
Clindamycin	<0.25	>16	<0.25
Tilmicosin	<4	>64	<4
Tulathromycin	8	>64	8
Tylosin Tartrate	1	>32	1
Tiamulin	1	8	1
Gentamicin	8	16	8
Florfenicol	4	>8	4
Sulphadimethoxine	>256	>256	>256
Chlortetracycline	<0.5	>8	<0.5
Oxytetracycline	<0.5	>8	1
Ceftiofur	>8	>8	>8

Assembly and multiple sequence alignment (MSA) of both isolates with *M. bovis* PG45 in Geneious 11(Biomatters, Auckland, New Zealand) (Figure 1) revealed that 2019-043682 had 91% sequence similarity to PG45. 1982-M6152 had 97.2% sequence similarity to PG4.

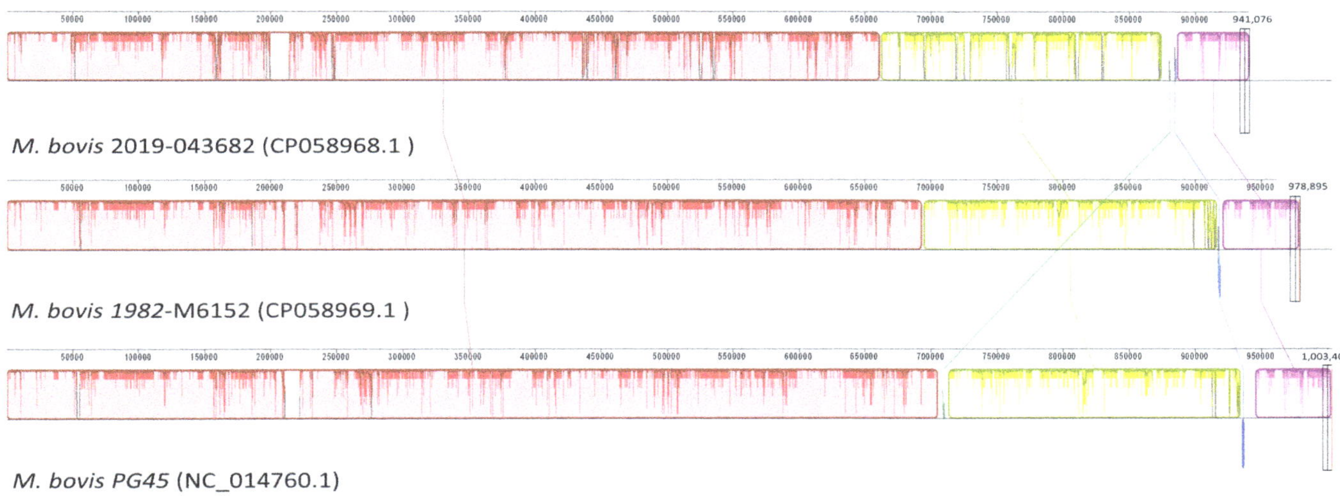

Figure 1. Graphical output of multiple sequence alignment (Mauve, Geneious 11) for *M. bovis* isolates 2019-43682, 1982-M6152 and *M. bvis* strain *PG45* with GenBank accessions displaying depth of sequencing and areas with large deletions.

Annotation of the MSA in MegAlign using feature data for PG45 identified 878 features (MegAlign's term: CDS, in more general usage) in strain PG45, with divergences by isolate summarized in Table 2. Features were reported as Identical by MegAlign if they were 100% identical to PG45, with 100% coverage. Features were reported as Not_Mapped by MegAlign if their % identity score fell below 95%. Unmapped features have been further categorized by the researchers as excised, truncated or highly variable based on their % coverage score (Table 2). Isolate 1982-M6152 had 696 features identical to PG45, 105 with substitutions, 37 with insertions or deletions and 39 reported as Not_Mapped.

Of these 39, 24 were excised, 11 truncated and 4 present but highly variable. Isolate 2019-043682 had 183 identical features, 471 with substitutions, 50 with insertions or deletions, and 173 reported as Not_Mapped. Of these, 81 were excised, 48 were truncated, and 44 were present but highly variable. Although several features were excised in the isolates relative to PG45, no unique features were identified in either isolate that were absent from PG45.

Table 2. Summary of variation of isolates from *M. bovis* PG45, by feature count (CDS), generated using MegAlign. v17 for multiple sequence alignment.

Genetic Events		1982-M6152	2019-043682
Variation types	Identical	696	183
	Deletion	8	18
	Deleted_end_3prime	3	3
	Deleted_end_5prime	1	3
	Indel	3	4
	Insertion	22	22
	Not_Mapped	39	173
	Substitution	105	471
	TOTAL	877	877
Unmapped features	Excised (<5% coverage)	24	81
	Truncated (5–95% coverage)	11	48
	Highly variable (>95% coverage)	4	44
	TOTAL	39	173

To determine which mutations could potentially alter gene function, further analysis of the two isolates using DNAStar's ArrayStar software revealed 3285 individual nonsynonymous mutations relative to *M. bovis* PG45 in total between the two isolates, across 513 genes and pseudogenes. Isolate 1982-M6152 contained 81 genes with non-synonymous mutations, 20 of which were disrupted. Isolate 2019-043682 contained 507 genes with non-synonymous mutations, with 67 genes disrupted. 17 genes with non-synonymous mutations were common to both isolate 1982-M6152 and isolate 2019-043682, with 14 of the mutations identical between the 2 isolates. Four genes with disrupting mutations were common to both isolates, with an insertion mutation in gene MBOVPG45_RS03940 (insertion TTGT, PG45 genome reference position 918372) identical between isolates. A subset of 55 genes (Table 3) containing NSMs was selected for further consideration based on the functional role of the genes and known mechanisms of antimicrobials, through consultation of the Comprehensive Antibiotic Resistance Database (CARD) and literature review [13]. Additionally, 22 genes were identified as ABC transporter system genes (Table 4) although the lack of available characterization has led to them being grouped separately for discussion. A full list of nonsynonymous mutations, their sequence and their positions is available as supplementary data (Supplementary Tables S1 and S2), as well as an expanded version of Table 3 (Supplementary Table S3) containing gene descriptions.

Table 3. Count of non-synonymous mutations (NSMs) relative to *M. bovis* PG45, by gene and by isolate, for a subset of NSM-containing genes identified as potentially associated with antimicrobial resistance.

Functional Role:	Gene:	1982-M6152	2019-043682	Associated AMR:	Reference:
Topoisomerases	gyrA	0	8	fluoroquinolones	[9]
	gyrB	0	6	fluoroquinolones	[9]
	parC	1 *	19 *	fluoroquinolones	[9]
	parE	0	4	fluoroquinolones	[14]
	topA	0	1 ^		

Table 3. *Cont.*

Functional Role:	Gene:	1982-M6152	2019-043682	Associated AMR:	Reference:
Protein Synthesis:					
Methyltransferases:	MBOVPG45_RS00465	0	2		
	MBOVPG45_RS00470	0	7		
	MBOVPG45_RS02280	0	4		
	rlmB	0	5	Predicted AMR	[15]
	rlmD	0	11		
	rlmH	0	1		
	rsmA	0	6	aminoglycosides	[16]
	rsmD	0	1	aminoglycosides	[16]
	rsmH	0	5	aminoglycosides	[16]
	rsmI	0	5	aminoglycosides	[16]
	trmB	0	4 ^		
30S Ribosomal Proteins	rpsB	0	3	aminoglycosides	[17]
	rpsC	2	1	tetracyclines	[18]
	rpsD	0	2		
	rpsE	1	2	aminoglycosides	[19]
	rpsH	0	1		
	rpsJ	1	0	tetracyclines	[20]
	rpsP	0	2		
	rpsS	0	1		
	rbfA	0	1		
50S Ribosomal Proteins	MBOVPG45_RS00445	0	1		
	rplB	0	1		
	rplC	0	1	pleuromutilins	[21]
	rplD	0	10	linezolid	[22]
	MBOVPG45_RS03525	0	2		
	rplV	0	1	macrolides	[23]
	MBOVPG45_RS01360	0	1		
	rpmE	0	1	MDR	[24]
tRNA ligases	alaS	1	8 ^	novobiocin	[25]
	MBOVPG45_RS01640	0	5		
	asnS	0	1	multi-drug resistance	[26]
	MBOVPG45_RS00205	0	9		
	MBOVPG45_RS01150	0	6 ^		
	MBOVPG45_RS02730	0	2		
	MBOVPG45_RS02640	0	1		
	ileS	1	5 ^	pseudomonic acid	[27]
	MBOVPG45_RS03145	0	1		
	MBOVPG45_RS02255	0	16		
	lysS	0	3	methicillin	[28]
	MBOVPG45_RS03150	0	10		
	pheS	0	2	MDR	[26]
	MBOVPG45_RS00380	0	18		
	serS	0	1		
tRNA ligases	MBOVPG45_RS02170	1	8 ^		
	trpS	0	1		
	MBOVPG45_RS04210	0	9 ^		
	MBOVPG45_RS00740	0	7 ^		
	tilS	0	8		
	thiI	0	4		
	mnmA	0	5		

* Identical NSM; ^ Contains a gene-disrupting NSM.

Table 4. Count of non-synonymous mutations (NSMs) relative to *M. bovis* PG45, by gene and by isolate, for ABC transporter system genes potentially linked to the bacterial efflux pump mechanism of AMR. ^Gene contains a disrupting mutation.

Gene:	1982-M6152	2019-043682	Description:
MBOVPG45_RS00090	0	1	ABC transporter ATP-binding protein
MBOVPG45_RS00180	0	2	ABC transporter permease
MBOVPG45_RS00555	0	2	ABC transporter permease
MBOVPG45_RS00570	0	4	ATP-binding cassette domain-containing protein
MBOVPG45_RS00600	0	1	ATP-binding cassette domain-containing protein
MBOVPG45_RS01485	0	2	energy-coupling factor transporter transmembrane protein EcfT
MBOVPG45_RS01540	0	1	sugar ABC transporter permease
MBOVPG45_RS01545	0	4	ATP-binding cassette domain-containing protein
MBOVPG45_RS01720	0	1	ABC transporter permease subunit
MBOVPG45_RS01770	0	1	ABC transporter ATP-binding protein
MBOVPG45_RS01775	1	7	ABC transporter permease
MBOVPG45_RS02005	0	5	ABC transporter ATP-binding protein
MBOVPG45_RS02710	0	1	ABC transporter permease subunit
MBOVPG45_RS02715	0	2	ATP-binding cassette domain-containing protein
MBOVPG45_RS02905	1	1	ABC transporter permease subunit
MBOVPG45_RS03425	0	1	ATP-binding cassette domain-containing protein
MBOVPG45_RS03465	0	4	ABC transporter ATP-binding protein
MBOVPG45_RS03470	0	6	ABC transporter ATP-binding protein
MBOVPG45_RS03705	0	6 ^	carbohydrate ABC transporter permease
MBOVPG45_RS03710	0	1	sugar ABC transporter permease
MBOVPG45_RS04310	0	5	ABC transporter ATP-binding protein
MBOVPG45_RS04315	1	89	ABC transporter permease

^ Contains a gene-disrupting NSM.

3. Discussion

The recent isolate 2019-043682 had significantly elevated MICs for multiple fluoroquinolones, macrolides and tetracyclines, as well as a lincosamide, a pleuromutilin, spectinomycin, and two inhibitors of protein synthesis (gentamicin and florfenicol), indicating multi-drug resistant *M. bovis* can emerge in the field.

Of the *M. bovis* genes previously linked by Sulyok et al. with AMR for various classes of antimicrobial, two sites linked with fluoroquinolone resistance (*gyrA* and *gyrB*) display multiple non-synonymous mutations (NSMs) for the high-MIC isolate 2019-043682 and no NSMs for the low-MIC isolate 1982-M6152. *ParC*, likewise associated with fluoroquinolone resistance, shows 18 unique NSMs in the isolate 2019-043682, and a single NSM in 1982-M6152, which is shared with the 2019-043682, therefore the shared single NSM is unlikely to be contributory to the elevated MICs. Although genes *rrs1-rrs2* and *rrl1-rrl2* were associated with AMR for tetracyclines, spectinomycin, macrolides, lincosamides and pleuromutilins, there are no NSMs for them in the isolate 2019-043682 despite the elevated MIC values, suggesting additional genetic events may be associated with AMR for these antimicrobials.

For antimicrobials where an observed increase in MIC was not matched with a previously identified *M. bovis* resistance-associated mutation, genes identified as AMR-associated in other species, as well as genes within the same functional groups are likely candidates for AMR association. Beyond the genes previously associated with AMR in *M. bovis*, an additional 510 features contain non-synonymous mutations. Assigning these genes to functional groups allowed us to exclude pseudogenes and genes coding for uncharacterized and hypothetical proteins. Also excluded were genes whose NSMs were identical between isolates 2019-043682 (high MIC) and 1982-M6152 (low MIC). Of the 149 genes remaining, we focused on a subset of 55 genes with nonsynonymous mutations within functional roles known to be involved in antimicrobial resistance [13]: protein synthesis and topoisomerases. Additionally, 22 genes with NSMs were identified as ATP binding cassette (ABC) transporter system genes. These genes, although lacking full characterization, are nonetheless included in the discussion as targets for future analysis, due to the role of efflux pumps, particularly ABC transporters, in AMR.

3.1. Protein Synthesis

Interference with protein synthesis is a primary method of action for the antimicrobials, with different antimicrobials interfering at different stages of synthesis, and at different locations within the ribosome complex.

3.1.1. Methyltransferases

RNA methyltransferases methylate specific bases within ribosomal RNA, altering the physical structure of binding sites and other active sites within the ribosomal subunits [16,29,30]. Mutations within the 16S RNA methyltransferase family are known to confer aminoglycoside resistance within other bacterial species [16], and five genes (*rsmA, rsmD, rsmH, rsmI* and MBOVPG45_RS02280, a 16S uracil methyltransferase) within isolate 2019-043682 contain NSMs not found in isolate 1982-M6152. The 23S methyltransferase *rlmA* has been associated with AMR for tylosin [29], and while *rlmA* is wildtype in isolate 2019-043682, the related 23S methyltransferases *rlmB, rlmD* and *rlmH* contain 5, 11 and 1 unique NSMs respectively. *RlmB* has also been identified as a potential site for AMR mutations based on an analysis of its structure [15], although no mutational studies have been conducted. For tRNA methyltransferases, *trmD* is implicated in multi-drug resistance [31]: it is wildtype in isolate 2019-043682, but two related tRNA methyltransferases (*trmB* and MBOVPG45_RS00465, a cytidine methyltransferase) contain NSMs, with *trmB* containing a gene disruption.

3.1.2. Ribosomal Proteins

Mutations in *rpsC* and *rpsJ*, components of the 30S ribosomal subunit, are known to confer tetracycline resistance [18,20]. *RpsC* contains a single NSM in isolate 2019-043682 that is unique from the two NSMs observed in isolate 1982-M6152, but *rpsJ* is wildtype in isolate 2019-043682 and contains a single NSM in isolate 1982-M6152 that is therefore unlikely to influence MIC values. *RpsB* and *rpsE* contain 3 and 2 NSMs in the 2019 isolate, with a single, separate NSM present for *rpsE* in the 1982 isolate: mutations in these genes have been linked with aminoglycoside resistance [17,19], Additionally, five other 30S ribosomal proteins (*rpsD, rpsG, rpsP, rpsS*, and *rbfA*) contain NSMs in isolate 2019-043682.

Of the 50S ribosomal proteins with observed NSMs, *rplD* and *rplV* have been previously associated with macrolide resistance in *Clostridium perfringens* and two *Campylobacter* species [22,23] with *rplD* containing ten separate NSMs in the isolate 2019-043682. The 50S subunit gene *rplC*, where mutation has been previously associated with pleuromutilin resistance [32], contains a single NSM in the 2019 isolate, unique from the two NSMs found in the 1982 isolate. 50S ribosomal proteins mutations have also been linked with resistance to lincosamides, macrolides and phenicols [32]: an additional five genes (*rplB, rpmE*, MBOVPG45_RS00445, MBOVPG45_RS03525 and MBOVPG45_RS01360) coding for 50S ribosomal proteins contain NSMs in isolate 2019-043682 while remaining wildtype in isolate 1982-M6152. Among these, *rpmE* has been linked with multi-drug resistance [24].

3.1.3. Aminoacyl-tRNA Synthetases

While none of the antimicrobials used in MIC testing in this study target them, aminoacyl-tRNA synthetases, also known as tRNA-ligases, are enzymes which attach individual amino acids to their corresponding tRNAs and are a target of interest for antimicrobial development [33]. Isolate 2019-043682 contains 22 tRNA-ligase genes with NSMs, of which ileS (a known target for pseudomonic acid) [27] is disrupted, as is alaS (a novobiocin target) [25], in addition to a glutamate-tRNA ligase (MBOVPG45_RSO1150) and a methionine-tRNA ligase (MBOVPG45_RS03150). *AsnS* and *pheS* have been linked with multi-drug resistance [26] and contain one and two unique NSMs in isolate 2019-043682, respectively. Three of these genes (alaS, ileS and MBOVPG45_RS02170, a threonine-tRNA ligase) contain different NSMs in isolate 1982-M6152, illustrating that the presence of an NSM on its own is not sufficient for AMR, and deeper investigation into changes in protein structure and function are required. LysS, containing 3 NSMs in isolate 2019-043682, has been identified as a gene contributing to methicillin resistance in MRSA [31]: as a β-lactam, methicillin is not used in the treatment of mycoplasma infections, but co-infection with *M. bovis* containing a potential AMR-associated mutation raises the possibility of horizontal gene transfer to a normally susceptible species.

3.2. Topoisomerases

In addition to *gyrA*, *gyrB* and *parC* discussed by Sulyok et al. (2017), *parE* mutations are also involved in fluoroquinolone resistance [14] and the isolate 2019-043682 contains four NSMs within the *parE* gene. While *topA*, a type I DNA topoisomerase, has not been linked with AMR previously, the gene, which is wildtype in isolate 1982-M6152, contains a single nucleotide "A" insertion at nt 1762 of the *topA* gene in isolate 2019-043682, which results in a *topA* (612–614 VK *) to *topA* (612–613 S *) mutation, likely a gene disrupting mutation. As bacterial topoisomerase I is a target of interest for antimicrobial development [34–36], screening for mutations affecting *topA* may be of future value to researchers and clinicians.

3.3. Bacterial Efflux Pumps: ABC Transporters

Bacterial efflux pumps are a class of membrane transport proteins whose role is the removal of toxic substances or metabolites from within the bacterial cell: It is estimated that 5–10% of all bacterial genes are involved in transport, with efflux pumps specifically comprising a large proportion of these transporters [37]. Of the two classes of efflux pump, primary and secondary, the primary transporters use ATP hydrolysis as an energy source, and are also known as ATP binding cassette transporters, or ABC transporters [38]. They are more commonly implicated in resistance to a single drug or category of drugs, although instances of multi-drug resistant ABC transporters have been described 200 [16,38].

As summarized in Table 4, 22 ABC transporter genes contain NSMs in isolate 2019-043682, one of which (MBOVPG45_RS03705) contains a gene-disrupting mutation. Three (MBOVPG45_RS01775, MBOVPG45_RS02905 and MBOVPG45_RS04315) also contain NSMs in isolate 1982-M6152. Although none are previously identified as SDR- or MDR- involved in *M. bovis*, the wide range of antimicrobials affected by efflux pumps suggests that this may be an area of interest for future research. While 8 non-ABC membrane transport proteins with NSMs were identified in isolate 2019-043682 (Supplementary Table S2), none has been characterized sufficiently to determine their potential as secondary efflux pumps and have thus been excluded from discussion.

3.4. Future Directions

Within the 55 genes selected for additional study based on functional role and the 22 ABC transporter genes, the 40 genes identified by their organism (eg., MBOVPG45_RS00380) rather than a common name limit the utility of a literature review or database search for assessing AMR potential. Although beyond the scope of the current study, a BLAST search for each gene to identify homology with other organisms could permit more detailed characterization of these genes and thus allow for a more thorough search of existing research into AMR. This would be of particular value for the ABC transporters, as all 22 identified as potential AMR associations due to their mutations are given *M. bovis*-specific identifiers. MBOVPG45_RS04315, with 89 separate NSMs in the high-MIC isolate, is a particularly strong candidate for a homology search.

As an initial foray by the research group into whole genome sequencing, the sequencing of a pair of high and low MIC isolates and the use of a fully-characterized reference strain (PG45) as a scaffold for assembly and annotation allowed us to determine which genes and which NSMs were non-contributory to the high MIC observed in the 2019 isolate, and allowed us to determine that no additional genes were present relative to the reference strain. Sequencing additional high-MIC strains of *M. bovis* as they arise in the future will allow us to develop further evidence in support of AMR association for the subset of genes identified and may uncover additional candidate genes for AMR association. Likewise, selecting historical strains for WGS that are high or low MIC for specific antimicrobials may allow for further refinement or expansion of the list of AMR-association candidates.

4. Materials and Methods

As a non-interventionary study, prior approval from the University of Guelph Research Ethics Board was not required for this research.

4.1. Culture & Isolation of Mycoplasmas

The body of a two-week old male Holstein calf was submitted to the Animal Health Lab in July of 2019 for post-mortem examination. Histologically, no lesions indicative of mycoplasma pneumonia were observed within the lungs. Culture and isolation of *M. bovis* AHL# 2019-043682 from the calf lung tissue was conducted as follows: The lung tissue submitted was perforated repeatedly using a sterile dry swab to collect sample material for broth (pig serum, horse serum and ureaplasma broths) and agar plate (pig serum agar, yeastolate agar, ureaplasma agar) culture [39]. Mycoplasma agar plates were incubated at 37 °C with 5–7% CO2 and 80–100% relative humidity. Ureaplasma agar plates ware incubated at 37 °C anaerobically. All broth cultures were incubated aerobically at 37 °C. Plates were read at 48–72 h intervals using a transilluminated stereomicroscope. Broth tubes were visually inspected for growth and pH change at 18–24 h intervals, and were subcultured twice, at 48–72 h growth and at 48–72 h following the first subculture. Agar plates were subcultured if suspicious growth was observed during reading. Following isolation, species identity as *M bovis* was confirmed using goat anti-rabbit/fluorescein isothiocyanate (GAR/FITC)-labelled antiserum fluorescent antibody staining [39]. Blocks of agar containing pure isolate were cut and stored at −80 °C for long term storage. Isolated 1982-M6152, an isolate of *M. bovis* from 1982 stored at −80 °C and identified in a previous study [3] as low MIC for most antimicrobials, was propagated and tested by WGS and MIC retesting.

4.2. MIC Testing

Minimum inhibitory concentration (MIC) testing was conducted on *M. bovis* isolates 2019-043682, 1982-M6152 and strain PG45 in triplicates for each isolate using previously described procedures [3], and using *M. bovis* isolate 227, an internal laboratory reference strain, as a control. Briefly: each isolate was first inoculated into 4 mL Mycoplasma MIC broth and incubated 48–72 h at 37 °C aerobically, before being frozen at −80 °C.

Following this incubation period, a colour-changing unit (CCU) and colony forming unit (CFU) count were setup to determine the number of CCU's in the frozen aliquots. A 10-fold serial dilution was prepared for each isolate using Mycoplasma MIC broth, with 200 µL total volume in each of 12 wells. 10µL of the first 6 dilutions were plated onto Hayflick's agar, and both the serial dilutions and agar plates were incubated for 48–72 h at 37 °C with 5–7% CO_2 and 80–100% relative humidity. Both serial dilutions (lowest serial dilution showing a blue-red colour change) and agar plates (colonies counted using a stereomicroscope) were read after 48–72 h, and the CCU and CFU counts of the isolates were calculated accordingly.

A frozen aliquot was thawed and diluted in tubes of Mycoplasma MIC broth in successively larger volumes so that at least 25 mL of a 103–105 CCU/mL dilution was achieved. MIC testing was setup by inoculating 200 μL of this dilution into every well of a Sensititre BOPO6F microtitre plate. The Sensititre plate was incubated at 37 °C with 5–7% CO_2 and 80–100% relative humidity for 24–72 h, until the positive control wells showed a blue-red colour change. At this point the Sensititre plate was read, and any wells showing a blue-red colour change were noted. The MIC for each antibiotic was calculated as the lowest concentration of drug that suppressed growth. After the Sensititre plate had been inoculated, the CCU and CFU counts of the inoculum were determined as previously described.

4.3. Nucleic Acid Extraction

For the isolates 1982-M6152, 2019-043682 and *M. bovis* PG45, 100 μL of a broth culture was extracted on the Applied Biosystems MagMAX 96 automated nucleic acid extraction platform (Applied Biosystems, Foster City, CA, USA) using the Low Cell Content protocol for the MagMAX Pathogen DNA/RNA kit (Applied Biosystems). Samples were eluted in a final volume of 90 μL, using the elution buffer provided with the kit, then held at −20 °C until prepared for WGS.

4.4. Whole Genome Sequencing & Bioinformatics

A 2 × 251 paired end sequencing reaction was conducted on the Illumina MiSeq platform (Illumina, San Diego, CA, USA) using a Nextera XT kit (Illumina) and associated protocols for whole genome sequencing (Illumina Custom Protocol Selector, Illumina Inc.) Quality filtering and assembly of FASTQ files was done on instrument and then uploaded to Illumina's BaseSpace storage and computing cloud. On BaseSpace, genome assembly was conducted using SPAdes Genome Assembler v3.9.0 [11], and MLST assignment of two isolates using the Bacterial Analysis Pipeline v1.0.4 [12].

The assembled FASTQ files were then downloaded from BaseSpace, the adapter for the Nextera XT Kit (CTGTCTCTTATACACATCT) trimmed, then the genomes were assembled using bioinformatics software DNAstar (V17) (DNASTAR, Madison, WI, USA) using NGS-Based Reference-guide (small genomes, contigs) of Hybrid reference-guide/de novo genome assembly function against and annotated with features from reference genome *M. bovis* PG45 (GenBank Accession: NC_014760.1). Multiple genome alignment was performed using Mauve Genome of Geneious v11 (Auckland, New Zealand) with automatically calculated seed weight and automatically calculated minimum LCB score. SNPs were analyzed with MegAlign, DNASTAR's ArrayStar v14 (DNASTAR, Madison, WI, USA), and Geneious v11 to identify deleted and truncated genes, SNPs and non-synonymous mutations relative to *M. bovis* PG45. Gene features were then tabulated in a spreadsheet (Supplementary Table S2) and further annotated by searching NCBI's Gene database to identify their functional roles where possible. Named genes with functional roles in protein synthesis and topoisomerase structure that contained NSMs or disruptions in the 2019 isolate were selected for additional study, using the CARD database [13] and literature review (Google Scholar, keywords used: "antimicrobial resistance", "antibiotic resistance", AMR, and the gene name or functional group, I.e. "rplD" "antimicrobial resistance") to identify mechanisms of antimicrobial resistance, and *M. bovis* gene homologues with AMR association in other organisms.

5. Conclusions

This study identified 55 genetic events of nonsynonymous mutations and gene disruptions linked to *M. bovis* AMR. Future studies are warranted to further analyze these candidate genes, identifying the effects of the altered amino acids on protein structure and their link to AMR. Additionally, mutated genes identified in this study but currently uncharacterized may be assigned to functional groups in future.

Author Contributions: Contributor roles for this publication are defined as follows: Conceptualization, H.Y.C; methodology, H.Y.C., J.E. and L.L.; software, H.Y.C.; validation, H.Y.C., L.L., J.E.; formal analysis, H.Y.C. and L.L.; investigation, J.E. and L.L.; resources, H.Y.C.; data curation, H.Y.C. and L.L.; writing—original draft preparation, L.L.; writing—review and editing, H.Y.C. and J.E.; visualization, L.L., H.Y.C.; supervision, H.Y.C.; project administration, H.Y.C.; funding acquisition, H.Y.C. All authors have read and agreed to the published version of the manuscript.

Acknowledgments: We greatly appreciate the technical support and advice on Illumina BaseSpace software provided by Aparna Krishnamurthy and Durda Slavic, Animal Health Laboratory, University of Guelph, Canada.

References

1. Caswell, J.L.; Bateman, K.G.; Cai, H.Y.; Castillo-Alcala, F. Mycoplasma bovis in Respiratory Disease of Feedlot Cattle. *Vet. Clin. N. Am. Food Anim. Pract.* **2010**, *26*, 365–379. [CrossRef]
2. Griffin, D.; Chengappa, M.M.; Kuszak, J.; McVey, D.S. Bacterial Pathogens of the Bovine Respiratory Disease Complex. *Vet. Clin. N. Am. Food Anim. Pract.* **2010**, *26*, 381–394. [CrossRef]
3. Cai, H.Y.; McDowall, R.; Parker, L.; Kaufman, E.I.; Caswell, J.L. Changes in antimicrobial susceptibility profiles of Mycoplasma bovis over time. *Can. J. Vet. Res.* **2019**, *83*, 34–41.
4. Byrne, W.J.; McCormack, R.; Egan, J.; Brice, N.; Ball, H.J.; Markey, B. Isolation of Mycoplasma bovis from bovine clinical samples in the Republic of Ireland. *Vet. Rec.* **2001**, *148*, 331–333. [CrossRef]
5. Rosenbusch, R.F.; Kinyon, J.M.; Apley, M.; Funk, N.D.; Smith, S.; Hoffman, L.J. In Vitro Antimicrobial Inhibition Profiles of Mycoplasma Bovis Isolates Recovered from Various Regions of the United States from 2002 to 2003. *J. Vet. Diagn. Investig.* **2005**, *17*, 436–441. [CrossRef]
6. Lysnyansky, I.; Ayling, R.D. Mycoplasma bovis: Mechanisms of Resistance and Trends in Antimicrobial Susceptibility. *Front. Microbiol.* **2016**, *7*, 595. [CrossRef]
7. Baym, M.; Stone, L.K.; Kishony, R. Multidrug evolutionary strategies to reverse antibiotic resistance. *Science* **2016**, *351*, aad3292. [CrossRef] [PubMed]
8. Owen, J.R.; Noyes, N.; Young, A.E.; Prince, D.J.; Blanchard, P.C.; Lehenbauer, T.W.; Aly, S.S.; Davis, J.H.; O'Rourke, S.M.; Abdo, Z.; et al. Whole-Genome Sequencing and Concordance Between Antimicrobial Susceptibility Genotypes and Phenotypes of Bacterial Isolates Associated with Bovine Respiratory Disease. *G3 Genes Genomes Genet.* **2017**, *7*, 3059–3071. [CrossRef] [PubMed]
9. Sulyok, K.M.; Kreizinger, Z.; Wehmann, E.; Lysnyansky, I.; Bányai, K.; Marton, S.; Jerzsele, Á.; Rónai, Z.; Turcsányi, I.; Makrai, L.; et al. Mutations Associated with Decreased Susceptibility to Seven Antimicrobial Families in Field and Laboratory-Derived Mycoplasma bovis Strains. *Antimicrob. Agents Chemother.* **2017**, *61*. [CrossRef] [PubMed]
10. Sato, T.; Higuchi, H.; Yokota, S.; Tamura, Y. Mycoplasma bovis isolates from dairy calves in Japan have less susceptibility than a reference strain to all approved macrolides associated with a point mutation (G748A) combined with multiple species-specific nucleotide alterations in 23S rRNA. *Microbiol. Immunol.* **2017**, *61*, 215–224. [CrossRef] [PubMed]
11. Nurk, S.; Bankevich, A.; Antipov, D.; Gurevich, A.; Korobeynikov, A.; Lapidus, A.; Prjibelsky, A.; Pyshkin, A.; Sirotkin, A.; Sirotkin, Y.; et al. Assembling Genomes and Mini-metagenomes from Highly Chimeric Reads. In *Proc Research Comp Molecular Bio*; Deng, M., Jiang, R., Sun, F., Zhang, X., Eds.; Springer: Berlin/ Heidelberg, Germany, 2013; pp. 158–170.
12. Thomsen, M.C.F.; Ahrenfeldt, J.; Cisneros, J.L.B.; Jurtz, V.; Larsen, M.V.; Hasman, H.; Aarestrup, F.M.; Lund, O. A Bacterial Analysis Platform: An Integrated System for Analysing Bacterial Whole Genome Sequencing Data for Clinical Diagnostics and Surveillance. *PLoS ONE* **2016**, *11*, e0157718. [CrossRef] [PubMed]
13. Alcock, B.P.; Raphenya, A.R.; Lau, T.T.Y.; Tsang, K.K.; Bouchard, M.; Edalatmand, A.; Huynh, W.; Nguyen, A.-L.V.; Cheng, A.A.; Liu, S.; et al. CARD 2020: antibiotic resistome surveillance with the comprehensive antibiotic resistance database. *Nucleic Acids Res.* **2020**, *48*, D517–D525. [CrossRef] [PubMed]
14. Perichon, B.; Tankovic, J.; Courvalin, P. Characterization of a mutation in the parE gene that confers fluoroquinolone resistance in Streptococcus pneumoniae. *Antimicrob. Agents Chemother.* **1997**, *41*, 1166–1167. [CrossRef]

15. Michel, G.; Sauvé, V.; Larocque, R.; Li, Y.; Matte, A.; Cygler, M. The Structure of the RlmB 23S rRNA Methyltransferase Reveals a New Methyltransferase Fold with a Unique Knot. *Structure* **2002**, *10*, 1303–1315. [CrossRef]
16. Fyfe, C.; Grossman, T.H.; Kerstein, K.; Sutcliffe, J. Resistance to Macrolide Antibiotics in Public Health Pathogens. *Cold Spring Harb. Perspect. Med.* **2016**, *6*, a025395. [CrossRef] [PubMed]
17. Feng, Y.; Jonker, M.J.; Moustakas, I.; Brul, S.; Ter Kuile, B.H. Dynamics of Mutations during Development of Resistance by Pseudomonas aeruginosa against Five Antibiotics. *Antimicrob. Agents Chemother.* **2016**, *60*, 4229–4236. [CrossRef]
18. Grossman, T.H. Tetracycline Antibiotics and Resistance. *Cold Spring Harb. Perspect. Med.* **2016**, *6*, a025387. [CrossRef]
19. Wang, Z.; Kong, L.C.; Jia, B.Y.; Liu, S.M.; Jiang, X.Y.; Ma, H.X. Aminoglycoside susceptibility of Pasteurella multocida isolates from bovine respiratory infections in China and mutations in ribosomal protein S5 associated with high-level induced spectinomycin resistance. *J. Vet. Med. Sci.* **2017**, *79*, 1678–1681. [CrossRef]
20. Hu, M.; Nandi, S.; Davies, C.; Nicholas, R.A. High-Level Chromosomally Mediated Tetracycline Resistance in Neisseria gonorrhoeae Results from a Point Mutation in the rpsJ Gene Encoding Ribosomal Protein S10 in Combination with the mtrR and penB Resistance Determinants. *Antimicrob. Agents Chemother.* **2005**, *49*, 4327–4334. [CrossRef]
21. Long, K.S.; Hansen, L.H.; Jakobsen, L.; Vester, B. Interaction of Pleuromutilin Derivatives with the Ribosomal Peptidyl Transferase Center. *Antimicrob. Agents Chemother.* **2006**, *50*, 1458–1462. [CrossRef]
22. Hölzel, C.S.; Harms, K.S.; Schwaiger, K.; Bauer, J. Resistance to Linezolid in a Porcine Clostridium perfringens Strain Carrying a Mutation in the rplD Gene Encoding the Ribosomal Protein L4. *Antimicrob. Agents Chemother.* **2010**, *54*, 1351–1353. [CrossRef] [PubMed]
23. Cagliero, C.; Mouline, C.; Cloeckaert, A.; Payot, S. Synergy between Efflux Pump CmeABC and Modifications in Ribosomal Proteins L4 and L22 in Conferring Macrolide Resistance in Campylobacter jejuni and Campylobacter coli. *Antimicrob. Agents Chemother.* **2006**, *50*, 3893–3896. [CrossRef] [PubMed]
24. Liu, A.; Tran, L.; Becket, E.; Lee, K.; Chinn, L.; Park, E.; Tran, K.; Miller, J.H. Antibiotic Sensitivity Profiles Determined with an Escherichia coli Gene Knockout Collection: Generating an Antibiotic Bar Code. *Antimicrob. Agents Chemother.* **2010**, *54*, 1393–1403. [CrossRef] [PubMed]
25. Milija, J.; Lilic, M.; Janjusevic, R.; Jovanovic, G.; Savic, D.J. tRNA Synthetase Mutants of Escherichia coli K-12 Are Resistant to the Gyrase Inhibitor Novobiocin. *J. Bacteriol.* **1999**, *181*, 2979–2983. [CrossRef]
26. Magalhães, S.; Aroso, M.; Roxo, I.; Ferreira, S.; Cerveira, F.; Ramalheira, E.; Ferreira, R.; Vitorino, R. Proteomic profile of susceptible and multidrug-resistant clinical isolates of Escherichia coli and Klebsiella pneumoniae using label-free and immunoproteomic strategies. *Res. Microbiol.* **2017**, *168*, 222–233. [CrossRef] [PubMed]
27. Yanagisawa, T.; Lee, J.T.; Wu, H.C.; Kawakami, M. Relationship of protein structure of isoleucyl-tRNA synthetase with pseudomonic acid resistance of Escherichia coli. A proposed mod of action of pseudomonic acid as an inhibitor of isoleucyl-tRNA synthetase. *J. Biol. Chem.* **1994**, *269*, 24304–24309.
28. Dordel, J.; Kim, C.; Chung, M.; Pardos de la Gándara, M.; Holden, M.T.J.; Parkhill, J.; de Lencastre, H.; Bentley, S.D.; Tomasz, A. Novel Determinants of Antibiotic Resistance: Identification of Mutated Loci in Highly Methicillin-Resistant Subpopulations of Methicillin-Resistant Staphylococcus aureus. *MBio* **2014**, *5*. [CrossRef]
29. Liu, M.; Douthwaite, S. Resistance to the macrolide antibiotic tylosin is conferred by single methylations at 23S rRNA nucleotides G748 and A2058 acting in synergy. *Proc. Natl. Acad. Sci. USA* **2002**, *99*, 14658–14663. [CrossRef]
30. Doi, Y.; Arakawa, Y. 16S Ribosomal RNA Methylation: Emerging Resistance Mechanism against Aminoglycosides. *Clin. Infect. Dis.* **2007**, *45*, 88–94. [CrossRef]
31. Masuda, I.; Matsubara, R.; Christian, T.; Rojas, E.R.; Yadavalli, S.S.; Zhang, L.; Goulian, M.; Foster, L.J.; Huang, K.C.; Hou, Y.-M. tRNA Methylation Is a Global Determinant of Bacterial Multi-drug Resistance. *Cell Syst.* **2019**, *8*, 302–314. [CrossRef]
32. Giguère, S. Lincosamides, Pleuromutilins, and Streptogramins. In *Antimicrobial Therapy in Veterinary Medicine*; John Wiley & Sons Ltd: Hoboken, NJ, USA, 2013; pp. 199–210. ISBN 978-1-118-67501-4.
33. Hurdle, J.G.; O'Neill, A.J.; Chopra, I. Prospects for Aminoacyl-tRNA Synthetase Inhibitors as New Antimicrobial Agents. *Antimicrob. Agents Chemother.* **2005**, *49*, 4821–4833. [CrossRef] [PubMed]

34. Tse-Dinh, Y.-C. Bacterial topoisomerase I as a target for discovery of antibacterial compounds. *Nucleic Acids Res.* **2009**, *37*, 731–737. [CrossRef] [PubMed]
35. Bansal, S.; Tawar, U.; Singh, M.; Nikravesh, A.; Good, L.; Tandon, V. Old class but new dimethoxy analogue of benzimidazole: A bacterial topoisomerase I inhibitor. *Int. J. Antimicrob. Agents* **2010**, *35*, 186–190. [CrossRef] [PubMed]
36. Nagaraja, V.; Godbole, A.A.; Henderson, S.R.; Maxwell, A. DNA topoisomerase I and DNA gyrase as targets for TB therapy. *Drug Discov. Today* **2017**, *22*, 510–518. [CrossRef]
37. Webber, M.A.; Piddock, L.J.V. The importance of efflux pumps in bacterial antibiotic resistance. *J Antimicrob. Chemother.* **2003**, *51*, 9–11. [CrossRef]
38. Marquez, B. Bacterial efflux systems and efflux pumps inhibitors. *Biochimie* **2005**, *87*, 1137–1147. [CrossRef]
39. Ruhnke, H.L.; Rosendal, S. Useful Protocols for Diagnosis of Animal Mycoplasmas. In *Mycoplasmosis in Animals: Laboratory Diagnosis*; Whitford, H.W., Rosenbusch, R.F., Lauerman, L.H., Eds.; Iowa State University Press: Ames, IA, USA, 1994; pp. 141–166.

17

Analysis of the Leukocyte Response in Calves Suffered from *Mycoplasma bovis* Pneumonia

Katarzyna Dudek [1,*], Dariusz Bednarek [1], Urszula Lisiecka [2], Anna Kycko [3], Michał Reichert [3], Krzysztof Kostro [2,†] and Stanisław Winiarczyk [2]

1 Department of Cattle and Sheep Diseases, National Veterinary Research Institute, 57 Partyzantów Avenue, 24-100 Pulawy, Poland; dbednarek@piwet.pulawy.pl

2 Department of Epizootiology and Clinic of Infectious Diseases, Faculty of Veterinary Medicine, University of Life Sciences in Lublin, 30 Głęboka Street, 20-612 Lublin, Poland; urszula.lisiecka@up.lublin.pl (U.L.); genp53@interia.pl (S.W.)

3 Department of Pathology, National Veterinary Research Institute, 57 Partyzantów Avenue, 24-100 Pulawy, Poland; anna.kycko@piwet.pulawy.pl (A.K.); reichert@piwet.pulawy.pl (M.R.)

* Correspondence: katarzyna.dudek@piwet.pulawy.pl

† This author has passed away in 2018.

Abstract: *Mycoplasma bovis* is known to be a cause of chronic pneumonia in cattle. To date, the disease pathomechanism has not been fully elucidated. Leukocytes play a key role in host antimicrobial defense mechanisms. Many in vitro studies of the effect of *Mycoplasma bovis* (*M. bovis*) on leukocytes have been performed, but it is difficult to apply these results to in vivo conditions. Additionally, only a few studies on a local immune response in *M. bovis* pneumonia have been undertaken. In this study, the experimental calf-infection model was used to determine the effect of field *M. bovis* strains on changes of the peripheral blood leukocyte response, including phagocytic activity and oxygen metabolism by cytometry analyses. An additional aim was to evaluate the lung local immunity of the experimentally infected calves using immunohistochemical staining. The general stimulation of phagocytic and killing activity of peripheral blood leukocytes in response to the *M. bovis* infection points to upregulation of cellular antimicrobial mechanisms. The local immune response in the infected lungs was characterized by the T- and B-cell stimulation, however, most seen in the increased T lymphocyte response. Post-infection, strong expression of the antigen-presenting cells and phagocytes also confirmed the activation of lung local immunity. In this study—despite the stimulation—both the peripheral and local cellular antimicrobial mechanisms seem to appear ineffective in eliminating *M. bovis* from the host and preventing the specific lung lesions, indicating an ability of the pathogen to avoid the host immune response in the *M. bovis* pneumonia.

Keywords: *Mycoplasma bovis*; cattle; leukocytes; phagocytosis; oxygen metabolism

---

1. Introduction

Mycoplasma bovis causes many disorders in cattle, such as pneumonia, arthritis, mastitis and keratoconjunctivitis, from which chronic pneumonia is one of the most diagnosed [1–3]. To date, the pathomechanism of *M. bovis* pneumonia has not been fully elucidated. One such mechanism is the ability of the pathogen to modulate the host immune response [4]. It has been previously confirmed that *M. bovis* possesses both immunostimulating and immunosuppressive properties, most demonstrated in vitro studies. *M. bovis* can induce strong TNF-α responses in the exposed macrophages isolated from mycoplasma-free bronchoalveolar lavages of adult cattle [5]. The ability of *M. bovis* to modulate different neutrophil functions has been demonstrated by Jimbo et al. [6]. After incubation of *M. bovis* with neutrophils isolated from clinically healthy animals the induction of the cell apoptosis and increased elastase production was observed. The same study showed upregulation of pro-inflammatory cytokines—i.e., TNF-α and IL-12—but with no effect on TGF-β production [6]. Otherwise, it was revealed that *M. bovis* can inhibit the oxygen-dependent microbicidal response of neutrophils isolated from the peripheral blood of adult cattle [7]. In vitro conditions, *M. bovis* is also able to suppress a phytohemagglutinin-induced stimulation of bovine peripheral blood lymphocytes, however with no cytotoxic effect [8]. Similarly, other in vitro study demonstrated the ability of *M. bovis* to inhibit a Concanavalin A-induced proliferation of peripheral blood lymphocytes isolated from *M. bovis* negative donor cattle [9]. Despite so many results, the data received is still not endless, especially since it is not often possible to interpret in vitro results for in vivo conditions. Additionally, only a few studies on the characterization of the local immune response in *M. bovis* pneumonia in calves were undertaken [10,11].

To better advance our knowledge of the disease pathomechanism, an in vivo study using the experimental animal model on calves was performed which evaluated the effect of *M. bovis* on bovine peripheral blood leukocytes. To better control the *M. bovis* infection, an additional aim was to evaluate the lung local immunity of calves experimentally infected with the pathogen.

2. Results

Infection efficacy in the experimental calves was confirmed by clinical, post mortem and histopathologic observations and the results of immunohistochemistry (IHC) and enzyme-linked immunosorbent assay (ELISA) analyses for *M. bovis* antigen were described previously by Dudek et al. [12]. Following the calf infection with *M. bovis*, extensive caseous necrosis and lobular consolidation were observed. The *M. bovis* antigen was detected in epithelial cells of bronchioli in the lungs of all experimental calves as opposed to the controls, which were negative. All detailed post mortem results were previously described by Dudek et al. [12].

2.1. Hematology

Following infection, the white blood cell (WBC) count was generally comparable to the control group throughout the study, with no significant differences ($p < 0.05$). However, the analysis of leucogram showed a comparable or lower percentage of the lymphocytes (LYM) in the experimental group throughout the study compared to the control group, with significantly lower values on Day 3 post the first infecting dose. In the experimental group, the monocyte (MON) percentage did not differ significantly ($p < 0.05$) from the control group throughout the study. However, the granulocyte (GRA) percentage was increased post the infection throughout the study compared to the control group and reached significantly ($p < 0.05$) higher values than the control group on Day 3 post the first infecting dose (Figure 1). Numerical values are presented in Figure S1.

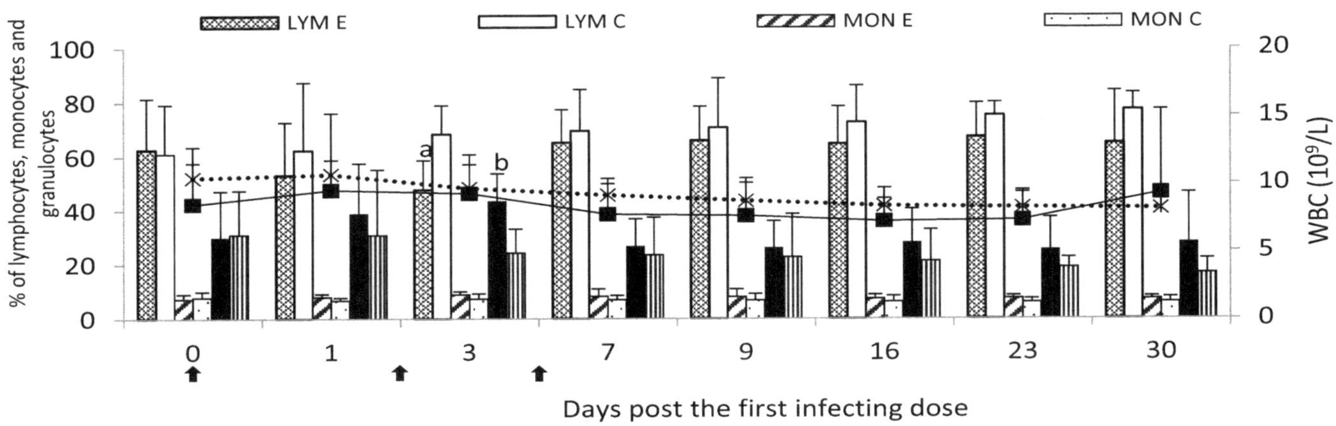

Figure 1. WBC count and a mean percentage of granulocytes, monocytes and lymphocytes in the peripheral blood of calves following infection with *M. bovis*. E—experimental group; C—control group; ⬆—single infecting dose of *M. bovis*; a—$p < 0.05$ between the experimental and control groups for lymphocytes; b—$p < 0.05$ between the experimental and control groups for granulocytes.

2.2. Flow Cytometry

2.2.1. Lymphocyte Phenotyping

There were no significant ($p < 0.05$) differences between the experimental and control groups in the percentage of $CD2^+$, $CD4^+$ and $CD8^+$ cells throughout the study. However, on Day 3 post the first infecting dose, the $CD4^+$ percentage was significantly lower ($p \leq 0.05$) than the control group (Figure 2). Numerical values were presented in Supplementary Figure S2.

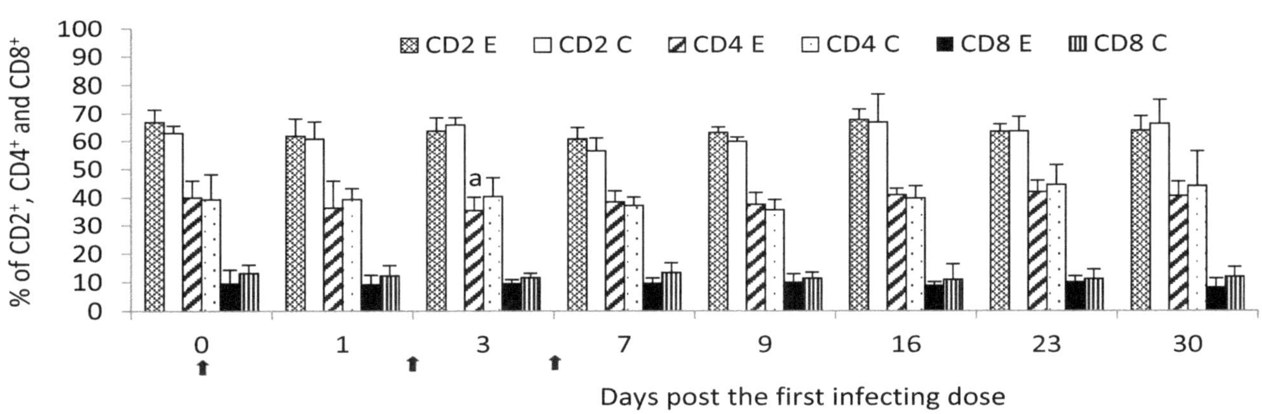

Figure 2. $CD2^+$, $CD4^+$ and $CD8^+$ mean percentage in the peripheral blood of calves following infection with *M. bovis*. E—experimental group; C—control group. ⬆—single infecting dose of *M. bovis*; a—$p < 0.05$ between the experimental and control groups for $CD4^+$.

2.2.2. Phagocytic Activity and Oxygen Metabolism of Leukocytes

The percentage of phagocytic granulocytes in the peripheral blood of the experimental group did not significantly differ ($p < 0.05$) from the control group throughout the study. However, the mean fluorescence intensity (MFI) for granulocytes visibly increased on Day 9 post the first infecting dose and it was statistically significantly higher ($p < 0.05$) than the control group on Day 16 (Figure 3). Numerical values were presented in Figure S3.

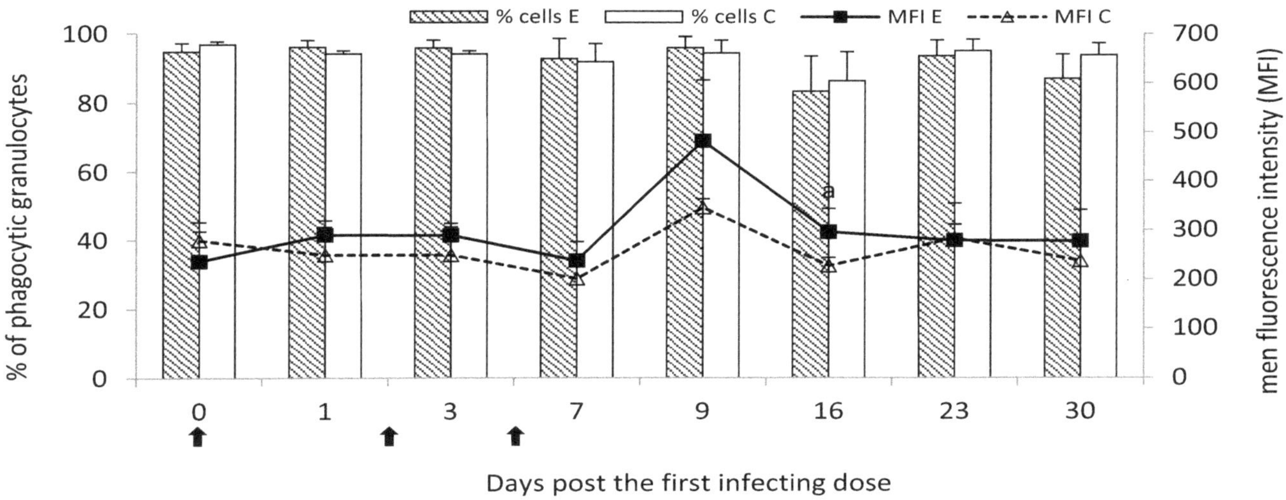

Figure 3. Phagocytic activity of granulocytes in the peripheral blood of calves following infection with *M. bovis* expressed as a mean percentage of phagocytic cells (bar graph) and mean fluorescence intensity (MFI; linear graph). E—experimental group; C—control group. ⬆—single infecting dose of *M. bovis*; a—$p < 0.05$ between the experimental and control groups for MFI.

Following the infection, the percentage of phagocytic monocytes was generally comparable to the control group throughout the study, with the exception of Day 9, when lower values were observed. However, on Day 23, a visible increase in the percentage in the experimental group was observed. Following the infection, the MFI for monocytes was generally slightly higher than the control group throughout the study, especially on Day one following the first infecting dose. However, no significant differences ($p < 0.05$) between the experimental and control groups on the phagocytic cell percentage and MFI were observed (Figure 4). Numerical values were presented in Figure S4.

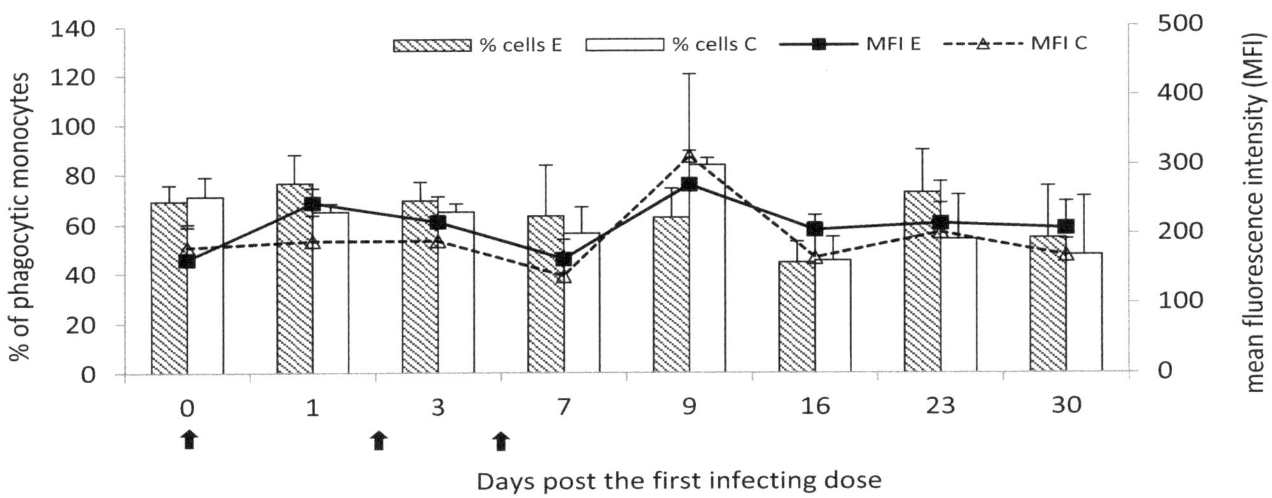

Figure 4. The phagocytic activity of monocytes in the peripheral blood of calves following infection with *M. bovis* expressed as a mean percentage of phagocytic cells (bar graph) and mean fluorescence intensity (MFI; linear graph). E—experimental group; C—control group. ⬆—single infecting dose of *M. bovis*.

For the oxygen metabolism, the percentage of activated leukocytes was significantly increased ($p < 0.05$) on Day one post the first infecting dose, however after that it suddenly decreased and had similar or lower values than the control group until the end of the study with significantly lower values ($p < 0.05$) on Day 23. The MFI was generally increased in the experimental group throughout the study when compared to the control group, however with no significant ($p < 0.05$) differences (Figure 5). Numerical values were presented in Figure S5.

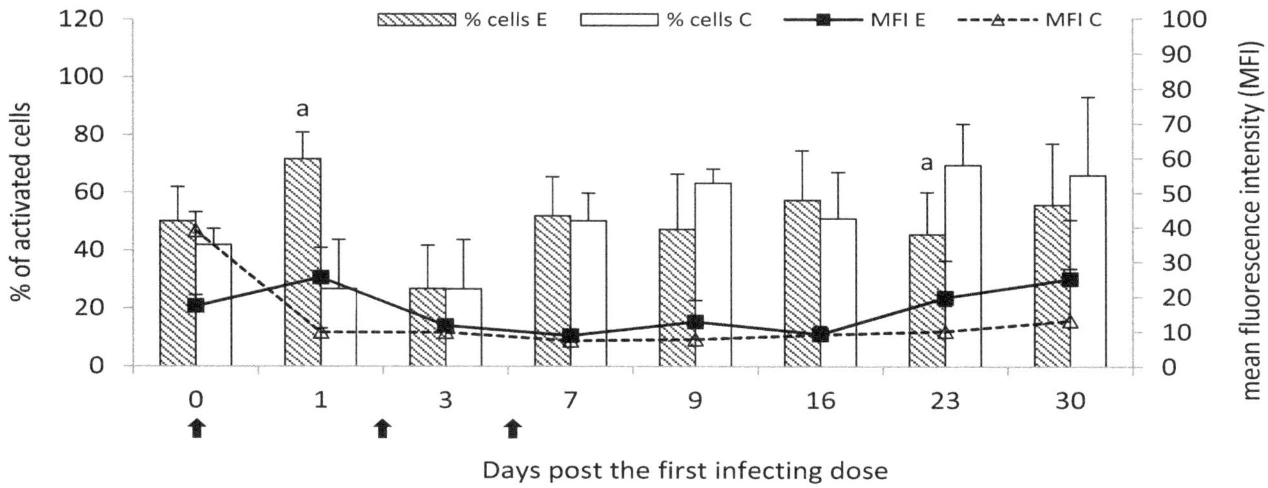

Figure 5. Oxygen metabolism of leukocytes in peripheral blood of calves following infection with *M. bovis* expressed as a mean percentage of cells (bar graph) and mean fluorescence intensity (MFI; linear graph) after activation by *E. coli*. E—experimental group; C—control group. ⬆—single infecting dose of *M. bovis*. a—$p < 0.05$ between the experimental and control groups for percentage of cells.

2.3. *Immunohistochemistry*

In the lungs of experimentally infected calves, multiple foci of CD3 positive cells were visible in the lung parenchyma, within the hyperplastic bronchus-associated lymphoid tissue (BALT) and peribronchiolar infiltrations (Figure 6A). In the control calves, the positive reaction for the CD3 antigen was visible in BALT (Figure 6B). The positive labeling for CD79a in the infected calves was present in the hyperplastic BALT and, to a lesser extent, in the cells around bronchioli or the cells infiltrating necrotic areas (Figure 6C). In the control animals, the reaction for the CD79a antigen was visible in BALT (Figure 6D). As a result of CD3 and CD79a quantification, the immunopositive cell counts determined as mean value ± standard deviation (SD) in the control group were 1408.8 ± 88.1 for CD3 and 1437.5 ± 267 for CD79a. In the experimental group the mean cell counts for CD3 and CD79a were 3823.7 ± 1551.3 and 2118.7 ± 730.18, respectively. Compared to the controls, the experimental group displayed a significant increase ($p < 0.05$) in the number of both CD3- and CD79a-positive cells, however within the group, the mean cell count value was significantly higher ($p < 0.05$) for CD3 than for CD79a.

In the lungs of the experimentally infected calves, the high concentration of MHC class II marker was found in the lymphoid cells infiltrating the granulomas, in BALT as well as in bronchiolar epithelium and the lymphoid cells in the alveolar walls (Figure 7A), while in the control animals the positive labeling for MHC class II was seen in BALT, the epithelial cells of bronchioli and in some lymphoid cells within the lung parenchyma (Figure 7B). When assessing the presence of S100 marker in the lungs of the infected calves, its high concentration was observed in vascular endothelial cells, as well as in some cells forming cellular infiltrates within granulomas (Figure 7C). In the control group, the positive IHC response was only demonstrated in vascular endothelial cells (Figure 7D).

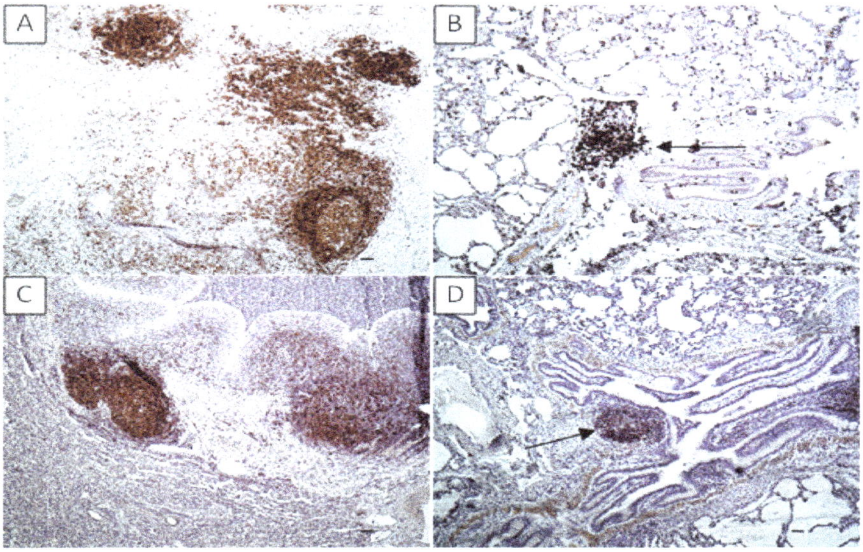

Figure 6. The lungs of the calves experimentally infected with *Mycoplasma bovis* (**A**,**C**), lungs of the control calves (**B**,**D**), IHC. (**A**) lung of an experimental calf. Positive immunolabeling of CD3 visible as dark brown staining in the hyperplastic bronchus-associated lymphoid tissue (BALT) and lymphoid cells scattered in the lung parenchyma. Bar = 50 μm; (**B**) lung of control calf. Positive immunolabeling of CD3 visible in BALT (arrow) and the single cells scattered in the lung parenchyma. Bar = 50 μm; (**C**) lung of an experimental calf. Positive immunolabeling of CD79a visible as dark brown staining in the hyperplastic BALT and lymphoid cells scattered in the lung parenchyma. Bar = 50 μm; (**D**) lung of control calf. Positive immunolabeling of CD79a visible in BALT (arrow). Bar = 50 μm.

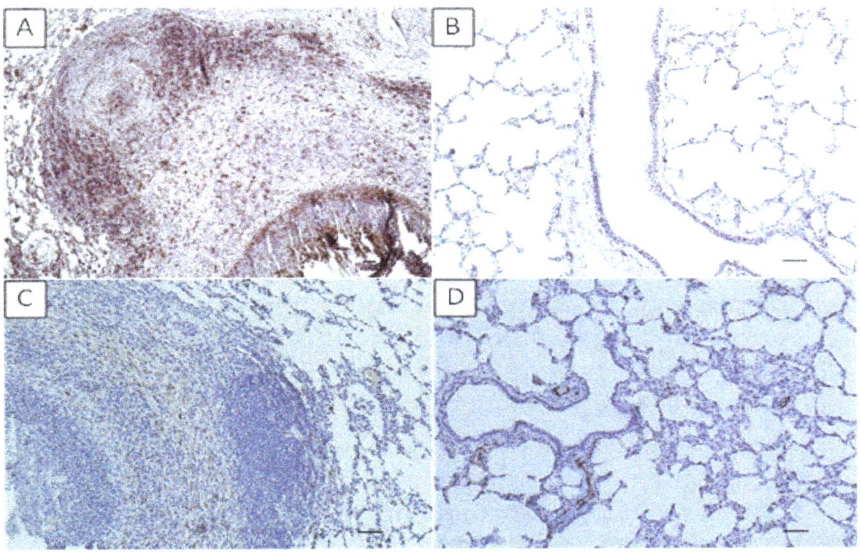

Figure 7. The lungs of the calves experimentally infected with *Mycoplasma bovis* (**A**,**C**), the lungs of the control calves (**B**,**D**), IHC. (**A**) lung of an experimental calf. Positive labeling of MHC class II visible as the brown staining in BALT, in the cells within the infiltrates surrounding the necrotic masses (right bottom) and in the single cells scattered in the lung parenchyma (left side). Bar = 50 μm (**B**) lung of control calf. Positive labeling of MHC class II visible as brown staining in the bronchiolar epithelial layer and the single cells around the bronchus. Bar = 50 μm; (**C**) lung of an experimental calf. Positive labeling of S100 visible as the brown staining in several cells within the granuloma. Bar = 50 μm; (**D**) lung of control calf. Positive labeling of S100 is visible in the endothelium of the blood capillaries. Bar = 50 μm.

3. Discussion

In the current study, the lung local immune response to *M. bovis* infection was characterized by the lymphocyte stimulation dependent on both the T- and B-cell responses, however, the most seen in the strong immunohistochemical labeling of T lymphocytes. It had a reflection in a general decrease in the percent of circulating lymphocytes, the most intensified post the second infecting dose of *M. bovis*. It was additionally confirmed by flow cytometry analysis which showed at the same time point a decline in the T-helper cell percentage. It was probably due to the migration of the lymphocytes from peripheral blood to sites of infection, including lung tissue. At the same point in time post the infection, a decrease in the percentage of circulating lymphocytes was compensated by the increased percentage of other leukocyte populations like granulocytes possibly indicating an enhancement production of these cells in the bone marrow and their release into the peripheral blood. Hermeyer et al. [11] examined the expression of CD3, CD79a, S100A8 and S100A9 markers within the lungs of the aborted bovine fetus and the newborn calf died with severe respiratory symptoms, both suffered from suppurative bronchointerstitial pneumonia due to *M. bovis* infection. The results of the study indicated the increased lymphocytic aggregates expressed CD3 and CD79a within the lung tissues of both animals confirming the presence of both T and B lymphocytes. All this suggests the activation of specific local immunity to *M. bovis* lung infection as was confirmed in the current study [11]. In another study, the identification and quantitative evaluation of $CD4^+$ and $CD8^+$ T lymphocytes using IHC staining in the chronic *M. bovis* pneumonia was performed. However, post the experimental infection of calves with *M. bovis*, no significant differences in the numbers of both cells in BALT of bronchioli were observed compared to the control [10].

Neutrophils and macrophages are known to be important in innate immune mechanisms in the lung, including bacteria recognizing and phagocytosis needed for the antigen presentation [4]. In the study of Hermeyer et al. [11], the increased number of macrophages expressed both S100A8 and S100A9 in the lung parenchyma of the aborted bovine fetus and neonatal calf affected with *M. bovis* was shown. Additionally, within the lung of aborted bovine fetus neutrophilic aggregates were presented [11]. In our *M. bovis* calf-infection model the increased S100 expression in the infected lungs was observed probably indicating the stimulation of phagocyte response according to Hermeyer et al. [11]. As previously proved, there is a phenomenon of *M. bovis* surviving nearby necrosis areas despite the presence of a large number of infiltrating cells like neutrophils and macrophages [13,14].

In the study of Hermeyer et al. [10] in the lungs of *M. bovis*-infected calves' immunoreactivity of MHC class II varied dependent on the affected area. The strong MHC class II expression was revealed on the lymphoid cells in hyperplastic BALT, whereas the weak immunoreactivity or negative reaction was observed in intra-alveolar as well as perinecrotic located macrophages and in areas near caseonecrotic lesions. According to the author, such location of MHC class II expression suggest on one hand, ongoing stimulation of the lung local immunity and on the other hand downregulation of the antigen-presenting mechanisms in chronic *M. bovis* pneumonia [10]. In the current study, the high concentration of MHC class II was found in both the BALT and within the infiltrates surrounding the necrotic masses indicating general upregulation of the antigen-presenting mechanisms in response to the *M. bovis* infection. All this seems to confirm the formation of antigen-MHC class II complexes in the infected lungs, their recognition by the activated T lymphocytes and further activation of B-cell dependent response to generate specific immunity.

It is well known that granulocytes—especially neutrophils—are crucial cells in host antimicrobial defense [15]. As a predominant population of circulating leukocytes, neutrophils play an important role in the first line of cellular defense of the host against invading pathogens by various functions, including phagocytosis and oxidative burst [6,16]. In the current study, the percentage of circulating granulocytes was increased post *M. bovis* infection. It had a reflection in the slight increase in the percentage of phagocytic granulocytes at the initial stage of the disease. As the disease progresses, the visible drop in the percentage of phagocytic cells was observed, the most seen at the end of the study (a chronic stage of the disease). However, the number of phagocytosed bacteria by granulocytes on Day

16 post the first infecting dose of *M. bovis* was significantly higher than the control despite the beginning of the decline in the percentage of phagocytic cells possibly indicating increased antimicrobial activity of the cells.

Marked, however not statistically significant stimulation of phagocytic activity at the most time points post the infection was observed for circulating monocytes. Unlike granulocytes, the percentage of phagocytic monocytes was visibly increased at the chronic stage of the disease.

In the current study, the analysis of oxygen metabolism of peripheral blood leukocytes showed the initial increase in the percentage of the activated cells to different extents, the most seen post the first infecting dose of *M. bovis*. It was reflected in the visibly increased killing activity of these cells. In turn, a further decline in the activated cell percentage probably resulted from the subsequent doses of *M. bovis* and the chronic stage of the disease. It was probably in favor of mobilizing these cells within the lungs against the persisting/survival of *M. bovis* antigen. However, the killing activity of circulating leukocytes at that time was enhanced, despite the decrease in the percentage of the activated cells, possibly indicating releasing of *M. bovis* from sites of the infection, including lung tissue. In the study of Wiggins et al. [17], the effect of multiple *M. bovis* isolates (field, clinical and high passage laboratory) on Reactive Oxygen Species (ROS) production by blood leukocytes isolated from six cattle using an oxidation of dihydrorhodamine 123 (DHR-123) was measured. The leukocyte incubation with both field and clinical *M. bovis* isolates generally impaired ROS production, as opposed to the laboratory ones. In this study, the leukocyte metabolic activity using the reduction of 3-(4,5-dimethylthiazol-2-yl)-2,5-diphenyltetrazolium bromide (MTT) was also determined. Mostly following the exposure to all *M. bovis* isolates no effect on cellular metabolism of the bovine leukocytes was shown, indicating that observed suppression of ROS generation was not dependent on the leukocyte impairment of metabolic functions [17].

In the current study, using the *M. bovis* calf-infection model, the changes in the phagocytic activity and oxygen-dependent killing in the peripheral blood leukocytes was related to the stage of *M. bovis* pneumonia. However, the general stimulation of phagocytic and killing activity of circulating leukocytes in response to the *M. bovis* infection points to the upregulation of cellular antimicrobial mechanisms. The general depletion in the percent of circulating lymphocytes supporting the ongoing infection with *M. bovis*. The lung local immune response to the *M. bovis* experimental infection was characterized by the lymphocyte stimulation, the most seen in the increased T-cell response. The calf infection with *M. bovis* also caused the increased expression of the antigen-presenting cells, as well as the phagocytes further confirming the activation of lung local immune response. Despite the general stimulation of both peripheral and local cellular antimicrobial mechanisms, their effectiveness appeared insufficient in eliminating the bacteria from the host and preventing specific *M. bovis* lesions, indicating the ability of the bacteria to avoid the host immune response in *M. bovis* pneumonia.

4. Materials and Methods

4.1. Animals

Experimental study on animals was carried out in accordance with the requirements of the Local Ethics Committee on Animal Experimentation of the University of Life Sciences in Lublin, Poland (Decision no. 102/2015 admitted 8 Dec 2015), which also meet the EU standards.

The study was performed on 10 four-week-old, clinically healthy female calves housed in the institute's vivarium. Before the proper study, the nasal swabs and blood samples were collected from the calves and examined for *Mycoplasma bovis* and other respiratory pathogens detection which was described previously by Dudek et al. [12]. After a three-week adaptive period, the calves were divided into two groups: experimental ($n = 6$) and control ($n = 4$).

All detailed information about the animals and methods used for confirmation of the infection efficacy was described previously by Dudek et al. [12].

4.2. Calf Challenge

The experimental calves were three times infected with 23 mL of inoculum containing the field *M. bovis* strain KP795974 suspended in sterile phosphate-buffered saline pH 7.2 (PBS), with a concentration of 1.5×10^8 CFU/mL. The inoculum was prepared as described previously [18] and given three times in total; for the first time on Day 0 of the study and then two times at 48 h intervals; twice intratracheally and once by a nasal aerosol application. Instead, the control animals were administered with sterile PBS. It was described previously in detail by Dudek et al. [12].

4.3. Sample Collection

Blood samples were collected in EDTA tubes (for hematology and CD marker detection) or standard heparinized tubes (concerning analyses of phagocytic activity and oxygen metabolism of leukocytes) on Days 0, 1, 3, 7, 9, 16, 23 and 30 post the first *M. bovis* infecting dose. At the end of the experiment on Day 30, all experimental and two control calves were euthanized to collect the lung samples for pathologic and immunohistochemical analyses.

4.4. Hematology

White blood cell (WBC) count and percentage of lymphocytes, monocytes and granulocytes were calculated in an automatic veterinary blood analyzer (Exigo, Boule Medical AB, Spånga, Sweden).

4.5. Flow Cytometry

4.5.1. Lymphocyte Phenotyping

Peripheral blood lymphocyte analysis using the CD markers for T-cells ($CD2^+$), T-helper cells ($CD4^+$) and T-cytotoxic suppressor cells ($CD8^+$) was performed by a flow cytometer (Coulter Epics XL 4C, Beckman Coulter Company, Brea, CA, USA) according to the method described previously by Dudek et al. [18].

4.5.2. Phagocytic Activity and Oxygen Metabolism of Leukocytes

Phagocytic activity and oxygen metabolism of peripheral blood leukocytes were evaluated according to the manufacturer's instructions of two separated commercial kits: Phagotest™ for leukocyte phagocytic activity and Phagoburst™ for oxygen metabolism analysis, both manufactured by Glycotope Biotechnology GmbH (Heidelberg, Germany) and analyzed using Epics XL flow cytometer (Beckman Coulter, Miami, FL, USA). The granulocyte and monocyte phagocytic activity was expressed as the percentage of cells that engulfed bacteria as well as mean fluorescence intensity (MFI) of the cells for estimating of phagocytosed bacteria amount. The oxygen metabolism of peripheral blood leukocytes was determined as the percentage of cells activated by *E. coli* as well as MFI for the measurement of phagocytic activity of leukocytes.

4.6. Immunohistochemistry

The collected lung samples were examined using an immunohistochemical staining for the detection of local immune response markers such as CD3 (T-cells), CD79 (B-cells), MHC class II and S100. Previously prepared sections were deparaffinized in xylene, rehydrated in descending ethanol concentrations, then incubated in 3% H_2O_2 diluted in methanol for 10 min and submitted to heat-induced epitope retrieval in citrate buffer (pH 6.0) using a pressure cooker for 20 min. Depending on the marker the slides were then incubated for one hour with primary antibodies as follows: rabbit anti-CD3 monoclonal antibody (A045201, DAKO, Glostrup, Denmark) at dilution 1:100 for CD3 detection; mouse monoclonal anti-CD79a antibody [HM57] (ab62650, Abcam, Cambridge, UK) at dilution 1:400 for CD79a detection; mouse anti-HLA-DR Antigen, Alpha-Chain, Clone TAL.1B5 (M074601-2, DAKO, Glostrup, Denmark) at dilution 1:40 for MHC class II detection and FLEX Polyclonal

Rb anti-S100, RTU (GA50461-2, DAKO) at dilution 1:1 for S100 detection. The antibody detection was performed using the Dako REAL EnVision Detection System, Peroxidase/DAB, Rabbit/Mouse (K5007, DAKO, Glostrup, Denmark), involving an incubation with a peroxidase-conjugated polymer as a secondary antibody (for 30 min) and DAB^+ Chromogen applied for a visualization of the reaction. Sections were counterstained with Mayer's hematoxylin, dehydrated and mounted. Sections incubated with PBS instead of the primary antibody were used to confirm the specificity of the staining. The tissues were analyzed under a light microscope (Axiolab, Zeiss, Oberkochen, Germany) for the presence of brown staining indicating positive labeling of *M. bovis*, CD3, CD79a, MHC class II and S100. To determine the difference between the number of T- and B-lymphocytes infiltrating the tissue in the examined sections of experimental group and to compare number of the two cell–type populations between the experimental and control groups, the CD3- and CD79a-positive cells were counted in 20 high power fields (400x) comprising the cell infiltrations and/or BALT in each slide.

4.7. Statistical Analysis

The results are presented as arithmetic means or mean percentage ± standard deviation. The differences between the mean values recorded in the E and C groups at the same time point were analyzed using *t*-test with a statistically significant level of $p < 0.05$. The same test and the *p*-value were applied to determine the difference between the mean values of summarized cell counts for the CD3 and CD79a markers analyzed with IHC in the experimental and control groups.

Author Contributions: Conceptualization, K.D. and D.B.; methodology, K.D., A.K., U.L., M.R.; formal analysis, K.D., A.K., U.L.; investigation, K.D., A.K., U.L., D.B. and technical staff; writing—original draft preparation, K.D. and partially A.K.; writing—review and editing, D.B. and U.L.; supervision, D.B., M.R., K.K., S.W.; project administration, K.D.; funding acquisition, K.D., D.B., K.K., M.R. All authors have read and agreed to the published version of the manuscript.

References

1. Adegboye, D.S.; Halbur, P.G.; Nutsch, R.G.; Kadlec, R.G.; Rosenbusch, R.F. *Mycoplasma bovis*-associated pneumonia and arthritis complicated with pyogranulomatous tenosynovitis in calves. *J. Am. Vet. Med. Assoc.* **1996**, *209*, 647–649. [PubMed]
2. Caswell, J.L.; Archambault, M. *Mycoplasma bovis* pneumonia in cattle. *Anim. Health Res. Rev.* **2009**, *8*, 161–186. [CrossRef] [PubMed]
3. Nicholas, R.A.; Ayling, R.D. *Mycoplasma bovis*: Disease, diagnosis, and control. *Res. Vet. Sci.* **2003**, *74*, 105–112. [CrossRef]
4. Srikumaran, S.; Kelling, C.L.; Ambagala, A. Immune evasion by pathogens of bovine respiratory disease complex. *Anim. Health Res. Rev.* **2008**, *8*, 215–229. [CrossRef] [PubMed]
5. Jungi, T.W.; Krampe, M.; Sileghem, M.; Griot, C.; Nicolet, J. Differential and strain-specific triggering of bovine alveolar macrophage effector functions by mycoplasmas. *Microb. Pathog.* **1996**, *21*, 487–498. [CrossRef] [PubMed]
6. Jimbo, S.; Suleman, M.; Maina, T.; Prysliak, T.; Mulongo, M.; Perez-Casal, J. Effect of *Mycoplasma bovis* on bovine neutrophils. *Vet. Immunol. Immunopathol.* **2017**, *188*, 27–33. [CrossRef] [PubMed]
7. Thomas, C.B.; Van Ess, P.; Wolfgram, L.J.; Riebe, J.; Sharp, P.; Schultz, R.D. Adherence to bovine neutrophils and suppression of neutrophil chemiluminescence by *Mycoplasma bovis*. *Vet. Immunol. Immunopathol.* **1991**, *27*, 365–381. [CrossRef]
8. Thomas, C.B.; Mettler, J.; Sharp, P.; Jensen-Kostenbader, J.; Schultz, R.D. *Mycoplasma bovis* suppression of bovine lymphocyte response to phytohemagglutinin. *Vet. Immunol. Immunopathol.* **1990**, *26*, 143–155. [CrossRef]
9. Vanden Bush, T.J.; Rosenbusch, R.F. Characterization of a lympho-inhibitory peptide produced by *Mycoplasma bovis*. *Biochem. Biophys. Res. Commun.* **2004**, *315*, 336–341. [CrossRef] [PubMed]

10. Hermeyer, K.; Buchenau, I.; Thomasmeyer, A.; Baum, B.; Spergser, J.; Rosengarten, R.; Hewicker-Trautwein, M. Chronic pneumonia in calves after experimental infection with *Mycoplasma bovis* strain 1067: Characterization of lung pathology, persistence of variable surface protein antigens and local immune response. *Acta Vet. Scand.* **2012**, *54*, 9–11. [CrossRef] [PubMed]
11. Hermeyer, K.; Peters, M.; Brügmann, M.; Jacobsen, B.; Hewicker-Trautwein, M. Demonstration of *Mycoplasma bovis* by immunohistochemistry and in situ hybridization in an aborted bovine fetus and neonatal calf. *J. Vet. Diagn. Investig.* **2012**, *24*, 364–369. [CrossRef] [PubMed]
12. Dudek, K.; Bednarek, D.; Ayling, R.D.; Kycko, A.; Reichert, M. Preliminary study on the effects of enrofloxacin, flunixin meglumine and pegbovigrastim on *Mycoplasma bovis* pneumonia. *BMC Vet. Res.* **2019**, *15*, 371–384. [CrossRef] [PubMed]
13. Khodakaram-Tafti, A.; López, A. Immunohistopathological findings in the lungs of calves naturally infected with *Mycoplasma bovis*. *J. Vet. Med. A Physiol. Pathol. Clin. Med.* **2004**, *51*, 10–14. [CrossRef] [PubMed]
14. Kleinschmidt, S.; Spergser, J.; Rosengarten, R.; Hewicker-Trautwein, M. Long-term survival of *Mycoplasma bovis* in necrotic lesions and in phagocytic cells as demonstrated by transmission and immunogold electron microscopy in lung tissue from experimentally infected calves. *Vet. Microbiol.* **2013**, *162*, 949–953. [CrossRef] [PubMed]
15. Gondaira, S.; Higuchi, H.; Nishi, K.; Iwano, H.; Nagahata, H. *Mycoplasma bovis* escapes bovine neutrophil extracellular traps. *Vet. Microbiol.* **2017**, *199*, 68–73. [CrossRef] [PubMed]
16. Howard, C.J.; Taylor, G.; Collins, J.; Gourlay, R.N. Interaction of *Mycoplasma dispar* and *Mycoplasma agalactiae* subsp. *bovis* with bovine alveolar macrophages and bovine lacteal polymorphonuclear leukocytes. *Infect. Immun.* **1976**, *14*, 11–17. [CrossRef] [PubMed]
17. Wiggins, M.C.; Woolums, A.R.; Hurley, D.J.; Sanchez, S.; Ensley, D.T.; Donovan, D. The effect of various *Mycoplasma bovis* isolates on bovine leukocyte responses. *Comp. Immunol. Microbiol. Infect. Dis.* **2011**, *34*, 49–54. [CrossRef] [PubMed]
18. Dudek, K.; Bednarek, D.; Szacawa, E.; Rosales, R.S.; Ayling, R.D. Flow cytometry follow-up analysis of peripheral blood leukocyte subpopulations in calves experimentally infected with field isolates of *Mycoplasma bovis*. *Acta Vet. Hung.* **2015**, *63*, 167–178. [CrossRef] [PubMed]

18

Serosurveillance and Molecular Investigation of Wild Deer in Australia Reveals Seroprevalence of *Pestivirus* Infection

Jose L. Huaman [1,2], Carlo Pacioni [3,4], David M. Forsyth [5], Anthony Pople [6], Jordan O. Hampton [4,7], Teresa G. Carvalho [2] and Karla J. Helbig [1,*]

1 Department of Physiology, Molecular Virology Laboratory, Anatomy and Microbiology, School of Life Sciences, La Trobe University, Melbourne 3086, Australia; j.huamantorres@latrobe.edu.au
2 Department of Physiology, Molecular Parasitology Laboratory, Anatomy and Microbiology, School of Life Sciences, La Trobe University, Melbourne 3086, Australia; t.carvalho@latrobe.edu.au
3 Department of Environment, Land, Water and Planning, Arthur Rylah Institute for Environmental Research, Heidelberg 3084, Australia; carlo.pacioni@delwp.vic.gov.au
4 School of Veterinary and Life Sciences, Murdoch University, South Street, Murdoch, WA 6150, Australia; jordan.hampton@murdoch.edu.au
5 NSW Department of Primary Industries, Vertebrate Pest Research Unit, Orange 2800, Australia; dave.forsyth@dpi.nsw.gov.au
6 Department of Agriculture and Fisheries, Invasive Plants & Animals Research, Biosecurity Queensland, Ecosciences Precinct, Brisbane 4102, Australia; tony.pople@daf.qld.gov.au
7 Ecotone Wildlife, P.O. Box 76, Inverloch, VIC 3996, Australia
* Correspondence: k.helbig@latrobe.edu.au.

Abstract: Since deer were introduced into Australia in the mid-1800s, their wild populations have increased in size and distribution, posing a potential risk to the livestock industry, through their role in pathogen transmission cycles. In comparison to livestock, there are limited data on viral infections in all wildlife, including deer. The aim of this study was to assess blood samples from wild Australian deer for serological evidence of exposure to relevant viral livestock diseases. Blood samples collected across eastern Australia were tested by ELISA to detect antigens and antibodies against *Pestivirus* and antibodies against bovine herpesvirus 1. A subset of samples was also assessed by RT-PCR for *Pestivirus*, Simbu serogroup, epizootic hemorrhagic disease virus and bovine ephemeral fever virus. Our findings demonstrated a very low seroprevalence (3%) for ruminant *Pestivirus*, and none of the other viruses tested were detected. These results suggest that wild deer may currently be an incidental spill-over host (rather than a reservoir host) for *Pestivirus*. However, deer could be a future source of viral infections for domestic animals in Australia. Further investigations are needed to monitor pathogen activity and quantify possible future infectious disease impacts of wild deer on the Australian livestock industry.

Keywords: Australia; deer; prevalence; *Pestivirus*; ruminants; serosurveillance; virology; wildlife disease

1. Introduction

Deer (family Cervidae) often attain high densities when introduced to new areas [1]. As cervids are ungulates and closely related to economically important livestock species including cattle, sheep and goats, it is unsurprising that they share many pathogens, including several of major agricultural relevance. Many viral pathogens of farm ruminants have been detected in wild cervids globally, the most important of which are bovine viral diarrhea virus (BVDV), bovine herpesvirus 1 (BoHV-1), epizootic hemorrhagic disease virus (EHDV) and bovine ephemeral fever virus (BEFV) [2–6].

In Australia, wild populations of six non-native deer species became established in the late 1800s and early 1900s. These populations have expanded in abundance and distribution [1,2]. Wild deer in Australia commonly share grazing areas with livestock, and their susceptibility to a wide range of viral infections of importance to the livestock industry has been demonstrated [2]. Hence, wild deer represent a significant potential source of pathogen transmission to livestock [1].

Australian agriculture is currently free from many viral diseases that impact livestock industries in other parts of the world, including foot-and-mouth disease (FMD) and louping ill virus. However, the issue of cervid-transmitted disease in Australia is important because incursions or outbreaks of emerging, exotic or endemic disease could cause serious production losses, resulting in substantial economic impacts for the livestock industry [1,2]. Transmission of disease by cervids could also prevent effective control, management or eradication of a livestock disease, resulting in prolonged epidemics [2].

There is currently limited information about the infection status of Australia's wild deer populations. A small number of studies assessed the distribution of BVDV in wild fallow (*Dama dama*) and red (*Cervus elaphus*) deer populations in the 1970s and 1980s [7,8], but these were conducted in small geographical areas. Moreover, serological studies of endemic livestock viruses including BEFV, EHDV and Simbu serogroup virus were performed in red deer from Queensland [9] and rusa deer (*Rusa timorensis*) from New South Wales [10]. Therefore, the role wild deer might play in the spread of diseases to livestock remains unclear. Addressing this knowledge gap is important for anticipating how viruses might be transmitted to other animals, and how diseases might be controlled. The objective of this study was to assess whether Australian wild deer populations are exposed to relevant viral livestock diseases by testing blood samples for antibodies and antigens or through detection of viral genetic material. Our results establish a baseline exposure level, and possible spreading patterns in Australia's wild deer.

2. Materials and Methods

2.1. Sampling

Blood samples were collected by recreational hunters and professional culling staff from deer populations across eastern Australia. Most of the sampling areas were located within a 1- to 10-kilometer radius from agricultural grazing areas (Table 1, Figure 1A). Samples were generally collected during field necropsies in cooler winter months (Table 1, Figure 1B), when most culling and hunting occurs in Australia. Blood was drawn from the jugular vein and/or the heart and thoracic cavity, and collected in tubes (Becton Dickinson, Franklin Lakes, NJ, USA) with and without anticoagulant (EDTA) to obtain plasma and serum, respectively. Collection tubes were immediately refrigerated and transported to the laboratory. At the laboratory, serum and plasma were separated by centrifugation (10 min at 2000 g), transferred to 1.5 mL screw capped vials and stored at −80 °C until assayed.

Table 1. Population characteristics and distribution of deer sampled and tested in this study.

States or Territory	Animals	Sampling Location	Species	Sex			Age Groups				Month of Sampling										No. Deer Tested by		
				M	F	N.r.	Ad	Yrl	Fw	N.r.	Feb	Mar	Apr	May	Jun	Jul	Aug	Oct	Nov	ELISA Ab	ELISA Ag	PCR
NSW	244	Liverpool Plains *	Fallow	74	52	0	74	47	5	0	0	0	0	0	39	0	87	0	0	126	126	42
		Eden *	Fallow	12	21	5	21	9	3	5	0	0	0	0	0	0	18	15	5	38	0	18
		Wollongong *	Rusa	69	11	0	68	12	0	0	43	0	14	0	13	0	0	10	0	80	66	7
ACT	34	Canberra *	Fallow	14	20	0	26	8	0	0	0	0	0	0	34	0	0	0	0	34	0	10
VIC	44	Alpine National Park	Sambar	17	14	1	19	6	6	1	10	0	15	7	0	0	0	0	0	32	16	17
		Upper Yarra Flats	Sambar	2	6	1	6	1	1	1	0	0	0	0	8	0	0	1	0	9	8	4
		Yellinbo	Sambar	0	1	0	0	0	1	0	0	0	0	0	0	1	0	0	0	1	0	1
			Fallow	0	2	0	1	0	1	0	0	0	0	0	0	2	0	0	0	2	0	2
QLD	110	North east Queensland *	Chital	41	69	0	90	20	0	0	0	47	0	0	5	0	0	0	58	110	105	43
Total	432			229	196	7	305	103	17	7	53	47	29	7	99	3	105	26	63	432	321	144

* Sampling was conducted in areas close to livestock farms; NSW: New South Wales; ACT: Australian Capital Territory; VIC: Victoria; QLD: Queensland; F: female, M: male, Ad: adult, Yrl: yearling, Fw: fawn, N.r.: Not recorded; chital deer (*Axis axis*), rusa deer (*Rusa timorensis*), sambar deer (*Rusa unicolor*), fallow deer (*Dama dama*).

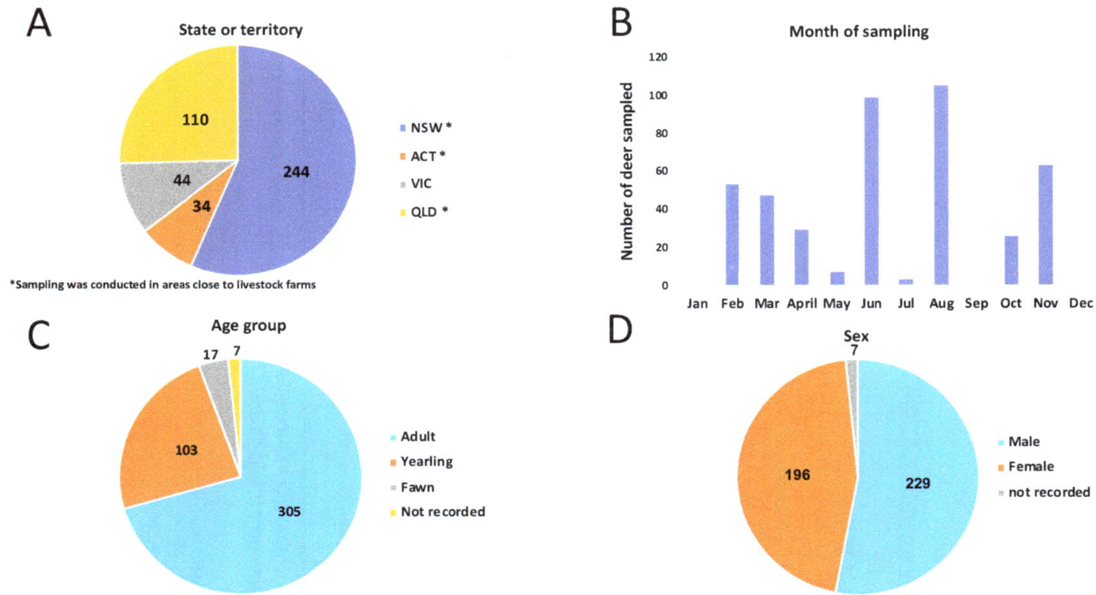

Figure 1. Population characteristics and distribution of deer sampled and tested in this study. Total numbers of deer sampled per region (**A**), per month (**B**), by age group (**C**) and by sex (**D**) are represented graphically.

2.2. Serological Methods

Serum and plasma were tested for *Pestivirus* antigen (Ag) and antibodies (Ab) against BoHV-1 and *Pestivirus* using the commercially available immunoenzymatic assay (ELISA) kits SERELISA® BVD p80 Ag Mono Indirect (Synbiotics SAS, Lyon, France), SERELISA BHV-1 Ab Mono Blocking ELISA (Synbiotics SAS, Lyon, France) and the PrioCHECK™ BVD & BD p80 Serum Kit (ThermoFisher Scientific, Rockford, USA) according to the manufacturer's instructions. For BoHV-1, samples with a ratio OD (optical density) sample/OD negative control ≤0.5 were classified as positive. This kit presents sensitivity (sn) of 96% and specificity (sp) 99%, according with the manufacturer. The *Pestivirus* kit detects antibodies targeted against the protein (p80/125), common to all BVDV and border disease virus (BDV) strains, with a manufacturer reported 97% sn and 98% sp for BVDV and 96% sn and 100% sp for BDV. Inhibition percentage (%INH) for each sample was calculated according to the manufacturer's kit insert.

Samples with a percentage inhibition (%INH) of <50 were classified as negative, those with 50 ≤ %INH < 80 as weak positive, and %INH ≥ 80 as strong positive. Results for the *Pestivirus* antigen detection kit are expressed as an index = 0.5 × OD sample−OD Positive control (P). Any sample having an index ≥(−0.15 × OD P) was considered positive, <(−0.3 × OD P) was considered negative and between (−0.15 × OD P) and (−0.3 × OD P) was considered doubtful according to the manufacturer's instructions.

Positive and negative controls were included in each run following the manufacturer's recommendations. Furthermore, all deer samples were initially tested in pools of three, with all serum samples in positive pools being additionally sampled individually and in duplicate. Optical density was measured using a plate reader (ClarioStar—BMG Labtech, Ortenberg, Germany) at 450 nm wavelength.

2.3. RNA Extraction and RT-PCR

Due to the large number of animals sampled, only a subset of 144 sera was selected across all sampled regions to be screened by PCR (Table 1) for four agriculturally relevant viruses (EHDV, BEFV, *Pestivirus* and Simbu serogroup). These included all the samples with ELISA-Ag positive and doubtful results. RNA was extracted from 140 μL of serum or cell culture supernatant (positive controls) using a QIAamp® Viral RNA Mini Kit (Qiagen, Valencia, CA, USA), according to the manufacturer's instructions. Viral RNA was reverse transcribed using a Tetro cDNA Synthesis Kit (Bioline, London, UK) using random hexamers according to the manufacturer's directions. RNA extracted from in vitro cultures for Akabane Virus, BEFV, EHDV and one bovine serum sample confirmed to be positive for BVDV, were used as positive controls. All culture material and BVDV positive sera were kindly donated by the Department of Jobs, Precincts and Regions, Victoria. PCR amplification was performed in a 25 μL reaction mixture containing 1× Green GoTaq Flexi buffer, 2 mM of $MgCl_2$, 10 mM of dNTPs, 0.2 μM of both forward and reverse primers (Table 2), 0.625 units of GoTaq G2 DNA polymerase (Promega, Madison, WI, USA) and 1 μL of total genomic DNA template. PCR primers were obtained from the literature for the four viruses included in this study (Table 2 and references therein). Amplification was carried out in a T100 thermal cycler (BioRad, Hercules, CA, USA), and amplification products visualized by gel electrophoresis, using 2% agarose gel, RedSafe™ (iNtRON Biotechnology, Gyeonggi-do, Korea), and a high-resolution imaging system—ChemiDoc™ MP Imaging System (Bio-Rad, Hercules, CA, USA).

2.4. Statistical Analysis

Samples were categorized as "positive" or "negative" based on the results of the ELISA-Ab. Seroprevalence was calculated from the proportion of seropositive results of those tested and is presented with 95% confidence interval (CI), calculated using the Wilson score interval (www.epitools.ausvet.com.au). Binary logistic regression models were used to evaluate the effect of the sex, age category and sampling site on the antibody status. Logistic regression was performed using R version 4.0.0 (R Development Core Team, Vienna, Austria). Due to the sparse nature of the data, we performed the logistic regression analysis only on fallow deer (in which most of the positive samples were detected). Lastly, we used the two-tailed Fisher's exact test to evaluate the hypothesis of non-random distribution of positive samples between fallow and rusa deer. $p < 0.05$ was considered statistically significant.

Table 2. List of oligonucleotides and PCR conditions used in this study.

Virus	Target Region	Primer Name	Sequence 5′–3′	Amplicon Length (bp)	PCR Condition	Reference
Pestivirus	5′UTR	324 326	ATGCCCWTAGTAGGACTAGCA WCAACTCCATGTGCCATGTAC	288	95 °C × 2 min 40 cycles (95 °C × 45 s, 52 °C × 45 s, 72 °C × 45 s) 72 °C × 5 min	[11]
Simbu Serogroup	Segment S	Uni-S-59F Uni-S-254R	GATGWCCWCAACGGAAT TGGGGAAAATGGTTATTAAC	215	95 °C × 2 min 40 cycles (95 °C × 45 s, 55 °C × 45 s, 72 °C × 45 s) 72 °C × 5 min	[12]
BEFV	Glucoprotein G	GF GR	ATGTTCAAGGTCCTCATAATTACC TAATGATCAAAGAACCTATCATCA	1871	95 °C × 2 min 40 cycles (95°C × 45 s, 52 °C × 45 s, 72 °C × 2 min) 72 °C × 5 min	[13]
EHDV	NS3	NS3F NS3R	CAGCGCYWTATWCGATATTG TCCGGAGATACCTCCATTAC	533	95 °C × 2 min 40 cycles (95 °C × 45 s, 55 °C × 45 s, 72 °C × 60 s) 72 °C × 5 min	[14]

3. Results

3.1. *Deer Sampling and Distribution*

During the sampling period, 432 wild deer were sampled encompassing four deer species (200 fallow deer, 110 chital deer (*Axis axis*), 80 rusa deer and 42 sambar deer (*Rusa unicolor*)) across eastern Australia (Table 1). Sampling was conducted from November 2017 to November 2019, with most samples (72%) collected between June and October (Table 1, Figure 1B). Slightly more females ($n = 229$) than males ($n = 196$) were sampled, while no information was available for seven animals (Table 1, Figure 1D). Individuals were classified in three age categories based on morphological characteristics, including body size, tooth wear and antler growth: fawn (<1 year), yearling (1 to <2 years) and adult (≥2 years). Most of the samples came from adult individuals ($n = 305$), followed by yearlings ($n = 103$) and fawns ($n = 17$). Information on age was not available for seven animals (Table 1, Figure 1C).

3.2. *ELISA Testing*

Sera and plasma samples from all 432 wild deer were screened by ELISA-Ab for *Pestivirus* and BoHV-1 (Table 1). All samples were negative for BoHV-1 antibodies. However, a total of 13 wild deer reacted positive for *Pestivirus* antibodies, resulting in an overall seroprevalence of 3.0%. Of the *Pestivirus* seropositive deer, 46.2% were sampled in June and 17.8% in August. Of the positive samples, 85% were obtained from adults. Additionally, all *Pestivirus* positive samples were collected from fallow and rusa deer, with a 5.5% and a 2.5% *Pestivirus*-seropositivity for each species, respectively (Figure 2).

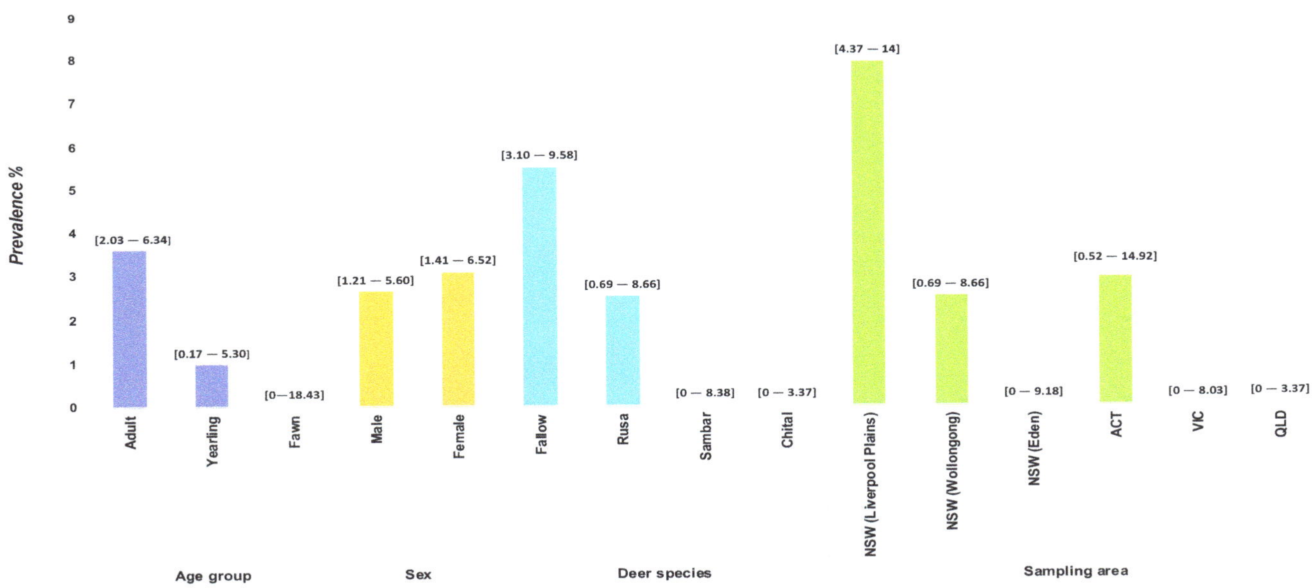

Figure 2. Prevalence of *Pestivirus* Antibodies: antibody prevalence was determined by ELISA and is represented as prevalence across age group, sex, species and sampling area. The 95% confidence interval is shown in brackets.

The animals positive for *Pestivirus* ELISA-Ab were sampled in Australian Capital Territory (ACT; 7.7%) and New South Wales (NSW; 92.3%). Two out of the three sampling areas from this last state showed seropositive deer with a local prevalence of 7.94% in central NSW (Liverpool Plains), and 2.5% in coastal NSW (Wollongong) (Figure 2). Five of the 13 wild deer reacted as strong positives with test values (%INH) ranging between 80–92%; the remaining eight wild deer were weak positives with percentages ranging between 51–79% (Table 3).

Table 3. Description of deer samples that tested positive for *Pestivirus* antibodies.

Sample	Species	Sampling Month	Sex	Age	Location	Anti-*Pestivirus* ELISA			
						Serum		Plasma	
						Result	%INH [a]	Result	%INH [a]
1	Fallow	June	F	Ad	New South Wales	WP	65	Neg	-
2	Fallow	June	F	Ad	New South Wales	SP	91.9	SP	91.4
3	Fallow	June	F	Ad	New South Wales	WP	73.7	WP	57.4
4	Fallow	June	F	Yrl	New South Wales	WP	73.6	WP	59.0
5	Fallow	June	F	Ad	New South Wales	WP	61.6	WP	67.0
6	Fallow	August	M	Ad	New South Wales	WP	71.6	WP	67.1
7	Fallow	August	M	Ad	New South Wales	SP	80.1	WP	79.4
8	Fallow	August	M	Ad	New South Wales	SP	84.4	SP	83.3
9	Fallow	August	M	Ad	New South Wales	SP	87.2	SP	80.1
10	Fallow	August	M	Ad	New South Wales	SP	87.2	WP	78.9
11	Rusa	February	ND	ND	New South Wales	WP	51.8	NS	-
12	Rusa	October	F	Ad	New South Wales	Neg	-	WP	60.1
13	Fallow	June	M	Ad	Australian Capital Territory	NS	-	WP	56.4

[a] %INH: percentage of inhibition obtained by ELISA; ND: no data, F: female, M: male, Ad: adult, Yrl: yearling; WP: weak positive, SP: strong positive, NS: no sample, Neg: negative.

Additionally, 321 out the 432 wild deer were also tested for *Pestivirus* antigens (see Table 1). Of the 321 deer tested, 278 (86.6%) showed a negative result, 24 (7.5%) revealed a doubtful result and 19 (5.9%) reacted positive. Additionally, only two of these positives overlapped with positive results shown for the ELISA-Ab screen.

Due to quasi-complete separation (i.e., most of the positives were in one category), we initially limited the predictors to the main effect of sex and age category (adult, yearling and fawn) or sex and location, and then tried to further simplify the model by considering sex only. In all models, the effect of the variables was not significant ($p > 0.05$). The proportion of seropositive *Pestivirus* results for fallow and rusa deer was similar ($p = 0.36$).

3.3. RT-PCR Screening

From the whole biobank of sera, 144 samples (see Table 1) were selected to be tested for *Pestivirus*, EDHV, BEFV and Simbu serogroup using previously validated RT-PCR primers sets [11–14]. These included all samples that had a doubtful or positive reaction for ELISA-Ag. Samples with hemolysis and insufficient volume were not included in the screening. No positive PCR amplification was obtained for any of the viruses screened, however, a positive result was obtained for all positive control samples in all runs.

4. Discussion

Australia's wild deer populations have increased in abundance and distribution during recent decades, and the close interaction between deer and livestock is a risk for pathogen transmission. However, little is known about the epidemiological role of wild deer in Australia. This study constitutes the largest number of deer, and deer species, sampled in Australia to date for viral pathogens, and complements a recent study performed on a similarly large number of animals across multiple geographic locations for the presence of parasitic infections [15]. Moreover, this study indicates exposure of deer to *Pestivirus* and is the first report of antibodies to ruminant *Pestivirus*es in rusa deer. This baseline information is of value for monitoring the status of endemic livestock pathogens in Australian deer, and for evaluating the risk of disease transmission between wild deer and livestock.

Although numerous pathogens have been detected in different cervids worldwide, including agriculturally relevant viruses [2], there is scarce knowledge about the viral infection status of Australian wild deer populations, with only four previous serosurveys being performed on red, fallow and rusa deer, but limited in their geographical coverage [7–10]. In contrast, the present study is based on the assessment of large sample sizes from four deer species collected throughout eastern Australia.

Our findings reveal the presence of antibodies in Australian wild deer species, against ruminant *Pestiviruses* (BVDV and BDV), which infect a variety of wild and domestic ungulate species and are associated with severe economic losses in livestock production worldwide [16]. In this study, positive serologic reactions were recorded in fallow and rusa deer at similar rates. Although the serosurveys have been proven to be a fundamental tool when it comes to disease surveillance, serological testing used in this study cannot distinguish between BVDV and BDV infections.

To our knowledge, this is the first report of *Pestivirus* antibodies in rusa deer. Additionally, in accordance with our findings, *Pestivirus* antibodies were identified previously in Australian fallow deer [7,8]. Seropositive fallow deer were first reported by Munday et al. (1972) [7] in Tasmania, with a prevalence of 14.5%. Ten years later, another serosurvey described a prevalence of 1.2% (1/86) in fallow deer sourced from New South Wales [8], in an area also included in our study. Moreover, McKenzie et al. [9] reported a prevalence of 4% in red deer sourced from 20 localities in eastern Australia. In comparison with the previous report for fallow deer from New South Wales [8], a higher seroprevalence is reported in the present study. The use of a different detection assay could have influenced the prevalence obtained. Compared with previous Australian serosurveys that used a virus neutralization test targeting only BVDV1, we used a more robust immunoassay that could detect antibodies against BVDV1, BVDV2 and BDV. The higher seroprevalence in this study might also reflect a real change in prevalence in the last 40 years, possibly due to an increase in deer density leading to greater interaction with livestock. Although samples from red deer were not included in our analyses, seroprevalence detected in fallow and rusa deer is comparable to that described in red deer by McKenzie et al. [9]. These findings may indicate that red, fallow and rusa deer are similarly exposed to *Pestivirus*.

Fallow deer, chital deer and, to a lesser extent, rusa deer, are gregarious, and hence, their transmission of pathogens would be expected to be higher compared to sambar deer, which are usually solitary [17]. No seroprevalence for *Pestivirus* was observed for sambar deer in this study, however, sampling numbers were low in comparison to other species. The sampling location for sambar deer in this study was composed of forested areas within mountain landscapes mostly distant from livestock grazing areas; however, the chital deer samples were collected from within pastoral areas where they are known to interact with cattle.

There is conflicting evidence in the literature surrounding prevalence of *Pestivirus* in cervids and known contact with cattle. Studies [18–20] have reported that close contact with cattle can induce high seroprevalence in wild cervids; however, a study by Frolich et al. [21] contrasted these findings and hypothesized an independent cycle as responsible for intrapopulation persistence. Additionally, the identification of persistently infected mule deer (*Odocoileus hemionus*) [22] and white-tailed deer (*Odocoileus virginianus*) [23–25] suggests that BVDV can sustain itself in deer populations without contact with cattle. The susceptibility of sambar and chital deer to BVDV has not been demonstrated, and we cannot completely discount the lack of susceptibility as a possible cause of these negative results. However, it is possible that mortality of persistently infected animals or differences in social behavior between chital and sambar deer with the other deer species, which could also explain these negative results.

Most of the seropositive *Pestivirus* outcomes were recorded in adult deer, which is not unexpected, as they constituted ~70% of the animals sampled in this study. Although antibody levels could be detected in the sampled deer, it is not possible to know when the animals were exposed to the virus. Seroconversion in cattle usually appears two weeks after infection, with the titer continuing to rise for 10 to 12 weeks; after this time, a plateau is reached [26,27]. Similarly, deer experimentally infected with BVDV exhibit a similar seroconversion course, developing antibodies at 8 to 15 days post infection [28,29]. However, antibodies against BVDV have been demonstrated to remain in serum for longer than three years [30].

Pestivirus antibody detection was performed in serum and plasma using a blocking ELISA kit with sensitivity and specificity comparable with other similar kits [31], also validated for non-bovine samples [32–34]. Concordance in results were found in eight overlapped specimens (serum and plasma), and two of the remaining overlapped specimens revealed positive outcomes only in one of the samples. Although this discrepancy is not enough to state which sample is better for *Pestivirus* antibody detection in deer, previous studies did not find variation between serum and plasma for viral antibody detection [35–37]. It is possible that other factors including the quality of the sample and antibody concentration could have affected the results in some samples.

Overall, the seroprevalence for *Pestivirus*es was 3%, considerably lower than the 52.6% observed in Australian cattle [16]. Similar findings were detected in European countries during serosurveys of *Pestivirus*es in deer to evaluate the epidemiological importance of deer in BVDV eradication programs: Belgium, 1.3% [38], Germany, 2% [39], Switzerland, 2.7% [3], and Italy, 4.5% [40]. The authors concluded that despite regular interactions with farmed ruminants, infection in deer was occasional with virus transmission from cattle to deer, and therefore, the possibility of deer being a source of infection for cattle was remote.

In contrast to other reports, we did not detect any infected deer by PCR, although the RT-PCR assay we used detects a broad range of *Pestivirus*es from pigs, cattle and sheep [11]. Thus, based on detection of a low seroprevalence for ruminant *Pestivirus*es in the deer population studied, the fact that we did not identify any persistently infected (virus positive, antibodies negative) deer, and given and the expected increase in distribution and abundance [1] (in the absence of substantial control), the high number of seropositive cattle in Australia, we consider it more probable that deer are an accidental spillover host rather than a reservoir host for ruminant *Pestiviruses*, and that persistently infected cattle could transmit these viruses to wild deer.

Pestivirus antigen detection by ELISA resulted in 5.9% and 7.5% of samples testing positive and doubtful, respectively. However, RT-PCR negative results were obtained in all the samples. The ELISA kit utilized is reported to detect *Pestivirus* antigens in ruminant samples, however, there is no published information about validation with cervid samples. A similar antigen detection methodology was previously used for roe deer (*Capreolus capreolus*) [41], with positive results obtained. However, those findings were not confirmed by RT-PCR. A possible explanation for the false positive antigen results could be variations in the primer target region not detectable by RT-PCR used. A second explanation is that there were unspecific cross-reactions, but further work is needed to determine the exact cause of the potential false positive antigen ELISA results obtained in this study.

We acknowledge that a limitation of this study is the type of tissue utilized for detection of BVDV genetic material. Although there are studies that used serum to detect BVDV by PCR [42,43], BVDV has trophism for epithelia of both the alimentary and integumentary systems [44], however, due to the collection strategies available to us during the sampling procedures, specimens that would be more reliable in detecting low levels of viral nucleic acid over a longer period of infection time, such as reproductive tissues [45,46] or spleen [47], were not available for testing.

BoHV-1 is the best characterized member of the subfamily *Alphaherpesvirus*, responsible for Infectious Bovine Rhinotracheitis (IBR), a cattle disease of major economic concern worldwide [48], and widespread in Australian cattle with a seroprevalence of 25–40% [49]. Susceptibility to BoHV-1 of wild cervids has previously been demonstrated [5,50], and additionally, several ruminant *Alphaherpesviruses* related to BoHV-1 have been isolated from cervids, including cervid herpesvirus 1 (CvHV-1) in red deer [51] and cervid herpesvirus 2 (CvHV-2) in reindeer (*Rangifer tarandus*) [52]. Our failure to detect antibodies against BoHV-1 is consistent with previous reports in Australia, which demonstrated an absence of BoHV-1 antibodies in fallow deer in Tasmania [7] and red deer in Queensland [9]. Furthermore, we can state that there is no evidence of cervid alphaherpesviruses in Australian wild deer, since serological cross reactivity by both virus neutralization and ELISA between ruminant alphaherpesviruses, including CvHV-1 and -2, is well documented [53–55].

The assessment of a subset of 144 serum samples by PCR also revealed no evidence of acute infection for the other viral livestock pathogens screened in this study. BEFV, EHDV and Akabane virus (a member of the Simbu serogroup) are endemic in Queensland and they have a seasonal spread in New South Wales [56–58]. Moreover, these viruses remain undetected in Victoria [57,58]. As they are vector-borne viruses, their occurrence is limited by the effect of cold weather, which restricts the distribution of their vectors. Previous studies performed in Australian deer reported serological evidence for BEFV, EHDV and Akabane virus in red deer from south-eastern Queensland [9]. Moreover, Moriarty et al. [10] found seropositive outcomes in a small sample of rusa deer in coastal central NSW for Akabane virus and EHDV. All the samples screened in the present study were negative for these viruses; however, the presence of vector species and previous evidence highlights the need for further serologic analysis to determine the role of deer as a spillover or reservoir host for these viruses, particularly in Queensland and New South Wales where BEFV, EHDV and Akabane virus are endemic. One limitation of this study was that all deer were sampled in the colder winter months, which would also lessen the activity of the vectors necessary for virus transmission.

5. Conclusions

Our findings provide an overview of the current *Pestivirus* infection status of wild deer in eastern Australia. The low prevalence of *Pestivirus* antibodies and negative findings for the viruses tested suggests that wild deer are an incidental spill-over host, and not a reservoir host. However, considering the substantial increase observed in fallow deer seroprevalence compared with a previous report [8], and the expected increase in distribution and abundance [1] (in the absence of substantial control), we cannot rule out the possibility that deer species sampled in this study could be a future source of infection for livestock.

Author Contributions: Conceptualization, C.P., T.G.C. and K.J.H.; methodology, J.L.H., C.P. and K.J.H.; formal analysis, J.L.H.; investigation, J.L.H., C.P. and K.J.H.; resources, C.P., D.M.F., A.P., J.O.H. and K.J.H.; data curation, J.L.H.; writing—original draft preparation, J.L.H. and K.J.H.; writing—review and editing, C.P., D.M.F., A.P., J.O.H., T.G.C. and K.J.H.; visualization, J.L.H. and K.J.H.; supervision, C.P., T.G.C. and K.J.H.; project administration, C.P., D.M.F., A.P., T.G.C. and K.J.H.; funding acquisition, C.P., D.M.F., A.P., T.G.C. and K.J.H. All authors have read and agreed to the published version of the manuscript.

Acknowledgments: We would like to thank Richard Francis (ABZECO), Jake Haddad (VPAC), Kirk Stone (Strathbogie Wildlife), Andrew Bengsen, Troy Crittle and Quentin Hart (all New South Wales Department of Primary Industries), Bob McKinnon and Amy Sheridan (North West Local Land Services), Michael Brennan and Matt Amos (Biosecurity Queensland) and the staff from Parks Victoria for assisting with sample collection. In addition, we thank Kim O'Riley and Peter Mee for technical support. Finally, we thank Tao Zheng, PhD and Stacey Lynch, PhD from the Department of Jobs, Precincts and Regions, Victoria, for providing samples and cell culture supernatant used as positive controls.

References

1. Davis, N.E.; Bennett, A.; Forsyth, D.M.; Bowman, D.M.J.S.; Lefroy, E.C.; Wood, S.W.; Woolnough, A.P.; West, P.; Hampton, J.O.; Johnson, C.N. A systematic review of the impacts and management of introduced deer (family Cervidae) in Australia. *Wildl. Res.* **2016**, *43*, 515–532. [CrossRef]
2. Cripps, J.K.; Pacioni, C.; Scroggie, M.P.; Woolnough, A.P.; Ramsey, D.S.L. Introduced deer and their potential role in disease transmission to livestock in Australia. *Mammal Rev.* **2019**, *49*, 60–77. [CrossRef]
3. Casaubon, J.; Vogt, H.R.; Stalder, H.; Hug, C.; Ryser-Degiorgis, M.P. Bovine viral diarrhea virus in free-ranging wild ruminants in Switzerland: Low prevalence of infection despite regular interactions with domestic livestock. *BMC Vet. Res.* **2012**, *8*, 204. [CrossRef] [PubMed]
4. Duncan, C.; Backus, L.; Lynn, T.; Powers, B.; Salman, M. Passive, opportunistic wildlife disease surveillance in the Rocky Mountain Region, USA. *Transbound. Emerg. Dis.* **2008**, *55*, 308–314. [CrossRef]
5. Graham, D.A.; Gallagher, C.; Carden, R.F.; Lozano, J.M.; Moriarty, J.; O'Neill, R. A survey of free-ranging deer in Ireland for serological evidence of exposure to bovine viral diarrhoea virus, bovine herpes virus-1, bluetongue virus and Schmallenberg virus. *Irel. Vet. J.* **2017**, *70*, 13. [CrossRef]
6. Roug, A.; Swift, P.; Torres, S.; Jones, K.; Johnson, C.K. Serosurveillance for livestock pathogens in free-ranging mule deer (*Odocoileus hemionus*). *PLoS ONE* **2012**, *7*, e50600. [CrossRef]
7. Munday, B.L. A serological study of some infectious diseases of Tasmanian wildlife. *J. Wildl. Dis.* **1972**, *8*, 169–175. [CrossRef]
8. English, A.W. Serological survey of wild fallow deer (*Dama dama*) in New South Wales, Australia. *Vet. Rec.* **1982**, *110*, 153–154. [CrossRef]
9. McKenzie, R.A.; Green, P.E.; Thornton, A.M.; Chung, Y.S.; MacKenzie, A.R.; Cybinski, D.H.; St George, T.D. Diseases of deer in south eastern Queensland. *Aust. Vet. J.* **1985**, *62*, 424. [CrossRef]
10. Moriarty, A. Ecology and Enviromental Impact of Javan Rusa Deer (*Cervus timorensis russa*) in the Royal National Park. Ph.D. Thesis, University of Western Sydney, Sydney, NSW, Australia, 2004.
11. Vilcek, S.; Herring, A.J.; Herring, J.A.; Nettleton, P.F.; Lowings, J.P.; Paton, D.J. Pestiviruses isolated from pigs, cattle and sheep can be allocated into at least three genogroups using polymerase chain reaction and restriction endonuclease analysis. *Arch. Virol.* **1994**, *136*, 309–323. [CrossRef]
12. Golender, N.; Bumbarov, V.Y.; Erster, O.; Beer, M.; Khinich, Y.; Wernike, K. Development and validation of a universal S-segment-based real-time RT-PCR assay for the detection of Simbu serogroup viruses. *J. Virol. Methods* **2018**, *261*, 80–85. [CrossRef] [PubMed]
13. Kato, T.; Aizawa, M.; Takayoshi, K.; Kokuba, T.; Yanase, T.; Shirafuji, H.; Tsuda, T.; Yamakawa, M. Phylogenetic relationships of the G gene sequence of bovine ephemeral fever virus isolated in Japan, Taiwan and Australia. *Vet. Microbiol.* **2009**, *137*, 217–223. [CrossRef]

14. Ohashi, S.; Yoshida, K.; Yanase, T.; Kato, T.; Tsuda, T. Simultaneous detection of bovine arboviruses using single-tube multiplex reverse transcription-polymerase chain reaction. *J. Virol. Methods* **2004**, *120*, 79–85. [CrossRef] [PubMed]
15. Huaman, J.L.; Pacioni, C.; Forsyth, D.M.; Pople, A.; Hampton, J.O.; Helbig, K.J.; Carvalho, T. Screening of Blood Parasites in Australian Wild Deer. *Authorea* **2020**. [CrossRef]
16. Scharnbock, B.; Roch, F.F.; Richter, V.; Funke, C.; Firth, C.L.; Obritzhauser, W.; Baumgartner, W.; Kasbohrer, A.; Pinior, B. A meta-analysis of bovine viral diarrhoea virus (BVDV) prevalences in the global cattle population. *Sci. Rep.* **2018**, *8*, 14420. [CrossRef]
17. Van Dyck, S.; Strahan, R. *The Mammals of Australia*; Reed New Holland: Sydney, NSW, Australia, 2008.
18. Aguirre, A.A.; Hansen, D.E.; Starkey, E.E.; Mclean, R.G. Serologic Survey of Wild Cervids for Potential Disease Agents in Selected National-Parks in the United-States. *Prev. Vet. Med.* **1995**, *21*, 313–322. [CrossRef]
19. Rodriguez-Prieto, V.; Kukielka, D.; Rivera-Arroyo, B.; Martinez-Lopez, B.; de las Heras, A.I.; Sanchez-Vizcaino, J.M.; Vicente, J. Evidence of shared bovine viral diarrhea infections between red deer and extensively raised cattle in south-central Spain. *BMC Vet. Res.* **2016**, *12*. [CrossRef]
20. Fernandez-Aguilar, X.; Lopez-Olvera, J.R.; Marco, I.; Rosell, R.; Colom-Cadena, A.; Soto-Heras, S.; Lavin, S.; Cabezon, O. Pestivirus in alpine wild ruminants and sympatric livestock from the Cantabrian Mountains, Spain. *Vet. Rec.* **2016**, *178*, U557–U586. [CrossRef] [PubMed]
21. Frolich, K. Bovine Virus Diarrhea and Mucosal Disease in Free-Ranging and Captive Deer (Cervidae) in Germany. *J. Wildl. Dis.* **1995**, *31*, 247–250. [CrossRef]
22. Duncan, C.; Van Campen, H.; Soto, S.; LeVan, I.K.; Baeten, L.A.; Miller, M.W. Persistent Bovine viral diarrhea virus infection in wild cervids of Colorado. *J. Vet. Diagn. Investig.* **2008**, *20*, 650–653. [CrossRef]
23. Passler, T.; Walz, P.H.; Ditchkoff, S.S.; Walz, H.L.; Givens, M.D.; Brock, K.V. Evaluation of hunter-harvested white-tailed deer for evidence of bovine viral diarrhea virus infection in Alabama. *J. Vet. Diagn. Investig.* **2008**, *20*, 79–82. [CrossRef] [PubMed]
24. Duncan, C.; Ridpath, J.; Palmer, M.V.; Driskell, E.; Spraker, T. Histopathologic and immunohistochemical findings in two white-tailed deer fawns persistently infected with Bovine viral diarrhea virus. *J. Vet. Diagn. Investig.* **2008**, *20*, 289–296. [CrossRef] [PubMed]
25. Passler, T.; Walz, P.H.; Ditchkoff, S.S.; Givens, M.D.; Maxwell, H.S.; Brock, K.V. Experimental persistent infection with bovine viral diarrhea virus in white-tailed deer. *Vet. Microbiol.* **2007**, *122*, 350–356. [CrossRef] [PubMed]
26. Collins, M.E.; Heaney, J.; Thomas, C.J.; Brownlie, J. Infectivity of pestivirus following persistence of acute infection. *Vet. Microbiol.* **2009**, *138*, 289–296. [CrossRef] [PubMed]
27. Howard, C.J. Immunological responses to bovine virus diarrhoea virus infections. *Rev. Sci. Tech.* **1990**, *9*, 95–103. [CrossRef]
28. Van Campen, H.; Williams, E.S.; Edwards, J.; Cook, W.; Stout, G. Experimental infection of deer with bovine viral diarrhea virus. *J. Wildl. Dis.* **1997**, *33*, 567–573. [CrossRef]
29. Tessaro, S.V.; Carman, P.S.; Deregt, D. Viremia and virus shedding in elk infected with type 1 and virulent type 2 bovine viral diarrhea virus. *J. Wildl. Dis.* **1999**, *35*, 671–677. [CrossRef]
30. Fredriksen, B.; Sandvik, T.; Loken, T.; Odegaard, S.A. Level and duration of serum antibodies in cattle infected experimentally and naturally with bovine virus diarrhoea virus. *Vet. Rec.* **1999**, *144*, 111–114. [CrossRef]
31. Hanon, J.B.; De Baere, M.; De la Ferte, C.; Roelandt, S.; Van der Stede, Y.; Cay, B. Evaluation of 16 commercial antibody ELISAs for the detection of bovine viral diarrhea virus-specific antibodies in serum and milk using well-characterized sample panels. *J. Vet. Diagn. Investig.* **2017**, *29*, 833–843. [CrossRef]
32. Morrondo, M.P.; Perez-Creo, A.; Prieto, A.; Cabanelas, E.; Diaz-Cao, J.M.; Arias, M.S.; Fernandez, P.D.; Pajares, G.; Remesar, S.; Lopez-Sandez, C.M.; et al. Prevalence and distribution of infectious and parasitic agents in roe deer from Spain and their possible role as reservoirs. *Ital. J. Anim. Sci.* **2017**, *16*, 266–274. [CrossRef]
33. Loeffen, W.L.; van Beuningen, A.; Quak, S.; Elbers, A.R. Seroprevalence and risk factors for the presence of ruminant pestiviruses in the Dutch swine population. *Vet. Microbiol.* **2009**, *136*, 240–245. [CrossRef] [PubMed]
34. Evans, C.A.; Lanyon, S.R.; Reichel, M.P. Investigation of AGID and two commercial ELISAs for the detection of Bovine viral diarrhea virus-specific antibodies in sheep serum. *J. Vet. Diagn. Investig.* **2017**, *29*, 181–185. [CrossRef] [PubMed]

35. Cherpes, T.L.; Meyn, L.A.; Hillier, S.L. Plasma versus serum for detection of herpes simplex virus type 2-specific immunoglobulin G antibodies with a glycoprotein G2-based enzyme immunoassay. *J. Clin. Microbiol.* **2003**, *41*, 2758–2759. [CrossRef]
36. Parra-Álvarez, S.; Coronel-Ruiz, C.; Castilla, M.G.; Velandia-Romero, M.L.; Castellanos, J.E. Alta correlación en la detección de anticuerpos y antígenos de virus del dengue en muestras de suero y plasma. *Rev. Fac. Med.* **2015**, *63*, 687–693. [CrossRef]
37. Lin, H.T.; Hsu, C.H.; Tsai, H.J.; Lin, C.H.; Lo, P.Y.; Wang, S.L.; Wang, L.C. Influenza A plasma and serum virus antibody detection comparison in dogs using blocking enzyme-linked immunosorbent assay. *Vet. World* **2015**, *8*, 580–583. [CrossRef]
38. Tavernier, P.; Sys, S.U.; De Clercq, K.; De Leeuw, I.; Caij, A.B.; De Baere, M.; De Regge, N.; Fretin, D.; Roupie, V.; Govaerts, M.; et al. Serologic screening for 13 infectious agents in roe deer (*Capreolus capreolus*) in Flanders. *Infect. Ecol. Epidemiol.* **2015**, *5*, 29862. [CrossRef]
39. Krametter, R.; Nielsen, S.S.; Loitsch, A.; Froetscher, W.; Benetka, V.; Moestl, K.; Baumgartner, W. Pestivirus exposure in free-living and captive deer in Austria. *J. Wildl. Dis.* **2004**, *40*, 791–795. [CrossRef]
40. Cuteri, V.; Diverio, S.; Carnieletto, P.; Turilli, C.; Valente, C. Serological survey for antibodies against selected infectious agents among fallow deer (*Dama dama*) in central Italy. *Zentralbl Veterinarmed B* **1999**, *46*, 545–549. [CrossRef]
41. Boadella, M.; Carta, T.; Oleaga, A.; Pajares, G.; Munoz, M.; Gortazar, C. Serosurvey for selected pathogens in Iberian roe deer. *BMC Vet. Res.* **2010**, *6*, 51. [CrossRef]
42. Decaro, N.; Lucente, M.S.; Lanave, G.; Gargano, P.; Larocca, V.; Losurdo, M.; Ciambrone, L.; Marino, P.A.; Parisi, A.; Casalinuovo, F.; et al. Evidence for Circulation of Bovine Viral Diarrhoea Virus Type 2c in Ruminants in Southern Italy. *Transbound. Emerg. Dis.* **2017**, *64*, 1935–1944. [CrossRef]
43. Fernandez-Sirera, L.; Cabezon, O.; Dematteis, A.; Rossi, L.; Meneguz, P.G.; Gennero, M.S.; Allepuz, A.; Rosell, R.; Lavin, S.; Marco, I. Survey of Pestivirus infection in wild and domestic ungulates from south-western Italian Alps. *Eur. J. Wildlife Res.* **2012**, *58*, 425–431. [CrossRef]
44. Bianchi, M.V.; Silveira, S.; Mosena, A.C.S.; de Souza, S.O.; Konradt, G.; Canal, C.W.; Driemeier, D.; Pavarini, S.P. Pathological and virological features of skin lesions caused by BVDV in cattle. *Braz. J. Microbiol.* **2019**, *50*, 271–277. [CrossRef] [PubMed]
45. Grooms, D.L.; Brock, K.V.; Ward, L.A. Detection of bovine viral diarrhea virus in the ovaries of cattle acutely infected with bovine viral diarrhea virus. *J. Vet. Diagn. Investig.* **1998**, *10*, 125–129. [CrossRef] [PubMed]
46. Givens, M.D.; Heath, A.M.; Brock, K.V.; Brodersen, B.W.; Carson, R.L.; Stringfellow, D.A. Detection of bovine viral diarrhea virus in semen obtained after inoculation of seronegative postpubertal bulls. *Am. J. Vet. Res.* **2003**, *64*, 428–434. [CrossRef]
47. Ohmann, H.B. Pathogenesis of bovine viral diarrhoea-mucosal disease: Distribution and significance of BVDV antigen in diseased calves. *Res. Vet. Sci.* **1983**, *34*, 5–10. [CrossRef]
48. Thiry, J.; Keuser, V.; Muylkens, B.; Meurens, F.; Gogev, S.; Vanderplasschen, A.; Thiry, E. Ruminant alphaherpesviruses related to bovine herpesvirus 1. *Vet. Res.* **2006**, *37*, 169–190. [CrossRef]
49. Gu, X.; Kirkland, P.D. Infectious Bovine Rhinotracheitis. In *Australian and New Zealand Standard Diagnostic Procedures*; The Department of Agriculture and Water: Canberra, ACT, Australia, 2008; pp. 1–18.
50. Lillehaug, A.; Vikoren, T.; Larsen, I.L.; Akerstedt, J.; Tharaldsen, J.; Handeland, K. Antibodies to ruminant alpha-herpesviruses and pestiviruses in Norwegian cervids. *J. Wildl. Dis.* **2003**, *39*, 779–786. [CrossRef]
51. Inglis, D.M.; Bowie, J.M.; Allan, M.J.; Nettleton, P.F. Ocular disease in red deer calves associated with a herpesvirus infection. *Vet. Rec.* **1983**, *113*, 182–183. [CrossRef]
52. Ek-Kommonen, C.; Pelkonen, S.; Nettleton, P.F. Isolation of a herpesvirus serologically related to bovine herpesvirus 1 from a reindeer (*Rangifer tarandus*). *Acta Vet. Scand.* **1986**, *27*, 299–301.
53. Lyaku, J.R.S.; Nettleton, P.F.; Marsden, H. A Comparison of Serological Relationships among 5 Ruminant Alphaherpesviruses by Elisa. *Arch. Virol.* **1992**, *124*, 333–341. [CrossRef]
54. Martin, W.B.; Castrucci, G.; Frigeri, F.; Ferrari, M. A Serological Comparison of Some Animal Herpesviruses. *Comp. Immunol. Microb.* **1990**, *13*, 75–84. [CrossRef]
55. Nixon, P.; Edwards, S.; White, H. Serological Comparisons of Antigenically Related Herpesviruses in Cattle, Red Deer and Goats. *Vet. Res. Commun.* **1988**, *12*, 355–362. [CrossRef] [PubMed]
56. Walker, P.J.; Klement, E. Epidemiology and control of bovine ephemeral fever. *Vet. Res.* **2015**, *46*, 124. [CrossRef] [PubMed]

57. Weir, R.P.; Agnihotri, K. Epizootic Haemorrhagic Disease. In *Australian and New Zealand Standard Diagnostic Procedures*; The Department of Agriculture and Water: Canberra, ACT, Australia, 2014; pp. 1–14.
58. Australia Animal Health. National Arbovirus Monitoring Program 2015–2016 Report. Available online: https://www.animalhealthaustralia.com.au/wp-content/uploads/2015/09/NAMP-Annual-Report_FA_print.pdf (accessed on 1 April 2020).

PERMISSIONS

All chapters in this book were first published by MDPI; hereby published with permission under the Creative Commons Attribution License or equivalent. Every chapter published in this book has been scrutinized by our experts. Their significance has been extensively debated. The topics covered herein carry significant findings which will fuel the growth of the discipline. They may even be implemented as practical applications or may be referred to as a beginning point for another development.

The contributors of this book come from diverse backgrounds, making this book a truly international effort. This book will bring forth new frontiers with its revolutionizing research information and detailed analysis of the nascent developments around the world.

We would like to thank all the contributing authors for lending their expertise to make the book truly unique. They have played a crucial role in the development of this book. Without their invaluable contributions this book wouldn't have been possible. They have made vital efforts to compile up to date information on the varied aspects of this subject to make this book a valuable addition to the collection of many professionals and students.

This book was conceptualized with the vision of imparting up-to-date information and advanced data in this field. To ensure the same, a matchless editorial board was set up. Every individual on the board went through rigorous rounds of assessment to prove their worth. After which they invested a large part of their time researching and compiling the most relevant data for our readers.

The editorial board has been involved in producing this book since its inception. They have spent rigorous hours researching and exploring the diverse topics which have resulted in the successful publishing of this book. They have passed on their knowledge of decades through this book. To expedite this challenging task, the publisher supported the team at every step. A small team of assistant editors was also appointed to further simplify the editing procedure and attain best results for the readers.

Apart from the editorial board, the designing team has also invested a significant amount of their time in understanding the subject and creating the most relevant covers. They scrutinized every image to scout for the most suitable representation of the subject and create an appropriate cover for the book.

The publishing team has been an ardent support to the editorial, designing and production team. Their endless efforts to recruit the best for this project, has resulted in the accomplishment of this book. They are a veteran in the field of academics and their pool of knowledge is as vast as their experience in printing. Their expertise and guidance has proved useful at every step. Their uncompromising quality standards have made this book an exceptional effort. Their encouragement from time to time has been an inspiration for everyone.

The publisher and the editorial board hope that this book will prove to be a valuable piece of knowledge for researchers, students, practitioners and scholars across the globe.

LIST OF CONTRIBUTORS

Andrew W. Byrne and Damien Barrett
One-Health Scientific Support Unit, Surveillance, Animal by-products, and TSEs (SAT) Division, Department of Agriculture, Food and the Marine, Agriculture House, Dublin 2 D02 WK12, Ireland

Philip Breslin, James O'Keeffe and Eoin Ryan
Ruminant Animal Health Division, Department of Agriculture, Food and the Marine, Backweston, Co. Kildare W23 VW2C, Ireland

Jamie M. Madden
Centre for Veterinary Epidemiology and Risk Analysis (CVERA), School of Veterinary Medicine, University College Dublin, Belfield, Dublin 4 D04 W6F6, Ireland

Wlaa Assi
Laboratory of Viral Infectious Diseases, Department of Computational Biology and Medical Sciences, Graduate School of Frontier Sciences, The University of Tokyo, 2-1 Hirosawa, Wako, Saitama 351-0198, Japan
Viral Infectious Diseases Unit, RIKEN, 2-1 Hirosawa, Wako, Saitama 351-0198, Japan
Photonics Control Technology Team, RIKEN Center for Advanced Photonics, 2-1 Hirosawa, Wako, Saitama 351-0198, Japan

Tomoya Hirose and Ryosuke Matsuura
Laboratory of Viral Infectious Diseases, Department of Computational Biology and Medical Sciences, Graduate School of Frontier Sciences, The University of Tokyo, 2-1 Hirosawa, Wako, Saitama 351-0198, Japan
Viral Infectious Diseases Unit, RIKEN, 2-1 Hirosawa, Wako, Saitama 351-0198, Japan

Satoshi Wada
Photonics Control Technology Team, RIKEN Center for Advanced Photonics, 2-1 Hirosawa, Wako, Saitama 351-0198, Japan

Shin-nosuke Takeshima
Laboratory of Viral Infectious Diseases, Department of Computational Biology and Medical Sciences, Graduate School of Frontier Sciences, The University of Tokyo, 2-1 Hirosawa, Wako, Saitama 351-0198, Japan
Viral Infectious Diseases Unit, RIKEN, 2-1 Hirosawa, Wako, Saitama 351-0198, Japan
Photonics Control Technology Team, RIKEN Center for Advanced Photonics, 2-1 Hirosawa, Wako, Saitama 351-0198, Japan
Department of Food and Nutrition, Jumonji University, Niiza, Saitama 352-8510, Japan

Yoko Aida
Laboratory of Viral Infectious Diseases, Department of Computational Biology and Medical Sciences, Graduate School of Frontier Sciences, The University of Tokyo, 2-1 Hirosawa, Wako, Saitama 351-0198, Japan
Viral Infectious Diseases Unit, RIKEN, 2-1 Hirosawa, Wako, Saitama 351-0198, Japan
Nakamura Laboratory, Baton Zone program, Riken Cluster for Science, Technology and Innovation Hub, 2-1 Hirosawa, Wako, Saitama 351-0198, Japan

Maria Grazia Amoroso, Barbara Degli Uberti, Francesco Serra, Giovanna De Luca, Sergio Brandi and Giovanna Fusco
Unit of Virology, Department of Animal Health, Experimental Zooprophylactic Institute of Southern Italy

Giuseppe Lucifora
Section of Vibo Valentia, Experimental Zooprophylactic Institute of Southern Italy, Contrada Piano di Bruno, 89852 Mileto, Italy

Giorgia Borriello, Maria Concetta Cuomo, Francesca Bove, Marita Georgia Riccardi and Giorgio Galiero
Department of Animal Health, Experimental Zooprophylactic Institute of Southern Italy, Via Salute 2, 80055 Portici, Italy

Alessandro De Domenico
Freelance Veterinary, Ordine dei Veterinari di Vibo Valentia, 89900 Vibo Valentia, Italy

Christiane Riedel, Hann-Wei Chen and Till Rümenapf
Institute of Virology, Vetmeduni Vienna, 1210 Vienna, Austria

Ursula Reichart
VetCore Facility for Research, Vetmeduni Vienna, 1210 Vienna, Austria

Benjamin Lamp
Institute of Virology, Faculty of Veterinary Medicine, Justus-Liebig University, 35392 Gießen, Germany

Vibor Laketa
Department of Infectious Diseases, Virology, University of Heidelberg, 69120 Heidelberg, Germany
German Center for Infection Research, 69120 Heidelberg, Germany

Luís Guilherme de Oliveira, Marina L. Mechler-Dreibi and Henrique M. S. Almeida
School of Agricultural and Veterinarian Sciences, São Paulo State University (Unesp), Jaboticabal. Via de Acesso Prof. Paulo Donato Castelanne s/n, Jaboticabal - SP 14884-900, Brazil

Igor R. H. Gatto
Ourofino Animal Health Ltda. Rodovia Anhanguera SP 330, Km 298. Distrito Industrial, Cravinhos - SP 14140-000, Brazil

Claire A.M. Becker, Chloé Ambroset, Agnès Tricot and Marie-Anne Arcangioli
UMR Mycoplasmoses des Ruminants, VetAgro Sup, Université de Lyon, 69280 Marcy-l'Etoile, France

Anthéa Huleux, Angélique Vialatte, Adélie Colin and Florence Tardy
UMR Mycoplasmoses des Ruminants, ANSES Laboratoire de Lyon, Université de Lyon, 69364 Lyon CEDEX 07, France

Bong-Kyun Park
Virus Disease Division, Animal and Plant Quarantine Agency, Gimchen, Gyeongbuk-do 39660, Korea
College of Veterinary Medicine, Seoul University, Gwanak-ro, Gwanak-gu, Seoul 08826, Korea

SeEun Choe, Gyu-Nam Park, Ra Mi Cha, Bang-Hun Hyun and Dong-Jun An
Virus Disease Division, Animal and Plant Quarantine Agency, Gimchen, Gyeongbuk-do 39660, Korea

Katie J. Knapek and Hana Van Campen
Department of Biomedical Sciences, Colorado State University, Fort Collins, CO 80523, USA
Department of Microbiology, Immunology and Pathology, Colorado State University, Fort Collins, CO 80523, USA

Hanah M. Georges, Jeanette V. Bishop, Natalia P. Smirnova and Thomas R. Hansen
Department of Biomedical Sciences, Colorado State University, Fort Collins, CO 80523, USA

Helle Bielefeldt-Ohmann
Australian Infectious Diseases Research Centre and School of Veterinary Science, The University of Queensland, St. Lucia, QLD 4072, Australia

Ana García-Galán, Antonio Sánchez and Christian de la Fe
Ruminant Health Research Group, Department of Animal Health, Faculty of Veterinary Sciences, Regional Campus of International Excellence "Campus Mare Nostrum", University of Murcia, 30100 Murcia, Spain

Laurent-Xavier Nouvel, Eric Baranowski and Christine Citti
IHAP, ENVT, INRAE, Université de Toulouse, 31300 Toulouse, France

Ángel Gómez-Martín
Ruminant Health Research Group, Department of Animal Health, Faculty of Veterinary Sciences, Regional Campus of International Excellence "Campus Mare Nostrum", University of Murcia, 30100 Murcia, Spain
Microbiological Agents associated with Reproduction (ProVaginBio) Research Group, Department of Animal Health and Public Health, Faculty of Veterinary Sciences, University CEU Cardenal Herrera of Valencia, CEU Universities, 46113 Valencia, Spain

Alais M. Dall Agnol, Alice F. Alfieri and Amauri A. Alfieri
Laboratory of Animal Virology, Department of Veterinary Preventive Medicine, Universidade Estadual de Londrina, Londrina, CEP 86057-970 Paraná, Brazil
Multi-User Animal Health Laboratory, Molecular Biology Unit, Department of Veterinary Preventive Medicine, Universidade Estadual de Londrina, CEP 86057-970 Paraná, Brazil
Rodovia Celso Garcia Cid Road-Campus Universitário, Londrina, CEP 86057-970 Paraná, Brazil

Andrew J. Read, Deborah S. Finlaison and Peter D. Kirkland
Virology Laboratory, Elizabeth Macarthur Agriculture Institute, Woodbridge Road, Menangle, New South Wales 2568, Australia

Salvatore Catania, Michele Gastaldelli, Eliana Schiavon, Andrea Matucci, Annalucia Tondo and Marianna Merenda
Istituto Zooprofilattico Sperimentale delle Venezie, viale Dell'Università 10, 371735 Legnaro, PD, Italy

Robin A. J. Nicholas
The Oaks, Nutshell Lane, Farnham, Surrey GU9 0HG, UK

Michael McGowan
School of Veterinary Science, The University of Queensland, Gatton, QLD 4343, Australia

Kieren McCosker
Department of Primary Industry and Resources, Katherine, NT 0851, Australia

Geoff Fordyce
Queensland Alliance for Agriculture and Food Innovation, Centre for Animal Science, The University of Queensland, St Lucia, QLD 4072, Australia

Peter Kirkland
Elizabeth Macarthur Agricultural Institute, PMB 4008, Narellan, NSW 2567, Australia

Victor Riitho and Rebecca Strong
Virology Department, Animal and Plant Health Agency, APHA-Weybridge, Woodham Lane, New Haw, Addlestone KT15 3NB, UK

Magdalena Larska
Department of Virology, National Veterinary Research Institute, Al. Partyzantów 57, 24-100 Puławy, Poland

Simon P. Graham
The Pirbright Institute, Ash Road, Pirbright GU24 0NF, UK
School of Veterinary Medicine, University of Surrey, Guilford GU2 7XH, UK

Falko Steinbach
Virology Department, Animal and Plant Health Agency, APHA-Weybridge, Woodham Lane, New Haw, Addlestone KT15 3NB, UK
School of Veterinary Medicine, University of Surrey, Guilford GU2 7XH, UK

Lisa Ledger, Jason Eidt and Hugh Y. Cai
Animal Health Lab, University of Guelph, 419 Gordon St., Guelph, ON N1H 6R8, Canada

Katarzyna Dudek and Dariusz Bednarek
Department of Cattle and Sheep Diseases, National Veterinary Research Institute, 57 Partyzantów Avenue, 24-100 Pulawy, Poland

Urszula Lisiecka, Krzysztof Kostro and Stanisław Winiarczyk
Department of Epizootiology and Clinic of Infectious Diseases, Faculty of Veterinary Medicine, University of Life Sciences in Lublin, 30 Głęboka Street, 20-612 Lublin, Poland

Anna Kycko and Michał Reichert
Department of Pathology, National Veterinary Research Institute, 57 Partyzantów Avenue, 24-100 Pulawy, Poland

Karla J. Helbig
Department of Physiology, Molecular Virology Laboratory, Anatomy and Microbiology, School of Life Sciences, La Trobe University, Melbourne 3086, Australia

Teresa G. Carvalho
Department of Physiology, Molecular Parasitology Laboratory, Anatomy and Microbiology, School of Life Sciences, La Trobe University, Melbourne 3086, Australia

Jose L. Huaman
Department of Physiology, Molecular Virology Laboratory, Anatomy and Microbiology, School of Life Sciences, La Trobe University, Melbourne 3086, Australia
Department of Physiology, Molecular Parasitology Laboratory, Anatomy and Microbiology, School of Life Sciences, La Trobe University, Melbourne 3086, Australia

Carlo Pacioni
Department of Environment, Land, Water and Planning, Arthur Rylah Institute for Environmental Research, Heidelberg 3084, Australia
School of Veterinary and Life Sciences, Murdoch University, South Street, Murdoch, WA 6150, Australia

David M. Forsyth
NSW Department of Primary Industries, Vertebrate Pest Research Unit, Orange 2800, Australia

Anthony Pople
Department of Agriculture and Fisheries, Invasive Plants & Animals Research, Biosecurity Queensland, Ecosciences Precinct, Brisbane 4102, Australia

Jordan O. Hampton
School of Veterinary and Life Sciences, Murdoch University, South Street, Murdoch, WA 6150, Australia
Ecotone Wildlife, Inverloch, VIC 3996, Australia

Index

www.ingramcontent.com/pod-product-compliance
Lightning Source LLC
Chambersburg PA
CBHW081416220926
51613CB00010B/248